Surgical Education

Advances in Medical Education

Volume 2

Series Editor

Stanley J. Hamstra, PhD
Academy for Innovation in Medical Education
University of Ottawa, Canada

For further volumes:
http://www.springer.com/series/8405

Heather Fry · Roger Kneebone
Editors

Surgical Education

Theorising an Emerging Domain

Springer

Editors
Heather Fry
Higher Education Funding Council
for England (HEFCE)
Northavon House
Coldharbour Lane
Bristol
BS1b 1QD
United Kingdom
h.fry@hefce.ac.uk

Roger Kneebone
Division of Surgery
Department of Surgery and Cancer
Faculty of Medicine
Imperial College London

Clinical Skills Centre
2nd Floor Paterson Building
St Mary's Hospital
Praed Street
London W2 1NY
United Kingdom
r.kneebone@imperial.ac.uk

ISSN 2211-1298 e-ISSN 2211-1301
ISBN 978-94-007-1681-0 e-ISBN 978-94-007-1682-7
DOI 10.1007/978-94-007-1682-7
Springer Dordrecht Heidelberg London New York

Library of Congress Control Number: 2011935997

Printed on acid-free paper

Springer is part of Springer Science+Business Media (www.springer.com)

Contents

Part I

Part I

Chapter 1
The Environment of Surgical Training and Education

Roger Kneebone and Heather Fry

1.1 Introduction

1.1.1 Focus

This book argues that surgical education is an emerging field, which is establishing its own identity. At present, however, the field's boundaries are not clearly drawn. This indistinctness is both problematic and productive. The book attempts to highlight the diversity of surgical education by bringing together a range of perspectives and viewpoints. Of course, these are only a selection of possible topics, since it is impossible to do more than scratch the surface in a book of this size. Yet, we hope to give an idea of the richness of a field which reaches out in many directions.

This chapter aims to introduce the reader to the scope, distinctiveness, and nature of surgical education, to show how and why areas of surgical education are of particular contemporary interest, and to indicate why the book and its chapters are organized the way they are.

The book distinguishes between 'doing' surgical education and engaging with it academically. While it is possible to be an excellent surgical teacher with only a rudimentary grasp of educational theory, effective academic engagement requires a sound grasp of educational ideas and a familiarity with relevant literature. Such an engagement is necessary for participation in high-level debate which can influence policy about training and standards, and for the innovative development

R. Kneebone (✉)
Surgical Education, Imperial College London, London, UK
e-mail: r.kneebone@imperial.ac.uk

H. Fry
Higher Education Funding Council for England (HEFCE), Bristol BS16 1QD, UK
e-mail: h.fry@hefce.ac.uk

H. Fry and R. Kneebone (eds.), *Surgical Education: Theorising an Emerging Domain*, Advances in Medical Education 2, DOI 10.1007/978-94-007-1682-7_1,

of educational structures and policy, which make both surgical and educational sense. It is also, for those who are already sound and interested surgical teachers, a way of extending educational repertoire and understanding. Much relevant literature comes from disciplines outside surgery – indeed, from outside medicine – and will probably be unfamiliar to those whose own education has taken place within a biomedical tradition. Making sense of this literature requires at least a nodding acquaintance with the ways in which educationalists and social scientists conduct research and present their ideas.

Because of surgery's multifaceted nature, no single field of enquiry can encompass it all. Education, social science, performing arts, and computer science may all have useful contributions to make – yet each of these speaks its own language, and each has its own literature and academic conventions. Indeed, education itself is a composite field that draws on history, economics, psychology, sociology, philosophy, and so on. Linking these disparate domains and functioning effectively across them is therefore a major challenge. In this book, we will try to show how this may be done. We will highlight the dangers of gleaning a superficial knowledge of many fields but gaining mastery of none, as well as pointing out some domains whose insights may be especially fruitful.

The decision to write this book was triggered by the authors' experience in jointly creating and establishing the UK's first Masters in Education (M Ed) in Surgical Education at Imperial College London in 2004. During the initial years of the programme, it became clear that surgical education does indeed have its own character, and that surgical practice is an underresearched and undertheorized area within healthcare. It became equally clear that many surgeons are unfamiliar with the wide range of theories, methodologies, and practices needed to do justice to this field.

The authors' academic backgrounds and interests have profoundly shaped this book's structure and approach. Heather Fry is an educationalist, with extensive experience in the study and practice of higher and professional education and in educational policy and strategy. Roger Kneebone is a clinician, with a background in surgery and in primary care, as well as an academic in the field of surgical education. Their shared experience in leading the Imperial M Ed has led to their conviction that surgical education requires a confluence of approaches and fields.

1.1.2 Organization and Perspective

The book is written by authors from several disciplines and countries and is intended for a wide readership. Most contributors draw examples from their own national context, but many themes of surgical education cross-national boundaries. As authors we have not attempted to homogenize context or language, but have allowed each perspective speak for itself. At a simple level, we have not attempted to insist on a single lexicon, considering that most readers are familiar enough with the variation of usage between, for example, the American operating room and the British theatre, for this to be unnecessary. Where there is a need for terminological explanation – from discipline or country – we have generally attempted to include this naturally within the text. We hope readers will not find this approach disconcerting.

Another issue worth drawing attention to at the outset is the use of the word 'training'. For most UK surgeons, the term 'surgical training' seems unexceptionable; for many educationalists, however, the term 'training' implies an activity that is aimed more at a technician, involving learning about limited tasks with clearly defined boundaries. There is thus from the outset the potential for considerable misunderstanding. We use the term training where it is the word an English surgeon would normally use. By that, we are describing in shorthand the arrangements and means by which the full panoply of surgical learning is acquired – this encompasses the gaining of specific technical skills, high levels of skill in diagnosis and patient management, autonomy of professional action based on evidence, interaction with patients and other healthcare professionals, coping with the complex and unexpected, and much else besides. We contrast this type of education (which is essential for the surgeon who is to become a UK consultant or equivalent) with the preparation required by a surgical assistant or technician. This latter is or might be of more limited scope, though still often going far beyond what educationalists might traditionally (and rather pejoratively) refer to as 'mere' training.

The first parts of this chapter provide a historical overview of the landscape of surgery from the perspectives especially of training, teaching, and learning. Our aim is to provide the reader with a map of the terrain. The chapter then outlines the structure of the book, providing a rationale for its design and introducing the areas which will be covered by its contributors.

1.2 Why Surgical Education

1.2.1 What is Surgical Education?

We start by considering what is meant by the term 'surgical education'. Of course, medical (as opposed to surgical) education is already firmly established throughout the world. So, it is legitimate to ask what makes surgery special, and whether there is really a need to consider surgical education as a branch of its own.

First, there arises an issue of terminology, as the word 'medical' is used in many senses. In the context of 'medical education', it traditionally refers to the education of doctors, distinguishing them from other professional groups such as lawyers, architects, or engineers. Used in this sense, the term encompasses undergraduate, postgraduate, and continuing professional education. 'Medical education' is thus a term often used to talk about the training of doctors up to initial registration, but also includes ongoing professional development for the purposes of further training, specialization, and keeping up to date. As a doctor gains experience, the training and learning may well become different in nature as well as content, taking into account more specialized and sophisticated needs and a wider and deeper background. This has many implications for the organization and 'delivery' of training – and for the learning which underpins it.

In another sense, 'medical' is used in contrast to 'nursing', say, or 'physiotherapy', marking out a particular set of professional boundaries. And in another sense again, 'medical' stands in contrast to 'surgical', referring to a group of clinical specialties which do not involve operating. In North American terminology, this corresponds broadly to 'internal medicine'.

In the context of this book, we are exploring the world of clinicians engaged in the practices of surgery, together with those from related disciplines (such as anaesthesia or the interventional specialties) where craft is a central element. Since most surgical training takes place at postgraduate level, the current use of the term 'surgical education' implies a primary postgraduate focus. Yet, undergraduate surgery is of great interest to educators too: it is here after all that students are first exposed to the operating theatre and start to learn simple technical skills. Moreover, while it may be tempting for an educationalist to view the whole of 'surgery' as a single field, surgeons see this differently. Plastic and orthopaedic surgeons, for example, can and do point out clear distinctions in the skills, expertise, and culture found in these two specialties.

For us as authors, surgical education stands at an intersection between several traditions of practice and enquiry. At one level, the issue is about ensuring that surgeons master their profession and provide the best possible care. From a surgeon's point of view, this is obviously of immediate interest and practical importance; from the patient's perspective, even more so. In the current climate of continual change and relentlessly increasing demands, finding the best ways for surgeons to learn and teach is clearly a priority. Yet, at another level, the *process* by which surgeons learn is also of great interest – not only to surgeons themselves but also to those outside surgery. For educationalists, for example, surgical learning is a special case, taking place within unique circumstances.

To make sense of such complexity, this book uses the primary lenses of surgery and education. But, these represent very different cultures and traditions, both of practice and of research (see Chap. 4). Few practitioners and scholars are fluent in the languages of both, and the ways of each often seem mysterious to an outsider. Moreover, surgical education (as with both surgery and education) must draw on other disciplines and practices for insight and illumination. Although no other profession has an identical profile to surgery, many involve parallel forms of expertise and may provide useful metaphors for exploring surgery (Reddy 1979). For example, surgeons and musicians both require high levels of dexterity and technical mastery; surgeons and motor racing teams both depend on expert team work; surgery and aviation both demand rapid, high stakes decision-making; and so on. This book draws on these wider fields to provide insight about surgical education.

1.2.2 What makes Surgery Special?

So, is there something unique about surgeons and surgical practice? In our view, the answer is yes. More than anything, it is *operating* which distinguishes surgeons from other clinicians. This apparent truism highlights that although surgery demands the integration of many skills and qualities, *craft* lies at the heart of what surgeons do. This craft is more than just another component of a surgeon's day – it is central to a surgeon's professional identity and to the mystique which to many still surrounds the surgical specialties (see Chaps. 6 and 11).

Yet although dexterity is crucial to any successful procedure, no operation takes place in isolation. Surgeons work within teams; operations take place within operating theatres; and, as we have already intimated, operative technique is inseparable from team working, communication, decision making, professionalism, and a host of other aspects which together constitute clinical expertise. Moreover, the process by which this expertise is mastered and maintained is highly complex. Much is tacit and implicit, and even more is explicit yet unspoken, taking place outside conscious awareness in ways which may seem mysterious or inaccessible even to those within the profession (see Chaps. 11 and 12).

Of course, education takes place in all of the many settings of surgical care – from the outpatient clinic to the bedside, from the operating theatre to the intensive care unit. In order to make our scope manageable, however, we will focus in this book on the learning that takes place in the operating theatre. This environment offers unique affordances, balanced by unique constraints. We acknowledge that this perspective privileges the surgeon's point of view, inevitably painting a partial picture where some voices in the theatre team (such as those of anaesthetists and nurses) are heard less clearly than others.

The book therefore posits that surgical education has its own identity, separate from the more widely established field of medical education, but of course sharing many common elements. As has already been suggested, there is probably more commonality between all branches of 'doctoring' at early, introductory levels than at more specialized and senior levels; this is true in terms of early acquisition of a broad palette of knowledge and skills, with the former often being considerably more and complex than the latter. But, as a trainee doctor specializes in surgery, distinctive elements emerge. Perhaps, most notably (and in contrast to the trainee physician), these include mastery of complex technical skills, detailed anatomical knowledge, a sense of 3D and spatial awareness, and adaptation to the operating theatre environment and culture.

Unravelling these processes and formulating them in educational terms is therefore a major challenge. The task requires a synergy between surgeons (and their teams) and those whose expertise lies in analysing educational activity within complex settings and making sense of what they see (Chap. 13). Especially for those who are familiar with the setting of surgery, much that happens is taken for granted and becomes invisible. Paradoxically, therefore, surgeons themselves may not be best placed to analyse their own educational practices. The 'new eyes' of an outsider may be needed to render visible what has disappeared from view.

Profound changes (in the practice of hospital medicine and the 'empowered patient', for example) are shaking long-established patterns of learning and forcing new approaches, and it is impossible to divorce local practices of education from such wider developments. These changes make it necessary to interrogate traditional educational practices and identify ways to make them more effective. To be constructive and rigorous, such interrogation requires a deep understanding of what surgical education is, and how it can evolve to meet the needs of a fluid and ever-shifting world.

1.3 A Historical Overview of Medical and Surgical Training in the UK

1.3.1 The Evolution of Surgical Training

The historical context of healthcare has exerted a powerful influence over more recent developments in surgical training. This historical background helps to explain a large part of why some features of surgical training (e.g., shorter training) are currently attracting more attention than others. Education may offer ideas and solutions that are helpful to surgery as it contemplates these changes. Educationalists may also look at the landscape of surgical training from the other end of the telescope, considering which educational ideas and theories might usefully be explored in a surgical context.

A brief historical overview may therefore be helpful here, especially for readers outside the UK and for those who are not surgeons. This initial scene setting provides a UK viewpoint, since that is the environment with which the authors are most familiar. It focuses on the training of hospital doctors (especially surgeons), as opposed to family physicians ('general practitioners' in UK terminology). In many cases, readers from other countries will be able to make comparisons and draw parallels with developments in their own settings. The account makes no claim to comprehensiveness, nor can it begin to do justice to a highly complex issue, but highlights what the authors see as some key factors affecting the topic of the book.

For centuries, surgical training in the UK was based on a traditional apprenticeship model. From the inception of the National Health Service (NHS) in 1948 until the 1980s, training was extremely protracted, often lasting up to 12 or 15 years after initial qualification as a doctor. During that time, trainees would be attached to a series of 'firms', in each of which they would join a clinical team led by a consultant surgeon (who had final clinical responsibility for all patients under his/her care). Attachments would often be in different parts of the UK, and might encompass a range of urban teaching hospitals as well as generally smaller and less specialized District General Hospitals (DGHs).

Training progressed through a series of training grades from Senior House Officer (SHO) to Registrar and Senior Registrar levels, with trainees assuming increasing levels of responsibility as they progressed. Until they were appointed to a consultant post, surgeons in training were referred to as 'junior doctors', even though many were extremely experienced clinicians in their thirties and even forties.

Within the system at that time, even relatively inexperienced trainees would be given high levels of practical responsibility, particularly at DGHs. Learning took place as part of the process of providing clinical care, usually on an opportunistic basis. This was especially so during the night and at weekends, where much of the operating was carried out by trainees without a consultant being present. The prevailing culture was physically demanding, with an expectation that junior doctors would work for many hours at a stretch without sleep. Firmly grounded in longstanding practice and hallowed by tradition, this arduous training was regarded as a rite of passage within the profession.

One consequence was that surgical trainees accumulated extensive experience and were exposed to a wide range of operations and associated complications. By the time they were appointed as consultants, many were extremely proficient operative surgeons. However, this learning was usually seen as a byproduct of the clinical job, without a clear educational framework. Assessment at this time was not formalized and was often idiosyncratic. Although trainee surgeons were required to pass the Fellowship of the Royal College of Surgeons (FRCS) diploma, this knowledge-based examination contained no assessment of operative ability. Judgements about trainees' skills were largely unstructured and opaque.

Although the benefits, drawbacks, and rigours were widely recognized within the profession, patients were generally unaware of the system's details. Rooted in an earlier age of deference, hierarchy and loyalty to the NHS, the *status quo* was generally accepted.

1.3.2 Changes Within the Profession

Under the system outlined above, the endpoint of training was marked by appointment to a consultant post, endowing considerable status and lifelong job security. Selection into such posts was underpinned by informal judgements by senior colleagues rather than on measurable performance within a transparent and explicit training programme. In particular, operative skill was never formally tested.

At that time, intake into surgical training was unregulated. A large number of SHOs with limited career prospects propped up the clinical service, while a bottleneck in the system developed at the Senior Registrar level. Limited consultant posts acted as a *de facto* brake, and many trainees found themselves after many years of surgical training in a position which many found demoralizing, being unable to achieve a consultant position but equally unable to move into a different specialty.

In the 1980s, Calman (the then Chief Medical Officer) introduced radical changes (Calman 1993, 2007; Calman and Downie 1988), aiming to rationalize the training structure across the whole of postgraduate training (including medicine and surgery). A new training grade was introduced – the Specialist Registrar (SpR) – with entry being strictly controlled through a competitive selection process, which aimed to align the numbers accepted for specialist training with projected consultant vacancies. Although reducing the number of 'perpetual Senior Registrars', this had the effect of shifting the bottleneck further down the system and creating even larger numbers of less experienced trainees at SHO level, with no clear career path ahead of them. The absence of clear progress markers, coupled with a lack of career counselling, resulted in a further drop in morale at the early stages of training.

In the twenty-first century, Donaldson (Calman's successor as Chief Medical Officer) introduced further changes, with the Foundation Programme and Modernising Medical Careers (MMC). This aimed to rationalize the early years of post-qualification training by providing a structured programme which would eliminate the so-called 'lost tribe' of SHOs and prepare trainees for specialist training. For the first time, a formal system of workplace-based assessment aimed to map and document clinicians' skills across a range of dimensions (Department of Health 2007). The introduction of MMC caused the surgical colleges in the UK to combine forces and draw on the combined expertise of their senior members to establish a curriculum for all the specialities of surgical training (the Intercollegiate Surgical Curriculum Project) (Surgeons 2010).

The introduction of MMC gave rise to much controversy and opposition, exacerbated by spectacular malfunctioning of the system for selection into training posts. This debacle triggered a widespread loss of public and professional confidence in the system of postgraduate education, culminating in an influential independent review by Tooke (2008). As well as identifying deficiencies of the newly introduced system, Tooke's review recommended a change in emphasis from competence to excellence, signalling an important philosophical shift. More recently, Collins' report on the Foundation Programme has highlighted both strengths and limitations of the initial 2 years after graduation (Collins 2010).

1.3.3 Wider Changes

At the same time as these events were taking place within the profession, a series of highly publicized cases began to shake public and professional confidence in the healthcare system as a whole, and to challenge long established patterns of care. These developments took place against a wider backdrop of profound social change and instability, detailed discussion of which lies outside the scope of this book. This discussion highlights a small number of landmark events which triggered major shifts in established practices and relationships relating to surgery.

As highlighted above, surgeons were traditionally held in high regard, both by the medical profession and the public (Becker et al. 1961; Cassell 1991; Katz 1999;

Ludmerer 1999; Millman 1976). For many years, a culture of individualism allowed surgeons to embrace and adopt new techniques with minimal accountability or external control.

The introduction of minimal access (keyhole) surgery (MAS) in the 1990s highlighted the perils of an unmonitored and unmanaged approach to new technology. MAS requires a completely different set of skills from 'open' operations. Although now firmly established within many branches of surgery, the difficulties and hazards of this new approach were insufficiently recognized at first (Surgeons 1991). Some practitioners embraced the new techniques without adequate formal training. During an initial flurry of uptake by enthusiastic but inadequately trained early adopters, patients were injured and many needless complications ensued. This led to a growing sense of unease within the profession at the uncritical pursuit of new techniques without adequate training or supervision.

Although this crisis of confidence in MAS was largely confined to the profession, a series of high profile incidents then began to erode the public's relationship of unquestioning trust. The case of the Bristol heart surgeons showed that some surgeons continued to operate, despite being known to have a higher mortality and complication rate than their colleagues (Smith 1998). The retention of children's body parts by pathologists at Alder Hey Hospital generated a perception that doctors' agendas were not always aligned with their patients' best interests. And the case of Dr Harold Shipman (a respected general practitioner who was found to have systematically murdered hundreds of patients over several decades) further shook the public's previously uncritical confidence in the medical profession.

At the same time, a growing awareness of patient safety began to permeate the debate on both sides of the Atlantic. A series of influential documents (Kohn et al. 2000; Vincent et al. 2001) highlighted the hazards of healthcare and the disturbingly high incidence of unintended harm, further challenging the *status quo*. All this contributed to a profound change in the dynamic between the public and the profession. Consequences have included greatly increased scrutiny of the processes of surgical training, increased attention to assessment, and a growing belief in the importance of educational design. As part of this process, the value of professional educational expertise started to become more evident.

1.3.4 Current Drivers

More recently, a series of powerful forces has fuelled further change. Crucially, the introduction of working hours restrictions across Europe has brought about a radical upheaval in professional practice in the UK, which is having profound educational repercussions.

As outlined above, a culture of personal responsibility for patients within a structure of surgical 'firms' was traditionally underpinned by extremely long working hours, especially for so-called 'junior' doctors. These long hours continued though the Calman changes and into the twenty-first century, with doctors regularly working more than 80 h/week and sometimes as much as 120 h. The phased introduction of the European Working Time Directive (and similar restrictions in other parts of the world) has brought about a major change in how care is provided. Further drastic reductions (culminating in a maximum 48 work week from 2009 in the UK) have disrupted continuity and triggered a change to shift working, eroding traditional 'firm' structures and profoundly altering the landscape.

Although offering clear benefits in terms of reducing fatigue and improving working conditions, this change is having far-reaching consequences in terms of education and training. A widely-quoted reduction in training from 30,000–6,000 h means that surgeons, when appointed to a consultant position, will have had much less clinical exposure than formerly (Chikwe et al. 2004). This is giving rise to considerable disquiet within the profession and beyond, raising the possibility that newly appointed consultants will no longer be confident and competent across a full range of clinical challenges and will be insufficiently experienced to cope with the unexpected.

At the time of writing, impassioned debate centres around the impact of reduced working hours upon the quality of surgical training. While the 2010 Temple Report concluded that high quality training can be delivered in 48 h/week, it highlighted the need for fundamental changes in the way training and service are delivered (Temple 2010). It remains to be seen how increasing financial austerity and radical funding cuts to public services will affect surgical education.

In the face of dwindling opportunities for clinical exposure, the case for a training structure which includes clear outcomes and endpoints is becoming increasingly compelling. Of course, much is already taking place, including extensive work on the assessment of a wide range of surgical skills and attributes. Formal training structures are well established and, as alluded to above, the Intercollegiate Surgical Curriculum Project now presents in detail what is required of trainees by the UK Royal Colleges of Surgeons.

At the same time, however, an extensive informal network of web-based learning resources is becoming available to surgical trainees at all stages. Much of this learning takes place outside the formal frameworks referred to above, constituting a parallel universe which reflects developments in the wider worlds of technology, education, and social networking. This learning operates 'below the radar' of more formal educational systems.

It is against this background that surgical education as a field is developing both an identity and a momentum. External events have ensured that surgeons' traditional ways of learning cannot survive unaltered, but must respond to a constantly changing environment whose hallmarks are instability and unpredictability. The question is not *if* surgical education should respond to this change, but *how* it should respond. Such uncertainty offers great opportunity, but also a need to ensure that any response is grounded in clear thinking, good science and a critical openness to new ideas.

1.4 Researching and Using Theory to Extend Knowledge and Innovation in Surgical Education

How then should the profession respond to such profound changes within and beyond its immediate scope? Perhaps even more importantly, how can surgeons (and others) establish a rigorous, scholarly basis for influencing policy as well as investigating specific questions of educational importance and interest?

We suggest that knowledge and research based within what is broadly called 'surgical education' can and does provide such a basis. Yet, conducting high quality surgical education in the face of such complexity and instability poses major challenges. Partly this is because the field is by nature composite and wide reaching. For example, there is no single database of literature that covers all relevant areas, and almost any question of interest may require the researcher to search the literatures of surgery, education, psychology, social science, and the humanities. But, on a wider canvas, there is a fundamental philosophical tension between biomedical research (with which surgeons are usually most familiar) and educational research. In the former, research questions are usually framed as hypotheses which can be tested. In the latter, the challenge is more often to *illuminate* an area of practice than to find 'the right answer'. Theory in education is not about establishing immutable laws, but about developing models with explanatory power. Indeed, the questions which are of most interest may resist being categorized in the manner of the so-called 'hard' sciences. There may not *be* a right answer, but rather a set of alternative viewpoints.

This raises important issues, which we address in detail in Chap. 4. In summary, because learning, teaching, and training have to do with human actions and responses, it is rarely possible to control variables as one would in the research laboratory. Even in apparently similar circumstances, it may be impossible to predict how different people (e.g., the learners and trainers that are at the heart of this book) will respond. Because of this variability and contingency, traditional notions of evidence-based practice have less purchase and surety in education than many might wish. Although 'theory' and 'evidence' may offer useful lines of explanation and suggestions for innovation and change, their nature and effects will be less certain and predictable than a natural scientist might expect.

In the complex unruly world of individuals, it may for example be impossible to tell if an educational approach 'works' or not – certainly not in the sense in which a new drug or operation may be said to 'work'. The principles of minimizing variables, generalizing to large populations by sampling, and generating and testing hypotheses may not be appropriate ways to address the questions which education most wants to answer (Regehr 2010).

A further challenge relates to accessing and making sense of work in fields outside surgery. A multidisciplinary approach can be extremely fruitful, especially when looking at how the cultural practices of surgery are built. Here, an exclusively 'insider' perspective may result in important practices being taken for granted and therefore overlooked (see Chap. 10). Yet, in order to make sense of what is written about these surgery-related activities and to understand how educational research can and does offer useful insights, knowledge is needed of the wider research traditions within such work is conducted and the methods which they employ.

Examples of boundary-crossing research include work on operative surgery (Koschmann et al. 2007; Lyon 2004; Schwind et al. 2004/2002), case presentations (Haber and Lingard 2001; Lingard and Haber 1999; Lingard et al. 2003a, b), the complexities of hospital communication (Iedema 2007) and the workings of academic seminars (Rendle-Short 2006). The challenges of integrating, interpreting, and making sense of research from disparate fields are considered in more detail in Chap. 4.

Any area of enquiry that tries to make sense of real world practice is beset with challenges. For example, many aspects of surgical practice change extremely fast, and new clinical technologies can be introduced at a dizzying speed. Some become established, while others fall by the wayside and are quickly replaced. Educational technologies demonstrate similar characteristics – innovations in simulation, for example, are apt to be taken up enthusiastically and equally readily discarded (see Chaps. 3 and 8). Fashion exerts a powerful influence, and there is often a mismatch between the adoption of new approaches and their systematic evaluation.

By contrast, educational evaluation moves at a much slower place than the innovations it is expected to judge. Evaluating impact requires protracted observation, and educational interventions may take years to evaluate – by which time the interventions themselves will have been superseded and become obsolete. In the rapidly changing environment of contemporary surgery, therefore, traditional approaches to evaluation may simply not be appropriate. A major challenge for surgical education is to address such tensions.

1.5 About this Book: Rationale and Organization

This book therefore frames questions rather than providing answers. Already it will be seen that this is not a textbook or a 'how to do it' manual. Rather, it is an attempt to highlight the diversity of surgical education by presenting a range of perspectives and viewpoints. Of course, in this short space, it is possible to provide only a selective introduction to the field, barely scratching the surface. Yet, we hope to give an idea of the richness of a field which extends in many directions. The book's structure is as follows.

Part One sets the book's frame, providing a general introduction to educational ideas, educational practice, and educational research. This part gives the authors an opportunity to contribute their personal views and expertise on areas they consider to be especially important.

The first part of Chap. 1 has already set out general points about surgical education as an emerging field, locating it within events and developments which affect contemporary healthcare. The chapter continues with an overview of how the book is arranged, outlining the broad terrain of each chapter.

In Chap. 2, Fry summarizes key theories of education which bear upon surgery. Building on her experience in various branches of higher and professional education, she identifies important currents of literature and thought. By encapsulating these theoretical positions and marshalling their arguments, Fry presents a background for the nonspecialist in education and a guidebook for making sense of what is to come.

In Chap. 3, Kneebone introduces concepts of simulation, which plays a key role in surgical education. In this chapter, he lays the foundations for more detailed consideration by other contributors later in the book. Rather than addressing the details of simulation design and implementation, Kneebone takes a philosophical standpoint and asks ‘what is simulation and how can it reflect the complexities of real world clinical care?’

In Chap. 4, the authors join with Sevdalis to examine the methodologies and methods which can be used for researching surgical education. The chapter aims to arm the reader with an understanding of the breadth of possible approaches, providing a compass for making sense of them and the types of knowledge and evidence they generate. Benefits and limitations of qualitative, quantitative, and mixed methodologies are outlined, putting the case for an integrative approach which uses the most appropriate tools for a given question.

Part Two consists of a series of chapters by invited scholars. Each was asked to give a personal perspective on a selected topic within their field of expertise. Most chapters link explicitly or implicitly to matters relating to learning and teaching surgery and developing surgical practice and expertise. Rather than imposing consistency, our aim as authors was to illustrate the wide range of approaches which surgical education can draw upon, courting controversy and stimulating debate. The contributors are international, chosen because of their expertise and the originality of their thinking. The authors have not aimed for comprehensiveness – that would be a hopeless task. The book’s intention is rather to illuminate selected aspects of surgical education, demonstrating the multifaceted nature of the field and illustrating a wide range of approaches and styles.

In Chap. 5, Schurwirth and Van der Vleuten consider surgical assessment from their perspective as psychometricians. They are among a handful of world leading experts in the assessment and measurement of medical education; here they use their knowledge to show the importance of key principles and methods to surgery.

In Chap. 6, Land and Meyer apply their work on threshold concepts to surgery. Based on recent interviews with a variety of surgeons, they explore the applicability of their innovative ideas (rooted in other professional domains) to surgeons and surgical practice, exploring issues around ontology and identity.

In Chap. 7, Ericsson brings his widely acknowledged experience in the field of expertise to bear upon surgical practice. In addition to summarizing the current state of knowledge about elite expert performance, he considers how the unique characteristics of surgical expertise are played out in a professional context.

In Chap. 8, Bello and Brenton consider simulation and e-learning technologies in detail, outlining the key characteristics of each. After describing a case study based on their own work, they elaborate the concept of a ‘simulation journey’ which progresses throughout medical and surgical training and brings together complementary elements of e-learning and simulation.

In Chap. 9, Nestel and Bentley address the central role of the patient in surgical education. After considering how the patient's perspective is (and is not) represented within current practice, they discuss how Simulated Patients (professional actors playing the role of patient) can be used within surgical and procedural simulation.

In Chap. 10, Moulton and Epstein explore the world of the autonomous surgeon, proposing self regulation and self monitoring as key to such autonomy, and to continued expertise and professional development. They introduce the idea of 'mindful practice' as an essential feature of self monitoring.

In Chap. 11, Bleakley examines how surgeons' identities are constructed. Drawing on a wide range of theoretical positions (including activity and actor network theory), he considers the complex area of surgical identity in an unstable and rapidly changing workplace.

In Chap. 12, Lingard postulates that communication is both descriptive and *constructive* of social settings, such as the surgical team in the operating theatre. This perspective, and her own research of communication in surgical teams, points to several implications for the concept of the expert surgeon, and for the associated training regimes, objectives, and curriculum designs aimed at their formation.

In Chap. 13, Kress writes from the perspective of a nonclinician who has been investigating the curriculum and pedagogy of the operating theatre from the viewpoint of social semiotics. He frames teaching and learning as social practice, exploring surgical education in terms of multiple modes and affordances. His controversial view of communication as interpretation of prompts highlights the responsibilities of teacher and learner.

In the Afterword, the authors attempt to make sense of these individual and divergent contributions, considering how they can shape a view of surgical education as a whole. The authors conclude by summarizing their views of surgical education, its emerging identity as a distinct field, and the challenges which it faces. They argue that progress will depend on a wide conceptual grasp, an openness to new ideas, and a sound footing in rigorous research.

References

Becker, H., Geer, B., Hughes, E., & Strauss, A. (1961). *Boys in white*. New Brunswick: Transaction Books.

Calman, K. (1993). *Hospital doctors: Training for the future. The report of the working group on specialist medical training*. London: Department of Health.

Calman, K. (2007). *Medical education past, present and future: Handing on learning*. Edinburgh: Churchill Livingstone Elsevier.

Calman, K. C., & Downie, R. S. (1988). Education and training in medicine. *Medical Education, 22*, 488–491.

Cassell, J. (1991). *Expected miracles surgeons at work*. Philadelphia: Temple University Press.

Chikwe, J., de Souza, A. C., & Pepper, J. R. (2004). No time to train the surgeons. *British Medical Journal, 328*(7437), 418–419.

Collins, J. (2010). Foundation for excellence an evaluation of the foundation programme. Medical Education England. http://www.mee.nhs.uk/pdf/401339_MEE_FoundationExcellence_acc.pdf. Accessed 22 July 2011.

Department of Health. (2007). Modernising medical careers foundation programme.

Haber, R. J., & Lingard, L. A. (2001). Learning oral presentation skills: A rhetorical analysis with pedagogical and professional implications. *Journal of General Internal Medicine, 16*(5), 308–314.

Iedema, R. (Ed.). (2007). *The discourse of hospital communication tracing complexities in contemporary health care organizations*. Basingstoke: Palgrave Macmillan.

Katz, P. (1999). *The scalpel's edge the culture of surgeons*. Needham Heights: Allyn and Bacon.

Kohn, L., Corrigan, J., & Donaldson, M. (Eds.). (2000). *To err is human: Building a safer health system*. Washington, DC: Institute of Medicine National Academy Press.

Koschmann, T., LeBaron, C., Goodwin, C., Zemel, A., & Dunnington, G. (2007). Formulating the triangle of doom. *Gesture, 7*(1), 97–118.

Lingard, L. A., & Haber, R. J. (1999). What do we mean by "relevance"? A clinical and rhetorical definition with implications for teaching and learning the case-presentation format. *Academic Medicine, 74*(10 Suppl), S124–S127.

Lingard, L., Garwood, K., Schryer, C. F., & Spafford, M. M. (2003a). A certain art of uncertainty: Case presentation and the development of professional identity. *Social Science & Medicine, 56*(3), 603–616.

Lingard, L., Schryer, C., Garwood, K., & Spafford, M. (2003b). Talking the talk: School and workplace genre tension in clerkship case presentations. *Medical Education, 37*, 612–620.

Ludmerer, K. (1999). *Time to heal*. Oxford: Oxford University Press.

Lyon, P. (2004). A model of teaching and learning in the operating theatre. *Medical Education, 38*(12), 1278–1287.

Millman, M. (1976). *The unkindest cut*. New York: William Morrow and Company.

Reddy, M. (1979). The conduit metaphor – A case of frame conflict in our language about language. In A. Ortony (Ed.), *Metaphor and thought*. Cambridge: Cambridge University Press.

Regehr, G. (2010). It's NOT rocket science: Rethinking our metaphors for research in health professions education. *Medical Education, 44*(1), 31–39.

Rendle-Short, J. (2006). *The academic presentation: Situated talk in action*. Aldershot: Ashgate.

Schwind, C. J., Boehler, M. L., Rogers, D. A., Williams, R. G., Dunnington, G., Folse, R., & Markwell, S. J. (2004/2002). Variables influencing medical student learning in the operating room. *American Journal of Surgery, 187*(2), 198–200.

Smith, R. (1998). All changed, changed utterly. British medicine will be transformed by the Bristol case. *British Medical Journal, 316*(27 June), 1917–1918.

Surgeons, Royal Colleges of. (2010). Intercollegiate surgical curriculum programme. https://www.iscp.ac.uk/Default.aspx. Accessed 22 July 2011.

Surgeons, Southern. (1991). A prospective analysis of 1518 laparoscopic cholecystectomies. The Southern Surgeons Club. *The New England Journal of Medicine, 324*(16), 1073–1078.

Temple, J. (2010). Time for training a review of the impact of the European working time directive on the quality of training. Medical Education England. http://www.mee.nhs.uk/PDF/14274%20Bookmark%20Web%20Version.pdf. Accessed 22 July 2011.

Tooke, J. (2008). Aspiring to excellence. Independent inquiry into modernising medical careers. http://www.mmcinquiry.org.uk/MMC_Inquiry_Launch_2.pdf. Accessed 22 July 2011.

Vincent, C., Neale, G., & Woloshynowych, M. (2001). Adverse events in British hospitals: Preliminary retrospective record review. *British Medical Journal, 322*(7285), 517–519.

Chapter 2
Educational Ideas and Surgical Education

Heather Fry

2.1 Introduction

Chapter 1 gave an account of the evolution of the arrangements for medical and surgical training in the UK. It also discussed the environment in which surgical training and education occur, with a focus on the surgical elements, such as the 'arena' of the operating theatre and the highly skilled technical nature of the craft of surgery. These features create a distinct educational environment. It also touched on some of the differences between the social sciences and science. This chapter focuses on key elements of one social science which can be brought to bear in the surgical environment, education. It attempts to outline several central educational ideas and practices, mainly drawn from higher, professional, vocational, and adult education, which are important to surgical education. These ideas are of value in their own right to the practice and understanding of surgical education. They are also used, underpin or implied in later chapters in this book. This chapter does not touch on aspects of education that relate more exclusively to simulation or learning technology as these are considered in Chaps. 3 and 8. Assessment is considered in much greater detail in Chap. 5.

2.2 Changing Educational Imperatives and Preferences

It is not only in the UK that medical and surgical education has changed beyond recognition in the last 25 years. This is not just because the context and practice of surgery have changed, but also because education as a discipline has evolved, and so have the specialist medical and surgical branches of it. Change is to be expected

H. Fry (✉)
Higher Education Funding Council for England (HEFCE), Bristol BS16 1QD, UK
e-mail: h.fry@hefce.ac.uk

H. Fry and R. Kneebone (eds.), *Surgical Education: Theorising an Emerging Domain*, Advances in Medical Education 2, DOI 10.1007/978-94-007-1682-7_2,

in a 25-year period, but its extent may be unusual. The two rapidly changing areas (surgery and education) have interacted with each other. It is this interaction that is responsible for most of the features that distinguish medical and surgical education today.

To a layperson, educational theory (i.e., the concepts and ideas that underpin the practice of teaching and learning) is perhaps an alien concept or almost a contradiction in terms. Non-educationalists may think that learning and teaching are some form of 'natural process' – a process about which there is no evidence as to the efficacy of one method or another, and where there is no need to question, probe and discover what is actually happening during teaching and learning, or theorise about it. But this is not the perspective educationalists take. For educationalists, trying to understand what is happening, so that explanatory models and theory can be developed, is the way in which the discipline of education moves on, and the practice of (surgical) education progresses. The practice, the doing, can be informed by theory; it can also be the basis from which educational theory develops. In these ways, educational theory and educational practice may evolve. Teaching and learning can be 'tested' for efficacy by collecting evidence about impact and experience, but such 'evidence' will frequently not be generalisable or robust because of the variability of context, learner, and teacher (Chap. 4 expands on some of these themes). Kennedy (2009) has been among others who have pointed to the relationships between educational practice and theory and their implications for post-registration training.

It is essential to be aware of and understand at least some key educational ideas to be able to make rational and informed educational choices about behaviour and organisation. It is possible to be a good teacher without such understanding, but only within limits. Being a good teacher can involve little more than having a 'flair' and repeating experienced good practice. But this is rarely a sufficient condition for educational innovation, learning from and building on the teaching practices of others, guiding curriculum change, or the development of educational policy. Often, it will be an understanding of the theory, combined with understanding of the context, that will lead to innovation and effectiveness in surgical educational practice; Kneebone's own work described in Chap. 3 illustrates this point. Moreover, even the good but limited trainer described above will meet situations in which they fail (e.g., the trainee who reacts in an unusual or unexpected way). They will then usually be unable to analyse what went wrong or know what corrective changes might work.

Educational situations are often not as directly comparable or replicable as scientists are used to, either at the bench, or, for example, when calculating the correct dosage of a drug. They have too many interacting variables that cannot be controlled and which do not react in predictable ways. This is one of the reasons why randomised control trials are not frequently used in education. Even when they are used, the results from them cannot necessarily be universally 'applied' with the same effect (as context and people will differ). For example, among any group of seemingly similar trainees, there will be different levels of knowledge, experience, and skill and each one will likely respond in different ways to stress, competition, etc. (see also Chap. 4). Rational and insightful choice about variation to enhance educational practice usually comes from the experience of teaching combined with understanding of learning and teaching theory, and usually also requires an appreciation of how to learn from and use relevant research.

Some examples may be useful to illustrate the points made above. Problem-based learning (PBL) is a method of teaching and learning which tries to put into practice a wide range of educational ideas tempered by contextual factors. But it can easily be less than optimally implemented due to a lack of understanding of the theory or the context of PBL, thus producing a mismatch between the two (a point returned to later in the chapter). Other fruitful examples that demonstrate a positive interaction between educational theory and practice include: ideas about coping with shorter trainer periods through using a more formal curriculum, and meeting demands from the lay person that trained doctors can be proved/guaranteed to be 'fit for practice' through more consistent and standardised assessment procedures.

Arguably, some of the major changes in medical and surgical education in recent years have been, especially at pre-registration level, a shift from a didactic approach based on subjects, teaching, and the teacher to more exploratory approaches that emphasise the learner and the nature of what is being learnt, or rather the nature of how that learning will need to be accessed and used in medical practice. Undergraduate curricula that are organised around body systems, link traditional disciplines together (e.g., learning about the cardiovascular system from a range of perspectives, including anatomy, biochemistry, etc.), introduce patients with relevant illnesses and symptoms, and bring in appropriate skills are characteristic of such approaches. They are designed to break down the old stereotype of the newly graduated doctor who may have a lot of knowledge but does not know how to use it. This shift has seen the virtual end of the separation of distinct underpinning sciences to their greater integration, relating them to clinical features, and the introduction of many new subjects borrowing from the social sciences, such as professionalism and communication (the latter of which is a theme in several chapters in this book, e.g., Chaps. 9–11).

Another shift has been the move from learning the practical skills of doctoring in the real world to learning them in the simulated world. At the same time, learning in the real world is happening earlier in training. In post-registration training, there has been a shift to more formal structures and a more obviously 'taught' period of training (see Chap. 1 for more detail). It is possible to see many of these changes as related to changes in the practice of medicine, and they are, but they equally relate to developing understanding and knowledge about learning and teaching. These changes are generally shifts in balance more towards one end of a spectrum than the other rather than complete revolutions.

2.3 Learning Theory and Surgical Education

Learning theory is a general term for many different concepts and ideas. Some theories are about the developmental stages of childhood (e.g., Piaget's work), others about learning in particular contexts. Six groups of widely used educational ideas of particular influence and currency in surgical education are introduced here; some reoccur or are an assumed underpinning of ideas in subsequent chapters.

2.3.1 Constructivism

Most contemporary learning theories are constructivist. Constructivist learning theories are based on the idea that, in sum, the individual 'stores' knowledge and understanding in unique ways that will in turn influence their recall and understanding of that knowledge and their creation of new knowledge. How knowledge is stored will be influenced by a number of factors, including how an individual first encounters that knowledge. Knowledge is said to be stored in schemata that can be more or less complex and that interconnect with each other. The acquisition of new knowledge and understanding needs to add to and change (i.e., transform) existing schemata if it is to become absorbed and accessible.

Constructivism is important not least because it is influencing a wide range of medical/surgical educational activity. For example, it has had a strong influence in pre-registration medical education in the move away from traditional subjects and several years of basic science before knowledge is used in the clinical context. Constructivist theory lies behind ideas such as that knowledge will be better retained and accessed when it has been learnt in context and has been better linked together during learning. The 'joined up' schemata will have been formed early on. It has also influenced our understanding of clinical reasoning and retention of information. However, like much learning theory, it cannot show/dictate an optimum way of putting the theory into practice.

2.3.2 Approaches to Learning

Ference Marton is the most influential figure in the development of a theory known as 'approaches to learning' (also known as approaches to study) (Marton and Booth 1997; Marton et al. 1997). His early work with Säljö has been subsequently expanded upon, but in essence postulates that learners who have different intentions when they set out to learn something will have different types of outcomes. This is an idea that is therefore particularly pertinent in post-compulsory education where learners are learning out of choice, have experienced much formal education, and might be thought to have a repertoire of responses available to them. However, research has shown that not all learners have such a wide repertoire and not all use that repertoire appropriately (e.g., see Biggs and Tang 2007). How someone is taught may influence which approach they use, with some methods of teaching and assessing likely to limit the approaches learners will feel encouraged to take.

Those taking a surface approach to learning tend to be intent on memorising isolated facts and see the learning task as being one of meeting external, short-term goals. Those who take a deep approach to learning are seeking to understand the larger picture and fundamental ideas. Thus, those taking a deep approach to study are more likely to have developed, complex, and linked schemata in which to hold their knowledge, and therefore be able to call upon it with greater longevity and to use it in different ways, from the much more isolated, and therefore, usually, more shortly retained, surface approach. 'Approaches to learning' is a constructivist theory.

John Biggs (1987) was largely responsible for elaborating on this theory and suggesting that when approaching a learning task, especially if assessment is involved, learners who have both approaches available to them can decide which is likely to be most successful for the task in hand; they can take a strategic or achieving approach. Thus, if they face a multiple choice test, they may feel rote learning of information is best, but if they face extended matching questions in a test and they have only rote learnt without understanding underlying principles, they are unlikely to succeed; when asked a complex clinical question, those primarily using a surface approach may give/access some information that is somewhat relevant, but struggle to apply their knowledge or reach a satisfactory synthesis or resolution (Chap. 5 explains the difference between different types of test, such as those referred to here).

Approaches to learning are considered to be engendered by a mix of things, including past educational experiences and the way teaching and assessment are organised. This idea thus has many implications for teaching and training, especially in surgery, as surgeons need a lot of factual (and procedural) knowledge but also have to see the bigger picture.

When a deep approach to learning is taken, learners are likely to retain knowledge for longer, because it has been fitted together, are more likely to be able to call on that knowledge when needed, and link together things learned in different contexts. These findings have profound implications for the training of doctors and surgeons. They have been part of the underpinning theory that has influenced a move away from a very didactic teaching style, based on transmission of information, and from assessment forms based on pure rote learning, to the introduction of a wider range of teaching and assessment forms.

2.3.3 Clinical Reasoning and Decision Making

Our understanding of clinical reasoning and decision making has changed hugely over the last 20 years. There has been a shift from the belief, put crudely, that it is about teaching a lot of fact in traditional disciplines and about learning a near universal method or series of steps through which diagnosis and decisions can be achieved. Our understanding now is that clinical reasoning is much more about recognising significant patterns. When this is not efficacious or the patterns cannot be discerned, it is about being able to go back to first principles and reason through what is happening. There are a handful of researchers who have worked in this area over many years and many of their ideas can be found in: Bordage (2007), Charlin et al. (2007), Norman et al. (2007) and Schmidt and Rikers (2007). The schemata of clinicians are often known as 'illness scripts', in which their knowledge about diseases and conditions are held and linked together. Swift, almost unconscious pattern recognition is often what distinguishes many expert clinicians. Better understanding of how clinical reasoning works has had an impact on curricula and methods of teaching (Bowen 2006; Del Mar et al. 2006). Chapter 10 takes readers through some of these arguments in more detail and from a particular perspective.

2.3.4 Social Theories of Learning

'Approaches to learning' and earlier ideas about clinical reasoning developed from the traditions of cognitive psychology with an emphasis on the individual and what and how they think and learn. However, over the last 20–30 years, *social* theories of learning have contributed as much or more that is of value to surgical education, as they do not take the individual as the centre of learning but focus more on the context, the impact of others on the processes and content of learning (Haggis 2009). Bandura (for example 1977) was a trail blazer in pointing to the way in which people learn from each other through a range of mechanisms that include imitation, observation, and modelling.

Social theories of learning have also interacted with and contributed to ideas about learning in and from the workplace (Eraut 1994, 2007; Evans et al. 2009; Lester and Costley 2010; Swanwick and Morris 2010). Ideas about workplace learning have developed in the UK not only in connection with the professions but also with the rise of a new type of vocational, associate degree (the foundation degree), which is intimately linked with the needs of employment and often incorporates large work-based elements – just as post-registration training for surgery does. Social theories are of particular interest in surgery where surgeons work in teams and within particular and very specialised cultures and contexts. Vygotsky and a number of his contemporaries who worked in Stalinist Russia are a main source of ideas for many variants of social learning theory. Their work is still being explored and developed in the contemporary era. These ideas are returned to in the next section and also figure prominently in Chap. 13.

Experiential learning (see later section) – simply put the idea that we can learn from and by doing things, that is, by 'having an experience' – started from a focus on the individual who reflects on and learns from that experience. But the development of these ideas, to consider, for example, feedback from others to aid reflection or the potential for a team to reflect collectively to learn about team activity, draws more on the social and cultural context and the roles of a social group in collective learning. An example from surgery (or anaesthesia) might be a reflection by a surgical team in the form of preparation before surgery and debriefing afterwards. A subsequent section of this chapter considers these ideas in more detail and they also reoccur in several others, for example, Bleakley in Chap. 11.

2.3.5 Activity Theory, Work-Based Learning, Situated Learning, and Communities of Practice

Lev Vygotsky who died in 1934 is the best known of an eminent group of Soviet psychologists who initiated work on an important and influential social theory of learning that has become known as activity theory (Vygotsky 1978). For many years, their work was little known outside Russia. Vygotsky described the cultural mediation of actions, and although he still focussed on the individual he gave consideration to the surrounding culture in the development of learning.

Unlike approaches to learning, activity theory, as developed by, for example, Engeström (1990), emphasises action rather than cognition and the interaction between the individual, the community, and the object or outcomes. The social context and community might be those of the surgical team and operating theatre who share the same object/outcomes of a successful operation. Activity theory is concerned with theorising and explaining 'doing', both by the individual (within a community) and by collectives of individuals. 'Tools' are used to produce an outcome. Using activity theory, the elements of activities may be 'plotted' and analysed in relation to each other, usually represented diagrammatically in a triangular format within which relationships can be shown and around which additional elements can be added. The whole system will usually include rules (implicit and explicit) about how the community works and interacts and understandings about how the object is achieved by the collectivity of people/settings involved. These ideas challenge the notion that *teachers teach* what is learnt. Here, it is only through participating in a context that certain things can be learnt. The relevance for surgical education is clear.

Engeström has studied many organisational and work contexts, using and developing activity theory as he did so, to explain/understand learning in such settings. This has included a study in a Finnish hospital (2001) during which he expanded on his idea of 'expansive learning', that is, that work contexts can, and do, themselves generate new practices and learning transformations. This may seem an obvious point to surgeons, but it is quite different from long-held academic scientific assumptions that knowledge is generated through hypothesis testing. It is important in showing how working contexts and practices generate/give rise to ideas that are later worked up and developed and trialled.

This whole area is important in developing theoretical understanding of how learning at work occurs. An area that was not theorised in the past, usually occurred effectively only due to the long duration of apprenticeship, but even then could be 'hit and miss' depending upon the natural skill, patience, judgement, knowledge, and expertise of the 'master' (in surgery, the consultant or experienced registrar).

In surgery, in many parts of the world, service pressures have removed/reduced the apprenticeship element of training, while new structures and shorter training have been put in place, and more formal assessment introduced as patients and governments demand greater accountability. Such structures may draw more and less fully and more or less successfully on newer ideas such as these outlined here, but where they do so it is mainly in the absence of an understanding from the surgical profession of what is happening and what is intended.

Further work by other activity theorists is extending ideas about, for example, the difference between creative and routine activity. Activity theory assumes that any 'community' will have tacit knowledge embedded within it – for example, norms of behaviour or understood practices which are not written up – which new entrants have to learn. Several other chapters in this book also refer to this aspect of learning surgery.

This is a theory therefore that is especially relevant to learning in, from and for the workplace. The attractiveness and applicability of these ideas to the surgical setting are clear to see, with obvious parallels to be drawn; Chaps. 3 and 10–12 in particular draw on this area.

Situated learning is a theory that explores the understanding of knowledge in context, in the sense of the social context in which that learning occurs and to which it relates (Lave and Wenger 1991). Situated learning and activity theory link back to the same Vygotskyian roots. Situated learning is the type of learning that can only occur through an individual (or team) being immersed in a specific environment, with a specific group or type of people. It relates too to acquiring the professional identity and perspective of the profession to which one is seeking entry. Key ideas, as indicated above, are that learning is or can be a social practice and that practice can generate knowledge. Situated learning does not emphasise the role of a teacher or trainer, or necessarily of a formal curriculum. It privileges context and is about learning at and through work (work-based learning) and gradually moving, in terms of learning and practice, from the periphery of a profession to its centre stage. The importance of this idea for surgery is considerable. Situated learning is increasingly drawn upon to help understand and integrate better teamwork and inter-professional working. It also relates to the development of professionalism and other more intangible areas. Individuals are said to work in a 'community of practice' (Wenger 1998), which contains knowledge within it and generates knowledge and knowledge-based practice. Chapter 6 draws extensively on these perspectives.

Apprenticeship ideals, about a long immersion in a context and learning on the job, could be theorised as a form of situated learning. While contemporary circumstances have generally reduced the apprenticeship aspect of surgical education, many would argue that the value of participating in a community of practice – meaning in the case of surgery, a work context and ethos of shared values, common actions and aims, and the understood, but usually implicit, norms – has not diminished. Thus, more conscious efforts are now made to invoke the learning power of the community of practice, for example, through using scenario training where parameters are more controlled than in the real world, by emphasising things such as the role and importance of team working and debriefing, and more consciously drawing on the power of role modelling (see Chaps. 3 and 10–13).

Although training time and real world exposure have typically diminished in surgical training, more conscious use of actions and practices which draw on this group of ideas, and which reinforce the opportunity for learning from and in the community of practice, can enhance learning. It can be suggested that their more conscious use to inspire compatible curriculum design and teaching and learning practices could make best use of scarce real world exposure and training time. As already mentioned, outside of surgical education the idea of work-based learning has been developing and growing in importance and there is still much to learn from drawing these strands together.

The challenge now is to seek to further test and understand how this group of theories can support and provide insight about surgical training, and to better acquaint surgeons, trainers, and learners with them.

2.3.6 Experiential Learning, Reflective Practice, and Feedback

Experiential learning is the term used to describe a particular way of learning from practice (Kolb 1984). It seems an obvious idea, in line with the truism that 'practice makes perfect'. But experiential learning is the theory that describes how this happens and how such learning can be optimised. This theory has also played a part in correcting the balance within formal education that favoured the idea that education and learning happen in places like lecture theatres, not in operating theatres or other complex clinical settings. This again, now, seems a very obvious statement, but it was not one that underpinned medical pre-registration curricula until comparatively recent times.

Many people trace experiential learning back to Kurt Lewin in the 1930s. He worked in Germany and the USA and was a contemporary of the Russian social learning theorists whose ideas were still confined to the USSR. Lewin's ideas have been taken up by many others, most notably David Kolb, who developed them further (1984); they are now referred to by the general term experiential learning and have already been mentioned in a section above. Experiential learning theory rests on the idea and potential of a four-stage process or a learning cycle:

- Of doing something (e.g., closing a wound);
- Reflecting actively upon that thing, re-forming, and reshaping thoughts and understanding through analysis and synthesis, preferably with the help of feedback (from peers, patients, and surgical outcomes);
- Identification of areas for change/adjustment;
- And putting these into action or using to solve problems, this last step thus being the one that sets off a new cycle of learning from (a now altered) experience.

This process is often represented schematically as a cycle of which the best known version is Kolb's learning cycle. Many clinicians see this process as comparable to an audit cycle. Thus, using experiential learning theory, one can hypothesise about learning from experience that is not about learning by accident, but about a process that will enhance/speed up learning if consciously used and incorporated into teaching and learning designs. Care is needed to remember, however, that in the real world learning is unlikely to progress smoothly or at an even pace – there will be reverses and jumps rather than smooth cyclical progression, a point also made in Chap. 6.

Experiential learning as a tool for consciously enhancing learning rests (as described above) on a very active, engaged, and consciously undertaken reflective step. This has given rise to the term reflective practice, that is, the idea that professionals enhance their expertise through actively considering it, often with input from others and from any available data, and acting upon the conclusions drawn (Boud et al. 1985). There are many variations and developments of this idea, from 'reflecting on practice' (i.e., after the event) to 'reflecting in action' – a form of simultaneous reflection and action (Schön 1987). The idea of reflective practice has been taken up in training, with efforts being made to teach learners how to reflect and consciously draw on it as a learning aid. This has often taken the form of encouraging reflective writing (De Cossart and Fish 2005), such as reflective elements in portfolios or log books. It remains to be seen how far written reflection engenders the 'habit' of reflection and whether it promotes a different type (e.g., more profound) of reflection from the well developed, if not always consciously named, reflective approach that many professionals have to developing their expertise.

Reflection and its role in learning are linked to contemporary ideas regarding the role of feedback in learning. Feedback is an important part of the reflective process and may give an insight beyond that of the learner. It is for this reason that many contemporary developments in assessment stress that feedback on performance, which also draws out the learner to assess their own performance, is crucial to the learning process (see the section below on assessment and also Chap. 5). Debriefing can also be considered to be a form of collective feedback and reflection. Chapters 7 and 10 among others draw on some of these ideas.

2.4 Curriculum Design and Learning Outcomes

Undergraduate (pre-registration) medicine has long had explicit curricula. Historically, these started much more as a syllabus (a list of content) linked with an examination schedule. Stenhouse's classic definition of curricula is that they are an 'attempt to communicate the essential principles and features of an educational proposal in such a form that it is open to critical scrutiny and capable of effective translation in practice' (Stenhouse 1975) Today, curricula are conceived and constructed as integrated wholes that consist of aims (what 'the course' – or work rotation – hopes to achieve in broad terms); statements about what 'students' – trainee surgeons – should learn (which are different from the content listing of traditional syllabi, as much content will be formulated as statements of what students are expected to be able to do/know as a result of their learning), which are known as learning outcomes; the teaching and learning methods to be used for different parts of the course; and the methods of assessment. These are regarded as interlocking elements that have to be consistent with each other and compatible with the educational context. The development of better understanding of these elements and their relationship with each other has evolved over several decades. John Biggs coined the term constructive alignment (Biggs and Tang 2007) to describe the complex relationships between these elements of curricula. Below, three important aspects of the evolution of curricula are mentioned in more detail.

Bloom famously developed taxonomies of learning of particular types, starting with the cognitive domain (Bloom 1956), that is, pertaining to knowledge and understanding. He developed a hierarchy for the domain, starting at the simplest level, which he regarded as memorisation of the parroting type, and moving upwards as understanding and reasoning grow to a more analytical stage, to the highest levels of evaluation and synthesis (an example of which is diagnosis). He and others later developed taxonomies of the affective (values) and psychomotor (skills) domains. These domains are each typically represented as pyramids which reach a pinnacle at the most complex level. Although there have been changes made to the hierarchy of each area and although fewer people nowadays explicitly use these ideas about domains and levels, they remain the foundation of much thinking about designing, learning, and formulating learning outcomes, as they are helpful shorthand ways of referring in an abstract/generalised manner to areas of learning and levels of difficulty. In recent years, Biggs has elaborated on the work of Bloom (for example Biggs and Tang 2007) by seeking to express hierarchies of learning difficulty in a different way, showing how each level is a foundation for the next and also, in the cognitive domain, linking this to the approaches to learning theory, suggesting that taking a surface approach to learning will inhibit or prevent learning at higher levels.

Learning outcomes are statements about what learners should be able to do as a result of learning. That learning can be classroom or practice based, or indeed home based. It may take place with the help of trainers, or independent of them. Learning outcomes are intimately linked to assessment, because the statements of what students should have learnt should also be a guide to what is assessed. Learning outcomes will generally be formulated to start with verbs (what the learners should be able to *do* after some learning). They can be formulated at different levels of specificity and detail. For example, a rather inadequate learning outcome might simply state that after a given amount of training the learner should be able to close a wound. The tendency of the 1970s and 1980s to use behavioural objectives rather than today's idea of learning outcomes resulted in some overly specified, detailed, and complex curricula that amounted to hefty volumes of minutely specified statements, which were then all supposed to be accurately assessed, but rarely could be. Learning outcomes are thus conceived as more flexible with regard to suiting the level of specification to the tasks in hand. One might want to add some conditions to the earlier example, such as the type of wound, using a particular knot, or in a particular part of the body, or using specific instruments – or simply using appropriate techniques. The degree of specificity has to be judged against the task, the possibility of assessment, and the importance of the skill or understanding concerned. It is also vital not to be so bound by overly specified learning outcomes that creativity and innovation are stifled, particularly if one is attempting to use them with (the learning of) senior practitioners.

Historically, post-registration education (in the UK) has not had a formal curriculum in Stenhouse's sense. It used an apprenticeship model where concepts such as a specified core of learning that had to be mastered or standardised levels of achievement that needed to be demonstrated were less formally construed, assessed, and regulated (see Chap. 1). The move to specify a curriculum at postgraduate levels is in part a reflection of standardisation, patient safety, and accountability, in part of shorter training, and in part a reflection of the evolution of education as a discipline and the use of understandings such as those indicated above about learning theory and curriculum design. It is worth noting that there is a long history in education of studies about the gap between the curriculum on paper, the curriculum as taught and experienced, and as assessed; ideas that have not yet been widely drawn on in relation to postgraduate surgical curricula.

2.5 The Role of Assessment and Psychometrics in Learning

Assessment is an important part of learning. Generally in this book, and always in the introductory four chapters, when assessment and evaluation are used in their specialist educational meaning, it is their UK usage that is adopted (rather than American English). In English educational terminology, the terms are clearly distinguished from each other. Assessment is concerned with judging the learner and evaluation with judging the teacher, course, or context in which that learning occurs.

Self-assessment is an important feature of surgical learning as it tends to be in many other professions. It frequently involves active reflection as to how well something was done, and thereby enhancement of performance (see earlier section and later chapters, especially Chap. 10). Self-assessment is less about external judgement and verification and more about self-regulation and continuous improvement. It has always been a feature of the professional practice of senior and expert surgeons who generally engage in it barely consciously. Self assessment should not be dismissed as a modern fad; its purposes and role in training and learning are quite different from 'big bang' assessment for the purpose of external regulation and verification.

Another important aspect of assessment and one that is closely linked to self assessment is the feedback of others – be they patients, senior surgeons, or other members of the surgical team. The main purpose of feedback is to provoke more learning through input from the perspective of someone other than the learner. Learning occurs both in reaction to positive feedback (the learner who is smart at picking up signals will think 'Ah, that's something that has worked that I should keep on doing and improve upon'), and to negative feedback, although in this case the feedback will rarely be positively received unless it contains suggestions about how to improve or change. Reflection and giving and receiving feedback are skills vital to all professions and experts, and part of a culture of learning from and through work.

Self-assessment and feedback are types of formative assessment, that is, assessment whose primary purpose is to aid learning rather than provide external validation of fitness to practice. Such external validation may come through many different types of test and examination whose primary purpose is summative, that is, to arrive at an overall external judgement at a standardised or externally imposed point in time. Of course in practice, any given assessment may be designed to achieve both purposes, as is the case with a considerable amount of assessment in the current UK integrated surgical curriculum (referred to in Chap. 1).

In formal learning, assessment tends to take on a more regulated external element. In medicine, this external element particularly relates to 'being fit to practise'. Medical and surgical assessment has always been more tightly controlled than most other university-taught courses. It has thus a much more developed understanding and use of psychometrics than many other disciplines and has evolved many types of assessment specific to itself. Nowadays, this tighter regulation is increasingly a feature also of post-registration assessment. From an educational perspective, this could be thought of as having both good and bad effects.

Medical assessment 50 years ago was very different from that of today. Then, at elementary levels, assessment was often not very appropriate, in that it did not always match what was intended to be assessed to the format used for assessing it (e.g., using essays to test recall of factual nuggets or long or short cases to test procedural proficiency). Validity and fidelity were lacking and reliability was poorly understood or exercised. Such assessment was often 'high stakes,' but was not suitably controlled and constrained to provide confidence in the reliability of judgements nor was it firmly linked to assessing the key parts of the curriculum that need to be tested to reassure patients and to ensure a satisfactory standard has been reached.

Chapter 5 describes in detail the key concepts that underpin effective medical and surgical assessment and also the main types of assessment in use today. It points firmly to the way in which assessment design is an integral part of curriculum planning, as we have already seen above. Changes have been introduced to improve reliability, validity, and fidelity. With the move away from behavioural objectives as a universal panacea, there is now a degree of fluidity which is occurring alongside firmer understanding and use of psychometrics, and a return to recognising the place of judgement within an overall assessment regime. (However, an exclusive emphasis on reliability does still on occasion lead to poor validity and to trivialised assessments that fail to make best use of the opinion and experience of expert surgeons.) This increased fluidity mirrors the way in which our understanding of curriculum development and learning theory has developed to be more complex, better able to cope with less rigid contexts, etc. As Chap. 5 explains, some assessments have high validity and poor reliability while others have the reverse properties. The key is appropriate selection for purpose.

One noticeable change being introduced to surgical assessment in some countries is the use of more workplace-based assessment and the return to realising the importance of feedback in professional development, with this being 'designed in' and specified rather than happening through an apprenticeship model of education. The rationale for some of these changes stems in part from trying to use educational theory to enhance educational practices in changing contexts.

2.6 A Case Study: Problem-Based Learning as an Example of Using Educational Theory to Drive Educational Change

Problem-based learning (PBL) is an interesting method of teaching and learning that is quite widespread in undergraduate medical education and that some argue is what naturally happens' in clinical practice. It divides opinion. Where it has failed or been rejected it is possible to argue it has done so because it was used in a way that so compromised its underlying rationales, which are based on educational theory, that it had little hope of success. Such compromises have sometimes arisen from lack of educational understanding and at others from practical pressures. It has also had many successes. It provides a salutary lesson about the need to understand and evaluate carefully how to use educational theory successfully.

PBL is also an interesting case study for surgical education because many medical students all over the world study using this system, and come, arguably, into post-registration training with a very different background and expectation from students used to more traditional processes.

PBL was initially described and used by Howard Barrows (Barrows and Tamblyn 1980), but has subsequently developed with many recognised variations. It is an integrated system of learning and teaching.

PBL, in its ideal, is about creating learners who take a deep approach and develop integrated and accessible knowledge that they can use in various ways. To achieve this, curriculum and teaching are, in an ideal world, organised to limit the effectiveness of surface approaches. Another feature of PBL is the attempt to learn in a context that mirrors the real world of medicine and thus, it is argued, starts to create more naturally pattern recognition and schemata in which knowledge is sorted in useful ways for practising medicine. If PBL is viewed in these ways, the roles of teaching, assessment, the integration of knowledge, and practice fall into place. It draws on motivation theory and, in its use in medicine, on a desire to start developing 'clinical thinking and practice' at an early stage. It is argued it achieves the latter through approaching problems 'in the round', much more like a practising doctor than as a student learning separate disciplines, or even learning from information organised in systems.

PBL is initiated through 'scenarios' or triggers that start the learning process; these triggers can be selected to focus on commonly presenting conditions, diseases, and situations (Mr X comes to your clinic complaining of ...). This is likely to be important to the development of clinical reasoning and illness scripts (see above). A common misunderstanding of PBL is that it has no curriculum and no learning outcomes. Just the reverse is true; PBL has to be highly designed to work well. The main point is that learners are not (initially) told what the learning outcomes are; part of motivating them to learn and to take a deep approach is that they have to determine what they need to learn to unravel the 'mystery of Mr X'. Such an approach can sound artificial; appear to waste time and to be paradoxical. When PBL is well designed, the huge proportion of students will rapidly access their existing knowledge about the scenario presented and effectively determine what they need to learn to understand it better; they may do this in various ways including self study and accessing more traditional forms of teaching. This process is at the heart of the method, but to achieve it triggers have to be piloted for efficacy and need not only to be tweaked in use, but also changed from time to time to remove the potential for students to take shortcuts by 'borrowing' work from earlier years. At the report-back stage of PBL (after students have researched and thought about what Mr X's problem might be), poorly implemented PBL can become little more than students reading from notes without interaction, understanding, or probing tutor input.

PBL is not a universal panacea and to best achieve its educational payoff, it is usually expensive as it is time hungry in terms of planning, training, and tutoring. Attempts have been made with mixed success to reduce some of its intensive use of resource, but doing this effectively requires an in-depth understanding of the theory behind it and the characteristics of the particular students being taught using it. Some medical schools have moved away from PBL because of its costs, staff failures to use it correctly, inadequate and ill-suited assessment strategies, student incomprehension with learners wanting more spoon feeding, etc. Simply having a PBL curriculum will not ensure it 'works' if teaching staff are still approaching it from a non-PBL mindset and students are not inducted into its use – or prove able to subvert its practices to reduce the input it requires from them. Numerous studies of functional PBL implementation have shown that its effect on learning is usually to reduce the depth of detail that students learn in the short term but to intensify retention, understanding, and recall of information in clinical settings (e.g., Schmidt et al 1987; Alabanese and Mitchell 1993; Dolmans and Schmidt 2006). It is worth noting this in terms of what can be expected of graduates from good PBL curricula. (See Feather and Fry 2009 for a discussion at greater length.)

2.7 Implications of Educational Ideas for Surgical Training

The development of educational ideas and understanding should have had an impact on surgical training. The danger is that insufficient numbers of surgeons are sufficiently acquainted with these ideas to be able to operate effectively in a system using them, and even fewer are able to effectively participate in decision making about education and training from a theoretically informed viewpoint. And of course educational ideas are only one of many factors that inform the development of training. Education as a discipline is so different from science-based disciplines that *how* its theories and ideas can be used is also misconstrued. There is thus much scope for misunderstanding and failure; a point we make repeatedly in these first four chapters and which can be seen in the PBL case study. It is also a misconception to see a lot of modern curricula for postgraduate training as overly influenced by educational theory. Shorter training times, fewer inpatient stays, public demands for practising doctors to be 'guaranteed' as reaching a satisfactory level of practice, etc. are nothing to do with education. But education does offer some ideas and hopefully some help about how to tackle these issues, from more formal and planned curricula that can maximise training time, through the use of simulation, to improved assessment practices.

Learners too need to grasp how they are expected to learn. Approaches that worked in school will not necessarily be effective in university education and strategies that worked at university may not be effective at post-registration level. Trainee doctors who can learn in different ways and from different circumstances are at an advantage over those who use a much more limited range of strategies. Doctors coming into clinical medicine who have not developed an 'independent learning' ethic will struggle. They will find they are no longer spoon fed, nor do they have many years in which they can demonstrate their ability to move to consultant level.

Designers of education – be they surgeons, educationalists, or policy makers – need to understand the overlapping worlds of surgical education. Educational designers need to take on board that not all educational practices work at all levels, or in all contexts.

Looking to the future, the contribution of educational ideas to surgical education will continue to be crucial. Surgical education in turn is well placed to contribute to the development of educational ideas, given its unique nature and practice-based training. One likely development is better understanding of how cognitive and social theories of learning fit together to explain learning.

References

Albanese, M., & Mitchell, S. (1993). Problem-based learning: A review of literature on its outcomes and implementation issues. *Academic Medicine, 68*(1), 52–81.

Bandura, A. (1977). *Social learning theory*. New York: General Learning Press.

Barrows, H. S., & Tamblyn, R. M. (1980). *Problem-based learning: An approach to medical education*. Heidelberg: Springer.

Biggs, J. (1987). *Student approaches to learning and studying*. Hawthorn: Australian Council for Educational Research.

Biggs, J., & Tang, C. (2007). *Teaching for quality learning at university: What the student does* (3rd ed.). Milton Keynes: Open University/Society for Research into Higher Education.

Bloom, B. (1956). *Taxonomy of educational objectives handbook 1: Cognitive domain*. New York: McGraw-Hill.

Bordage, G. (2007). Prototypes and semantic qualifiers: From past to present. *Medical Education, 41*(12), 1117–1121.

Boud, D., Keogh, R., & Walker, D. (Eds.). (1985). *Reflection: Turning experience into learning*. London: Academic.

Bowen, J. L. (2006). Educational strategies to promote clinical diagnostic reasoning. *The New England Journal of Medicine, 355*(21), 2006.

Charlin, B., Boshuizen, H. P., Custers, E. J., & Feltovich, P. J. (2007). Scripts and clinical reasoning. *Medical Education, 41*(12), 1178–1184.

De Cossart, L., & Fish, Della. (2005). *Cultivating a thinking surgeon. New perspectives on clinical teaching, learning and assessment*. Shrewsbury: TFM Publishing Ltd.

Del Mar, C., Doust, J., & Galsziou, P. (2006). *Clinical thinking. Evidence, communication and decision-making*. Oxford: Blackwell/BMJ.

Dolmans, D. H., & Schmidt, H. G. (2006). What do we know about cognitive and motivational effects of small group tutorials in problem-based learning? *Advances in Health Sciences Education, 11*(4), 321–336.

Engeström, Y. (1990). *Learning, working and imagining: Twelve studies in activity theory*. Helsinki: Orienta-Konsultit.

Engeström, Y. (2001). Expansive learning at work: Towards an activity theoretical consideration. *Journal of Education and Work, 14*(1), 133–156.

Eraut, M. (1994). *Developing professional knowledge and competence*. London: Falmer.

Eraut, M. (2007). Learning from other people in the workplace. *Oxford Review of Education, 33*, 403–422.

Evans, K., Guile, D., & Harris, J. (2009). *Putting knowledge to work*. London: Institute of Education.

Feather, A., & Fry, H. (2009). Key aspects of teaching and learning in medicine and dentistry. In H. Fry, S. Ketteridge, & S. Marshall (Eds.), *A handbook for teaching and learning in higher education. Enhancing academic practice* (3rd ed., pp. 424–448). London: Routledge. chapter 26.

Haggis, T. (2009). What have we been thinking of? A critical overview of 40 years of student learning research in higher education. *Studies in Higher Education, 34*(4), 377–390.

Kennedy, T. J. F. (2009). Towards a tighter link between supervision and trainee ability. *Medical Education, 43*(12), 1126–1128.

Kolb, D. A. (1984). *Experiential learning*. Englewood Cliffs: Prentice-Hall.

Lave, J., & Wenger, E. (1991). *Situated learning: Legitimate peripheral participation*. Cambridge: Cambridge University Press.

Lester, S., & Costley, C. (2010). Work-based learning at higher education level: Value practice and critique. *Studies in Higher Education, 35*(5), 561–575.

Marton, F., & Booth, S. (1997). *Learning and awareness*. Mahwah: Lawrence Erlbaum Associates.

Marton, F., Hounsell, D., & Entwistle, N. (1997). *The experience of learning* (2nd ed.). Edinburgh: Scottish Academic Press.

Norman, G., Young, M., & Brooks, L. (2007). Non-analytical models of clinical reasoning: The role of experience. *Medical Education, 41*(12), 1140–1145.

Schmidt, H. G., & Rikers, R. M. (2007). How expertise develops in medicine: Knowledge encapsulation and illness script formation. *Medical Education, 41*(12), 1133–1139.

Schmidt, H., Dauphinee, W., & Patel, V. (1987). Comparing the effects of problem-based learning and conventional curricula in an international sample. *Journal of Medical Education, 62*, 305–315.

Schön, D. (1987). *Educating the reflective practitioner: Toward a new design for teaching and learning in the professions*. San Francisco: Jossey-Bass.

Stenhouse, L. (1975). *An introduction to curriculum research and development*. London: Heinemann.

Swanwick, T., & Morris, C. (2010). Shifting conceptions of learning in the workplace. *Medical Education, 44*(6), 538–539.

Vygotsky, L. (1978). *Mind in society: The development of higher psychological processes*. Cambridge: Harvard University Press.

Wenger, E. (1998). *Communities of practice. Learning, meaning and identity*. Cambridge: Cambridge University Press.

Chapter 3
Simulation

Roger Kneebone

3.1 Introduction

The starting point for this chapter is that simulation already occupies a central position in surgical education, both at undergraduate and postgraduate levels, and that this role seems certain to expand. The preeminence of craft within surgical practice means that simulation has traditionally played a more prominent role there than in other specialities.

Many of the other contributors to the book allude to simulation, and some (especially Chap. 8) consider selected aspects in great detail. This chapter takes a more philosophical perspective, highlighting some issues that are often overlooked during discussions of specific simulation approaches and challenging some assumptions that are implicit in current strategies.

First of all, it will outline the place of simulation in current surgical practice before going on to consider some more innovative applications. The discussion will focus on the use of physical simulation applied to surgical procedures, recognising but leaving aside for the moment other uses of simulation in healthcare education (such as the use of Simulated Patients to practise history taking). A detailed account of simulator and e-learning design is presented by Bello and Brenton in Chap. 8, highlighting potential synergies between these approaches. The current chapter does not address issues of e-learning.

To many people, simulation implies using inanimate models and mannequins for gaining procedural skills, offering a safe alternative to carrying out procedures on real patients. I will argue that although necessary, this aspect of simulation is not sufficient to satisfy the growing demand for alternatives to traditional clinical learning. As highlighted by other contributors to this book (see Chaps. 11–13),

R. Kneebone (✉)
Surgical Education, Imperial College London, London, UK
e-mail: r.kneebone@imperial.ac.uk

H. Fry and R. Kneebone (eds.), *Surgical Education: Theorising an Emerging Domain*, Advances in Medical Education 2, DOI 10.1007/978-94-007-1682-7_3,

learning is a social activity which takes place within and alongside the highly complex processes of clinical care. From this perspective, simulation should recreate sociocultural practice rather than focusing exclusively on the acquisition of component skills.

This is not to belittle the value of simulation in practising procedural skills. Of course, such approaches are not new – generations of medical students have honed their skills by suturing blankets and giving injections into oranges. In recent years, a range of inanimate models and computers of varying levels of sophistication have emerged, allowing learners to practise a widening array of techniques. Indeed, dedicated 'skills centres' form an essential part of any contemporary medical school. In such centres, students can practise how to take blood, insert urinary catheters, set up intravenous infusions, and give injections. Benchtop models or 'part task trainers' offer deliberately simplified, decontextualised versions of clinical tasks, allowing learners to become familiar with techniques before trying to apply them to real patients (Issenberg et al. 2005/1; McGaghie et al. 2010). The key aim is to reduce the pressures of clinical practice as well as eliminating the potential for causing harm.

Yet, this view of simulation privileges inanimate models and a task-focused view of procedural skills. Although the case for acquainting novices with the basics of a new procedure in a safe setting is compelling, such an approach carries a number of assumptions. This chapter tests some of these assumptions, viewing simulation through a critical lens and attempting to tease out and examine key concepts. The aim is to scrutinise established practices, examining how they fit the needs of surgical education at postgraduate level. In the process, some controversial views will be advanced.

3.1.1 Simulation as a Mirror for Clinical Care

A widely held view is that surgical training should be based on the progressive acquisition of propositional and procedural knowledge and the mastery of operative skills, initially 'straightforward' but moving to increasing levels of difficulty. By simplifying these skills and stripping away the distractions of context, simulation (the argument goes) allows first things to be mastered first.

An alternative view, however, is that the most important aspect of any operation is not a surgeon's technique, but their ability to function effectively in a setting where members of a team share responsibility for the care of the patient undergoing surgery. In a sense, the operating theatre functions as an ecosystem, whose inhabitants function individually but in a profoundly interrelated way. The survival of the whole depends on the interlocking of its parts. From this perspective, communication, professionalism, and the ability to work collectively to solve problems are not extras to be added once technique has been mastered, but constitute the essential attributes of safe practice.

These elements of surgical practice are more complex, more subtle, and far harder to define than specific operative techniques. When working well, they are invisible, and it is only when things go wrong that they become evident. Yet, if simulation is to be effective, it must address these complexities and render them visible.

A more satisfactory conception of simulation might therefore be as part of a spectrum of resources drawn up alongside clinical care in order to complement its richness. Acknowledging that learning must be rooted in the complex and unruly world of actual care, a menu of additional resources (including e-learning and simulation) provides additional support to be used selectively when needed. Bello and Brenton develop the concept of the Simulation Journey in Chap. 8.

3.1.2 Drivers for Simulation

Chapter 1 highlighted some key drivers that are changing the landscape of clinical care. From a surgical perspective, these include reductions in working hours, dwindling opportunities for hands-on experience in the operating theatre, a changing ethical climate, and an unstoppable rise in the role played by technology in surgical care. Dwindling opportunities for clinical exposure are affecting undergraduate and postgraduate education alike, and there is growing concern that clinicians will not have gained adequate experience by the time they complete their training. Simulation offers an attractive solution. Until relatively recently, however, simulation was regarded as the province of a minority of enthusiasts – of clear benefit in specific settings (such as resuscitation and anaesthesia training), but peripheral to mainstream training.

Simulation has a particular resonance in the case of surgeons, as it seems ideally suited to their particular needs. In particular, it appears to allow them to master their operative craft through repeated practice without endangering patients. Current developments in health policy are throwing simulation into even sharper focus and profoundly altering its position on the stage. The Chief Medical Officer's 2009 report (CMO 2009) highlighted the centrality of simulation within healthcare training of a multiprofessional workforce. More recently, the Temple Report has identified simulation as a key plank in addressing the challenges of providing effective education within a limited working week (Temple 2010). Implicit in these reports is a need to make simulation-based education widely available – yet it is not obvious how this might be achieved, especially within increasing resource constraints.

On closer inspection, moreover, fault lines appear in this apparently self-evident view of simulation's benefits. In spite of a growing acceptance in many quarters of simulation's key role, there remains confusion about exactly what simulation is and how best to use it. In the current financial climate, established approaches to so-called 'immersive' simulation (focusing on a small number of extremely expensive, resource-intensive specialised centres) seem unsustainable. And with the increasing prominence of simulation has come mistrust of its rise and resistance to what is sometimes perceived as its centralised imposition.

Even the word 'simulation' itself is not neutral, but carries many meanings and holds many resonances. Simulation activity, although widespread, frequently takes place without a clear definition or theoretical framework. To some, simulation is synonymous with simple benchtop models as described above. Others think of sophisticated mannequins and 'drills' for practising emergency procedures. To others again, Simulated Patients (professional actors) provide opportunities to explore subtleties of consultation dynamics and technique. Given this variety of meanings, it is not surprising that misunderstandings sometimes arise.

This chapter explores some of those meanings, attempting to set out such a framework for debate. It will distinguish between *simulation* (in the wider sense of a means of safely recreating elements of a complex clinical reality) and *simulators* (the use of models, mannequins, or computers for learning specific tasks) – a distinction also drawn by Bello and Brenton in Chap. 8. It will argue for simulation to be grounded in relevant theory, underpinned by a sound knowledge of education and related fields as well as a deep understanding of clinical care. Crucially, it will argue that simulation should address the conditions of clinical practice (with all its complexity, uncertainty, and contingency) rather than only focusing on selected components.

Elsewhere (Kneebone 2005), the author has brought together key theories relating to the acquisition and retention of expertise; ways in which knowledge and skill are learned and taught (proposing a Vygotskian conception of simulation as a resource within an individual's Zone of Proximal Development) (Wertsch 1985); the relationship between formal teaching and the workplace-based communities of practice where such knowledge is applied (drawing on contemporary apprenticeship theory); and the affective or emotional climate of learning and teaching. Such an overview must now be extended to take into account societal changes such as the widespread adoption of social networking and the impact of Web 2.0 technology on e-learning.

3.2 What is Simulation About?

This chapter asserts that simulation, if is to be meaningful, must reflect clinical practice, and that this involves far more than dexterity or technique. At the heart of any clinical encounter stand two people: a patient and a clinician, linked in a relationship of care. Such care consists of many elements, sometimes (though not always) including invasive procedures or operations. But always the anchor is a personal relationship, one which develops and unfolds within the complexity and unpredictability of people's lives. In real-world clinical care, there is a sense of uniqueness, of contingency, and of 'unruliness'. No person is exactly like another, and everyone brings to a clinical encounter their own history and experience as well as their body. Working with this complexity is an essential part of becoming a clinician. The application of knowledge and skills in the context of individual care is a key element of effective practice.

Box 3.1: Limitations of Simulation

Alongside the benefits of simulation centres mentioned above, key limitations include the following:

- The primary relationship is between a learner and a machine/model, rather than between two human beings (a clinician and a patient).
- Skills are learned within the confines of a dedicated simulation centre, where the primary activity is seen to be simulation rather than clinical care and where a clinical context is absent.
- The horizon of learning is confined to component tasks, often without a sense of progression or an awareness of the wider context of team work and communication. Skills acquired in a simulation centre are treated as snapshots rather than building a progressive trajectory of clinical expertise.
- Simulation centre activity often carries a sense of imposition and of external control which may generate resistance and impede widespread acceptance. Simulation centres can be driven by agendas (such as the need to achieve throughput targets and ensure financial viability) that do not mesh with the expectations of learners.
- Simulation centres may carry connotations of assessment, kindling memories of summative examinations and being placed under scrutiny. An undue focus on reliability can detract from validity.

The argument for acquiring and refining clinical skills in a simulated environment before using them in real life is compelling. But in order to make sense educationally, such learning needs to resonate with the conditions of clinical care. At present, a narrow definition of simulation seems widely prevalent. According to this view, simulation offers a way of practising individual tasks and procedural skills, as outlined above. Simulators are seen as central to this activity and range from simple benchtop models to sophisticated mannequins and virtual reality computer programs.

This primacy of simulators immediately raises the important issue of authenticity. Of course, there are obvious benefits in mastering the essential constituents of a clinical task before trying to apply it to a real patient. It clearly makes no sense to attempt a procedure without understanding the equipment which must be used to perform it or the aims that it must achieve. But frequently within task-based simulation there is a lack of realism, a sense that the simulation is taking place in a separate universe that is somehow disconnected from the real world. This disconnection is accentuated by the fact that simulation activity commonly takes place within dedicated facilities or simulation centres, as described above. Box 3.1 outlines some limitations of current approaches to simulation.

By their nature, simulation centres do not deal with real patients. Instead, they deal with representations of patients (usually inanimate models or computers) which allow clinicians to 'do things;' that is, to invade without the normal consequences of invasion. Simulation centres provide a space within which such invasion can be practised in safety, using inanimate simulators as proxies for real patients.

The core relationship is therefore between a person (the learner) and an object or machine (the simulator). But a machine, however sophisticated, must remain a machine. The human-machine relationship will always be qualitatively different from the relationship between two people. Increasing the complexity and sophistication of the machine will not address this fundamental limitation. Paradoxically, indeed, efforts to increase the sophistication of a mannequin may result in a *reduction* in perceived realism. Highlighting the physicality of the simulator may interfere with participants' internal imaginative processes, forcing the artificial nature of the encounter into the foreground. This is especially evident in surgical procedures, where simulator representations of tissues and organs are seldom sufficiently realistic to overcome a natural disbelief.

The lens of critical discourse analysis is helpful here (Hodges et al. 2008). The context and environment described above might be summarised as a *discourse of the simulation centre*. This discourse frames simulation itself as the primary activity, and highlights the benefits of abstracted, depersonalised training. The vocabulary of the simulation centre includes words such as assessment, reliability, validation, and other terminology that can seem alien to clinicians whose primary aim is to learn. Within this discourse, a powerful voice is that of simulator developers. Often rooted in engineering and software design, such developers may lack understanding of the clinical issues within which learning is embedded.

The term 'discourse of the simulation centre' is not used in a pejorative sense in this chapter. On the contrary, abstraction of the kind which simulation centres provide offers immense power and great benefit. But a conflation of ideas around simulation has muddied the waters of debate. This chapter proposes that another discourse must underpin that of the simulation centre – a *discourse of clinical care*. These discourses are often divided from one another, and the relationship between them is problematic. A major challenge for simulation is to reconcile the two discourses while preserving the essentials of both.

3.3 Conceptualising Simulation

There is an obvious tension here. In one sense, too much abstraction can lead to a lack of realism and authenticity. Yet, surgical operations have characteristics which surgeons are required to master, irrespective of the patients upon whom the operations are performed. An appendicetomy is definable as a procedure, without having to be linked to an individual who undergoes it. Moving beyond the care of one individual person to gain widely applicable knowledge and skill therefore demands a simplification, a reduction, a boiling down – in other words, a *representation* of care which moves away from the particularity of an individual patient. So, how can this circle be squared, ensuring that abstracted knowledge and skill are always placed at the service of real-world clinical care?

It is worth trying to elucidate the relationship between the real world of clinical care and the world of simulation a little further. In his recent book *The Master and his Emissary: the divided brain and the making of the Western world*, McGilchrist offers an interesting viewpoint that may help to crystallise the issue (McGilchrist 2009). McGilchrist takes the title of his book from a story by Nietsche of a powerful ruler who dispatches an emissary to distant parts, entrusting him with powers to rule on his behalf. The emissary gradually takes over the functions of the ruler himself, with disastrous consequences for both. McGilchrist uses this as a metaphor for the relationship between the cerebral hemispheres.

> There are two fundamentally opposed realities, two different modes of experience; each of is ultimate importance in bringing about the recognisably human world; and their difference is rooted in the bihemispheric structure of the brain (p. 3).

Although not writing with simulation in mind, he argues that a central difference in the functioning of the two hemispheres underlies two different yet complementary views of the world which, if out of balance, create major problems. McGilchrist proposes that the world of the left hemisphere depends on abstraction and the ability to manipulate things out of context. This provides great analytical power, but is ultimately lifeless and self-referential. The world of the right hemisphere, on the other hand, is the messy and unpredictable world of real life – unimaginably complex and impossible to tie down or precisely define, but the only mediator of directly lived experience.

Drawing extensively on evidence from psychiatry and the neurosciences, McGilchrist describes a *reverberative* relationship between the two hemispheres. The left hemisphere selects, abstracts, and generalises from what the right hemisphere feeds it – but must then return what it has processed to be subsumed by the right hemisphere. Both these realities are critically important, but they must be interwoven. Undue dominance of either leads to a destructive imbalance. But this crucial final stage of synthesis does not occur when the left hemisphere holds sway.

The concept of an emissary who arrogates to himself the wider functions which he should serve offers a cautionary tale for the relationship between the simulated and the real. Without wishing to overstretch the argument, McGilchrist's view offers a helpful metaphor for the relationship between clinical reality and simulation, highlighting the crucial importance of reintegration. The touchstone must be actual clinical care, with all its individuality and unruliness (a right hemisphere world). To achieve the educational objectives of institutions and society (such as learning, assessment, or certification), this reality must be counterbalanced by abstraction into a setting where variables can be controlled, safety ensured, and performance measured (a left hemisphere world). To remain effective, the outcomes of this left hemisphere process must be fed back directly into the everyday world of care (Kneebone et al. 2004).

The reverberative process can work in two ways. If well adjusted and mutually respectful, abstraction works in the service of care. The learning of those aspects which lend themselves to abstraction is temporarily brought into a brightly-lit world where edges are hard and there are few shadows. Specific elements can be practised and assessed. But these activities must remain part of a bigger picture; soon they are 'returned' to their natural setting where the lights are dimmer and the shadows begin to emerge.

If ill-adjusted, however, the circle can become vicious. Approaches which are appropriate in the simulation centre do not always transfer to real people. If decontextualised simulation becomes the dominant discourse, learners' *clinical* behaviour can be moulded by the world of impersonal abstraction and the tail wags the dog. Procedures (rather than the patients who need them) can become ascendant, and the technical can come to dominate the human. If that happens, clinicians may start to treat real patients as 'procedures' ('the appendix in Bed 3').

According to this view, the key issue is the relationship between the clinical and the simulated. If the two worlds are aligned effectively, each enriches the other. If the alignment fails, the activities of the simulation centre do not mesh with the everyday world of work in which clinicians are immersed and simulation becomes detached from its roots (Bligh and Bleakley 2006). How then can we frame simulation so that it meets these demands for alignment? In Chap. 8, Bello and Brenton develop the concept of a 'simulation continuum', where a wide range of simulations, simulators, and e-learning resources support each learner's trajectory as it unfolds.

3.4 Authenticity, Expertise, and Dexterity

A key issue here is the extent to which simulation can capture real world practice. Writing in 1993, Grant Wiggins wrote:

> If we want competent performance later, we need to introduce novices to that performance from day one. Only a deep and ancient prejudice about academic learning keeps us thinking that intellectual competence is achieved by accretion of knowledge and movement through simple logical elements to the complex whole – instead of movement from a *crude* grasp of the whole to a *sophisticated* grasp of the whole (Wiggins 1993b) p. 202.

But intellectual competence is only one component of surgery. Amongst many others, dexterity skills are central to the surgeon's craft (Sennett 2008). It is clear from the extensive literature on expertise that such mastery requires many years of sustained deliberate practice (Ericsson chapter & refs) (Ericsson 2004; Ericsson et al. 2006, 2007; Ericsson and Charness 1994; Guest et al. 2001) – a case made by Ericsson himself in Chap. 7. In the case of surgical procedures, the acquisition of technical mastery requires repeated practice, allowing fundamental skills to become part of the surgeon's unconscious repertoire. From there, they can be called into play whenever needed. Many such techniques, especially at an early stage of training, lend themselves well to simulation-based practice. In both open and minimal access surgery, basic skills of handling instruments, tying knots, dissecting tissues, and performing anastomoses can be effectively practised in a simulation centre setting.

Yet craft skills are always applied within a specific context, where each work is unique and outcomes cannot be guaranteed. Pye distinguishes between the workmanship of certainty and the workmanship of risk (Pye 1968). The former implies a factory-like process, where the result is predetermined and unalterable once production begins. In the latter, however, the quality of the result is not predetermined, but depends on the judgement, dexterity, and care which the maker exercises during the process of making. In the case of a surgeon, this workmanship of risk requires an interplay between human tissues and manipulative skill in a setting whose complexity defies predictability (Heidegger 1968). This need to adapt, to respond appropriately to the unexpected, becomes especially evident in complex operations on sick patients.

But dexterity is not only an indispensable attribute of surgeons for the obvious reason of being able to perform operations safely. It is also crucial to the formation of a surgeon's identity *as a surgeon*, to the kind of professional they are or want to become. To surgeons, deftness and precision are not just desirable skills to have, but are central to who they are.

At first glance, simulation centres seem ideally suited to support the acquisition of expertise, as they allow component skills to be performed as often as required. Yet, as outlined above, surgical expertise is not confined to procedural dexterity. Indeed, there is far more to surgery and being a surgeon than what takes place in the operating theatre. A surgical patient's trajectory encompasses many elements, including preoperative diagnosis, the operation itself, the postoperative phase, and preparation for discharge. Every stage requires an amalgam of complex and highly demanding professional qualities and skills, including communication, leadership, decision making, and team work, as well as the obvious need for technical mastery.

The concept of routine and adaptive expertise is useful here, and is explored further by Epstein and Moulton in Chap. 10 (Bereiter 2002; Bereiter and Scardamalia 1993; Mylopoulos and Regehr 2007). Routine experts become highly proficient in dealing with similar tasks repeatedly. Although this is very effective when all goes well, such experts tend to frame unexpected problems according to solutions they have already determined. Adaptive experts, on the other hand, generate new solutions for every situation, deliberately challenging themselves by working outside their comfort zone. Each type of expertise is valuable, and both are required within surgical practice. If successful, simulation can provide the conditions for acquiring both – for acquiring that 'sophisticated grasp of the whole' which allows a range of integrated qualities to be tested within conditions of uncertainty (Wiggins 1993a).

Rather than defining an individual's expertise as falling into one category or another, it may be more helpful to think in terms of *dimensions* of expertise, which everyone possesses to a greater or lesser extent. From this perspective, the challenge becomes how to recognise and apply the most appropriate dimension in a given set of circumstances. Simulation has much to offer here.

3.4.1 *Risk and Safety*

A key requirement of clinical care is to ensure the safety of patients. In surgery, this concern is especially well founded. The dangers of operative surgery are plainly evident, and a botched operation causes immediate damage. At an obvious level, simulation centres offer insulation from harm, ensuring that even novices can practise without jeopardising patients.

Yet, here again, the case is not as simple as it first appears. It is an inescapable reality that surgery involves risk, and that part of surgeon's role is managing that risk responsibly. This involves learning how to recognise and deal with dangerous clinical situations, functioning as an effective team member under conditions of uncertainty, and coming to terms with the consequences of error. For a surgeon, encountering the unexpected or making a mistake can generate high levels of stress which in turn can affect judgement, performance, and effective communication.

If simulation is to be effective, it must somehow allow learners to 'experience danger safely' – not provide a setting where all semblance of danger has been stripped out. Unless this can be achieved, simulation will only offer a pale representation of the real world. Worse, it may encourage complacency and a misplaced overconfidence. This resonates with Meyer and Land's identification of *uncertainty* as a threshold concept within surgery (Chap. 6) – the need for continual reading and reframing of a situation as it develops.

3.5 New Directions for Simulation

Simulation offers the opportunity to abstract from a complex reality, to generalise from the particular, and to create conditions for repeated practice which minimise any potential for harm. Yet, common themes running through the arguments outlined above are complexity, nonlinearity, and the need to 'think clinically'. It follows that any simulation should recreate these conditions of clinical practice, helping learners to think like clinicians (not technicians) while preserving the centrality of the relationship of care. This is a tall order.

3.5.1 *Placing the Patient at the Centre*

When practising a procedural skill on an isolated benchtop model in a simulation centre or skills lab, it is extremely difficult to 'imagine oneself into' the clinical situation which this exercise represents. Partly, this is due to a lack of contextual cues – simulation centres seldom recreate the conditions of clinical practice in a way which appears convincing. But largely this is caused by the absence of a human patient. This absence places an inanimate model at the centre of the learner's focus.

Work by our group has developed the concept of hybrid or patient-focused simulation, where a simulator (usually a benchtop model) is attached to or aligned with a real person (usually a Simulated Patient or professional actor) (Kneebone 2009a; Kneebone et al. 2002, 2003, 2005, 2006, 2007). This brings about a powerful shift in perception, compelling the learner to relate to the patient as a human being at the same time as performing the procedure. By having to respond to the 'patient's' questions during a procedure, for example, the clinician has to bring into play a wide range of key skills and behaviours. This concept is described further by Nestel and Bentley in Chap. 9.

Initial work aligning existing models with Simulated Patients (SPs) was technically crude, though it provided surprisingly high levels of perceived realism and engagement. Yet there are obvious limitations to scenario design if models have to be contrived so as to conceal a join. Current work within our group is using prosthetics expertise from film and television to create 'seamless simulation' – highly realistic yet relatively low-cost models which are attached to a person in such a way that the join cannot be seen. Preliminary studies have demonstrated very high levels of engagement by participants and we are currently exploring this concept systematically.

3.5.2 Heightening Realism for Surgeons

A particular issue with surgical simulation is that current models and programs are seldom convincing enough to overcome the scepticism of participants. This is especially the case with experienced surgeons, who have already mastered the preliminary stages of technique and whose challenges have moved to a different level.

Historically, immersive simulation has been spearheaded by anaesthetists, for whom simulation-based crisis training has become an integral component of learning (Gaba et al. 2001, 1998/7; Gaba 2004; Gaba and DeAnda 1988; Holzman et al. 1995/12). For anaesthetic teams, the anaesthetic machine acts as a crucial mediator between the world of the patient and the world of the clinician (Goodwin 2008; Hindmarsh and Pilnick 2002, 2007). This is especially the case in scenarios involving a general anaesthetic, where many of the characteristics of authentic practice (including physiological monitoring and the administration of drugs) can be convincingly recreated by means of such a machine, in the absence of a real patient. In a sense, communication with the anaesthesised patient takes place 'through the machine', reflecting pathophysiological responses generated by a mannequin.

For the surgeon, however, the picture looks very different. As outlined above, dexterity and operative skill are key to a surgeon's professional identity. Crucially, these involve interacting with human tissue. Although effective team work is indispensable, the ability to 'do' the operation is a primary focus. Indeed, the operating theatre is designed so surgeons can give their undivided attention to what they are looking at, without having to raise their eyes from the brightly lit operative field. The special social practices of surgery allow the surgeon to demand an instrument and expect it to be placed in his/her hand immediately, bypassing completely the usual conventions of eye contact and polite phraseology (see Chap. 10).

If the surgeon's primary focus is the operative field, any simulation which does not recreate that field realistically will impose considerable demands in terms of willing suspension of disbelief. Yet, most current surgical simulators are strikingly unrealistic, both in appearance and behaviour. Inanimate models are insufficiently subtle to recreate the nuances of human tissue, while dead animal parts cannot recreate the characteristics of living organs. Crucially, perhaps, bleeding is usually absent and anatomical variation is seldom seen. Although in some countries, live animals are used for surgical training, in many parts of the world (including the UK) this is not possible. All too often, therefore, the impact of simulation is of a predetermined, formulaic exercise which is more realistic for other team members than for the surgeons themselves and which fails to capture the uniqueness of individual operations.

3.5.3 Creating an Effective Simulation

A central question is therefore *what* should be simulated and what level of detail is required in order to provide authenticity and to secure engagement. In many simulation centres (especially those catering to postgraduate surgical training), much attention is paid to the replication of a whole environment such as an operating theatre or intensive care unit. As many elements as possible of the original setting are provided, including operating lights and tables, anaesthetic machines and storage facilities. Such simulations allow clinical teams to take part in scenarios based around common or important clinical situations.

Yet, the central issue concerns function rather than structure. What must be recreated for the clinician is a sense of being involved in an operation. The challenge is to ensure that simulation *works* at the appropriate levels. From this perspective, simulation is more like a painting than a photograph, recreating those elements which are functionally most important rather than attempting to replicate every detail. In fact, attention is not uniform and unselective – clinicians see most clearly what is most important to them, and the rest becomes blurred. And where this focus is directed will depend on the clinician's specialty.

Elsewhere, the author has used an image of concentric 'circles of focus' to describe a gradient of perceived realism (Kneebone 2010). Applying this model to the surgeon, the primary focus of attention in the operating theatre is the operative field. In this central circle, every detail is of interest and importance. Around this is another circle – the setting within which the operation is taking place. Although this too is crucial, what takes place here registers at a lower level of awareness. This circle relates to *context* – the setting where the operation occurs and the people who take part in it. Within this second circle, a general sense of being in an operating theatre is supported by a complex combination of sights, sounds, and sensations – the noises of the monitor and the buzz of muted conversation; an awareness of the anaesthetic machine and the team around it; the bright light overhead; and the sensation of being gowned and gloved. Because the surgeon is focusing so intently on the primary circle, however, events and objects in this second circle are less distinct. This blurring is both physical and metaphorical. Components of this circle register at a less conscious level – some elements indeed are only noticeable if they are not there.

These two circles are embedded within a third – the wider picture of the clinical scenario that is unfolding, the tapestry of events from which the operation is constituted. Anaesthetic decisions are made, drugs are fetched and administered, instruments are requested – and sometimes problems arise and stressors are introduced. But again, this activity takes place outside the surgeon's primary focus.

If this model of circles of focus has authenticity, then, it can form the basis for a different approach to simulation design. Instead of simple *replication* of an operating theatre, the process becomes one of active *recreation*. And at the heart of this lies *selective abstraction*, the identification of what are the crucial elements required for belief in a simulation as a mirror of reality. In this way, resources can be employed selectively, achieving the greatest realism at the lowest cost.

3.5.4 Widening Access to Simulation Centre Facilities

Providing and maintaining dedicated simulation environments on a wide scale are costly, resource intensive, and probably unaffordable in the current financial climate. Largely because of their cost and scarcity, such centres are only available to a limited number of potential users. How then might immersive simulation be made widely accessible? One possibility is the concept of 'in situ simulation' – where simulators and simulated scenarios are taken to actual clinical settings (Allan et al. 2010; LeBlanc 2008; Rall et al. 2008; Weinstock et al. 2005, 2009). Although this approach offers obvious attractions and is gaining ground, the practical difficulties of aligning such simulations with service demands have led us to explore other avenues.

The selective approach outlined above has practical implications for simulation design and for addressing the challenges of making effective simulation available on a wide scale in austere times. We have developed the concept of *Distributed Simulation (DS)* (Kneebone et al. 2010). The underlying philosophy of DS is to provide simulation facilities that are 'good enough' to engage participants and achieve learning goals, yet are low cost, portable, and able to be erected in a variety of clinical or nonclinical locations. Using the principles outlined above, only salient features are selected and recreated.

Engagement within the first circle is achieved by creating realistic prosthetic models of human tissue, drawing advanced techniques from film and television.

The aim is to minimise the need for 'imaginative work' on the part of surgeons by creating tissues that look and feel as real as possible. In order to develop the DS framework for the outer circles of focus, a team of industrial engineers was given the brief of identifying and recreating key triggers for perceived realism from the surgeon's perspective. During an extended period of observation in actual operating theatres and in-depth discussions with surgical teams, the engineers (who had no previous exposure to clinical settings) selected key components which constitute a surgical setting (e.g., operating lamp; ambient sounds; monitor beep; anaesthetic machine; and equipment trolleys).

The first function was to establish a physical boundary. Drawing on terminology from theatre studies, we framed simulated clinical activity as taking place within a conceptual enclosure (a 'space'), which is independent of its actual geographical location (the 'place') (Balme 2008; McAuley 2000). In order to function effectively, this space must be delimited from its surroundings, so that those within it can perform without distraction from the world outside – as they would within the walls of a real operating theatre, where access is restricted and authorisation required. DS provides a portable simulation space which can be quickly erected in any available location, using an inflatable circular 'igloo' to 'shut out' external surroundings. This creates an 'impression' of a clinical environment which can then be populated by a variety of scenarios, people, and 'props', depending on specific need.

Next, this delimited space is furnished with simplified representations of equipment, for example, a lightweight, tripod-mounted operating lamp constructed from moulded plastic, and a life-size photograph of an anesthetic machine. Preliminary studies with surgeons confirmed our belief that equipment and activity beyond the first circle was perceived as real, even when represented by low-cost models and pictorial representations. Feasibility and validation studies have confirmed that the concept has potential, and further studies are in progress.

The creation of a convincing environment for simulated care, although necessary, is not a sufficient condition for authentic simulation. The next requirement is to provide *experiences* that reflect clinical practice, and allow educational goals and outcomes to be achieved. The construction of simulations (scenarios) must of course be based on actual clinical experience. As discussed above, this requires the relationship of care between patient and clinician to be established. But again, this is a process of recreation rather than replication – although in this case a functional rather than a structural recreation. Here, the process of selective abstraction results in a dynamic 'performance'. If successful, the means by which this performance is achieved will fall out of conscious awareness, and participants will experience it 'as if' it were the real thing (Dieckmann et al. 2007).

Current work is widening the focus to anaesthetists, using a similar approach to develop apt simulations which can recreate the key elements of the anesthetist's practice, while the theatre nurse's perspective forms another essential component of this complex picture.

3.5.5 *Rehearsal*

Much of the above discussion has focused on mirroring clinical performance, using simulation as a means of practising component skills. Yet, performance is more than the sum of component parts.

There are interesting parallels between instrumental musicians and surgeons, both of whom display high levels of dexterity within a complex matrix of other skills (Kneebone 2009b; Lehmann et al. 2007; Parncutt and McPherson 2002; Williamon 2004). Both professions require *performance* – an operation in the case of surgeons, a public performance in the case of musicians. Both professions rely on *practice* – in simulation centres in the case of surgeons, in solitary practice rooms in the case of musicians (Chaffin et al. 2002). But musicians – especially those playing in small ensembles – include an intermediate stage of *rehearsal*. Here, they come together as a group, having perfected their parts as individuals, to put together what they have learned. During rehearsal, they negotiate a shared interpretation of the piece, discuss issues of speed and timing, and work on how they want the music to sound before committing themselves in front of the public where there is no going back. The crucial elements appear to be the *context* of rehearsal (approaching it as if it were performance) and working with the *people* who will perform.

For surgeons, however, rehearsal is still relatively rare. Of course it is true that surgeons build up extensive experience through operating, but this does not provide the combination of safety and realism which rehearsal implies. In some centres, VR computer programs allow surgeons to 'run through' demanding minimal access procedures before the actual operation, using that patient's imaging data to recreate the conditions of surgery. But most surgical learning still takes place within performance, supplemented by increasing reliance on task-based practice in simulation centres. Newer concepts of contextualised simulation therefore offer opportunities for surgeons at all levels systematically to rehearse what they have practised before operating on a real patient.

3.6 Where Next?

It is tempting to speculate what the future may hold for simulation within surgery. In this chapter, some examples from the author's own research have provided a lens for examining current approaches. However, such ideas are constantly in flux. Moreover as highlighted in Chap. 1, predictions are likely to be proved wrong within the cycle of a book's production. As with any fast moving field where technology plays a major part, any discussion about simulation is doomed to seem quaintly outdated by the time it comes to print.

Yet, we seem to be on the threshold of major changes in how simulation is viewed and used, especially in a climate of increasing financial constraint. The low cost, portable yet immersive simulation environments described above raise the possibility of widespread access to immersive simulation within any hospital or institution, without requiring investment in fixed facilities or dedicated staff. This could change current approaches to simulation-based education, allowing static centres to focus on the activities that require full-scale clinical environments (such as anaesthetic team training) while opening up new possibilities at a local level. In particular, such developments could allow a shift in focus from tasks to the environment, exploring the notion of a 'surgical ecosystem' as outlined above.

Seen from this perspective, simulation offers a means of making visible the shared 'atmosphere' within which surgery takes place and which is essential for safe practice. An understanding of how this atmosphere works, of what is required to sustain it, and of how to recognise and remedy early signs of dysfunction is probably one of the most important attributes of any member of the surgical team. Yet a hegemony of the technical threatens to overshadow these crucial attributes.

3.7 Conclusion

This chapter started by proposing that simulation is much more than simulators. To be effective, simulation must capture the essence of real-world practice, with all its complexity and variation. The chapter outlined a theoretical model for the mutually dependent relationship between the simulated and the real, proposing that each can immeasurably enrich the other when the balance is right. After highlighting some limitations of current simulation approaches, the argument puts forward a case for heightening authenticity by actively and selectively *recreating* the settings of clinical care rather than simply *replicating* them.

Simulation seems set to play a steadily increasing role in surgical education. It is therefore crucial to retain a critical stance to what simulation can and cannot offer, using the tools of educational research and analysis to illuminate this challenging, complex, and underresearched field. Building a robust evidence base, grounded in methodologies which are both rigorous and apt, will develop a theoretical infrastructure which is sorely needed but often missing.

References

Allan, C. K., Thiagarajan, R. R., Beke, D., Imprescia, A., Kappus, L. J., Garden, A., et al. (2010). Simulation-based training delivered directly to the pediatric cardiac intensive care unit engenders preparedness, comfort, and decreased anxiety among multidisciplinary resuscitation teams. *The Journal of Thoracic and Cardiovascular Surgery, 140*(3), 646–652.

Balme, C. (2008). *The Cambridge introduction to theatre studies*. Cambridge: Cambridge University Press.

Bereiter, C. (2002). *Education and mind in the knowledge age*. Mahwah: Lawrence Erlbaum Associates.

Bereiter, C., & Scardamalia, M. (1993). *Surpassing ourselves: An enquiry into the nature and implications of expertise*. Chicago/La Salle: Open Court.

Bligh, J., & Bleakley, A. (2006). Distributing menus to hungry learners: Can learning by simulation become simulation of learning? *Medical Teacher, 28*(7), 606–613.

Chaffin, R., Imreh, G., & Crawford, M. (2002). *Practicing perfection: Memory and piano performance*. Mahwah: Lawrence Erlbaum Associates.

CMO. (2009). 150 years of the annual report of the chief medical officer: On the state of public health 2008.

Dieckmann, P., Gaba, D., & Rall, M. (2007). Deepening the theoretical foundations of patient simulation as social practice. *Simulation in Healthcare, 2*(3), 183–193.

Ericsson, K. A. (2004). Deliberate practice and the acquisition and maintenance of expert performance in medicine and related domains. *Academic Medicine, 79*(10), S70–S81.

Ericsson, K. A., & Charness, N. (1994). Expert performance. Its structure and acquisition. *The American Psychologist, 49*(8), 725–747.

Ericsson, K. A., Charness, N., Feltovich, P., & Hoffman, R. (Eds.). (2006). *The Cambridge handbook of expertise and expert performance*. Cambridge: Cambridge University Press.

Ericsson, K. A., Prietula, M. J., & Cokely, E. T. (2007). The making of an expert. *Harvard Business Review, 85*(7–8), 114–121. 193.

Gaba, D. M. (2004). The future vision of simulation in health care. *Quality & Safety in Health Care, 13*(Suppl 1), 2–10.

Gaba, D. M., & DeAnda, A. (1988). A comprehensive anesthesia simulation environment: Recreating the operating room for research and training. *Anesthesiology, 69*, 387–394.

Gaba, D. M., Howard, S. K., Flanagan, B., Smith, B. E., Fish, K. J., & Botney, R. (1998/7). Assessment of clinical performance during simulated crises using both technical and behavioral ratings. *Anesthesiology, 89*(1), 8–18.

Gaba, D., Howard, S., Fish, K., Smith, B., & Sowb, Y. (2001). Simulation-based training in anaesthesia crisis resource management (ACRM): A decade of experience. *Simulation and Gaming, 32*(2), 175–193.

Goodwin, D. (2008). Refashioning bodies, reshaping agency. *Science, Technology & Human Values, 33*(3), 345–363.

Guest, C. B., Regehr, G., & Tiberius, R. G. (2001). The life long challenge of expertise. *Medical Education, 35*(1), 78–81.

Heidegger, M. (1968). *What is called thinking?* New York: Harper & Row.

Hindmarsh, J., & Pilnick, As. (2002). The tacit order of teamwork: Collaboration and embodied conduct in anaesthesia. *The Sociological Quarterly, 43*(2), 139–164.

Hindmarsh, J., & Pilnick, A. (2007). Knowing bodies at work: Embodiment and ephemeral teamwork in anaesthesia. *Organization Studies, 28*(9), 1395–1416.

Hodges, B. D., Kuper, A., & Reeves, S. (2008). Discourse analysis. *British Medical Journal, 337*, a879.

Holzman, R. S., Cooper, J. B., Gaba, D. M., Philip, J. H., Small, S. D., & Feinstein, D. (1995/12). Anesthesia crisis resource management: Real-life simulation training in operating room crises. *Journal of Clinical Anesthesia, 7*(8), 675–687.

Issenberg, S. B., McGaghie, W. C., Petrusa, E. R., Gordon, D., & Scalese, R. J. (2005/1). Features and uses of high-fidelity medical simulations that lead to effective learning: A BEME systematic review. *Medical Teacher, 27*(1), 10–28.

Kneebone, R. L. (2005). Clinical simulation for learning procedural skills: A theory-based approach. *Academic Medicine, 80*(6), 549–553.

Kneebone, R. (2009a). Perspective: Simulation and transformational change: The paradox of expertise. *Academic Medicine, 84*(7), 954–957.

Kneebone, R. L. (2009b). Practice, rehearsal, and performance: An approach for simulation-based surgical and procedure training. *Journal of the American Medical Association, 302*(12), 1336–1338.

Kneebone, R. (2010). Simulation, safety and surgery. *Quality & Safety in Health Care, 19*(Ergonomics & Safety Supplement), i47–i52.

Kneebone, R., Kidd, J., Nestel, D., Asvall, S., Paraskeva, P., & Darzi, A. (2002). An innovative model for teaching and learning clinical procedures. *Medical Education, 36*(7), 628–634.
Kneebone, R., Nestel, D., Moorthy, K., Taylor, P., Bann, S., Munz, Y., et al. (2003). Learning the skills of flexible sigmoidoscopy – The wider perspective. *Medical Education, 37*(Suppl. 1), 50–58.
Kneebone, R. L., Scott, W., Darzi, A., & Horrocks, M. (2004). Simulation and clinical practice: Strengthening the relationship. *Medical Education, 38*(10), 1095–1102.
Kneebone, R., Kidd, J., Nestel, D., Barnet, A., Lo, B., King, R., et al. (2005). Blurring the boundaries: Scenario-based simulation in a clinical setting. *Medical Education, 39*, 580–587.
Kneebone, R., Nestel, D., Wetzel, C., Black, S., Jacklin, R., Aggarwal, R., et al. (2006). The human face of simulation: Patient-focused simulation training. *Academic Medicine, 81*(10), 919–924.
Kneebone, R. L., Nestel, D., Vincent, C., & Darzi, A. (2007). Complexity, risk and simulation in learning procedural skills. *Medical Education, 41*(8), 808–814.
Kneebone, R., Arora, S., King, D., Sevdalis, N., Kassab, E., Aggarwal, R., et al. (2010). Distributed simulation – Accessible immersive training. *Medical Teacher, 32*(1), 65–70.
LeBlanc, D. (2008). Situated simulation: Taking simulation to the clinicians. In R. Kyle & W. Murray (Eds.), *Clinical simulation: Operations, engineering and management*. Amsterdam: Elsevier.
Lehmann, A., Sloboda, J., & Woody, R. (2007). *Psychology for musicians: Understanding and acquiring the skills*. Oxford: Oxford University Press.
McAuley, G. (2000). *Space in performance making meaning in the theatre*. Ann Arbor: University of Michigan Press.
McGaghie, W. C., Issenberg, S. B., Petrusa, E. R., & Scalese, R. J. (2010). A critical review of simulation-based medical education research: 2003–2009. *Medical Education, 44*(1), 50–63.
McGilchrist, I. (2009). *The master and his emissary. The divided brain and the making of the Western world*. New Haven/London: Yale University Press.
Mylopoulos, M., & Regehr, G. (2007). Cognitive metaphors of expertise and knowledge: Prospects and limitations for medical education. *Medical Education, 41*(12), 1159–1165.
Parncutt, R., & McPherson, G. (Eds.). (2002). *The science and psychology of music performance: Creative strategies for teaching and learning*. Oxford: Oxford University Press.
Pye, D. (1968). *The nature and art of workmanship*. Cambridge: Cambridge University Press.
Rall, M., Stricker, E., Reddersen, S., Zieger, J., & Dieckmann, P. (2008). Mobile 'in Situ' simulation crisis resource management training. In R. Kyle & W. Murray (Eds.), *Clinical simulation: Operations, engineering and management*. Amsterdam: Elsevier.
Sennett, R. (2008). *The craftsman*. London: Allen Lane.
Temple, J. (2010). Time for training. A review of the impact of the European working time directive on the quality of training. Medical Education England. http://www.mee.nhs.uk/PDF/14274%20Bookmark%20Web%20Version.pdf. Accessed 22 July 2011.
Weinstock, P. H., Kappus, L. J., Kleinman, M. E., Grenier, B., Hickey, P., & Burns, J. P. (2005). Toward a new paradigm in hospital-based pediatric education: The development of an onsite simulator program. *Pediatric Critical Care Medicine, 6*(6), 635–641.
Weinstock, P. H., Kappus, L. J., Garden, A., & Burns, J. P. (2009). Simulation at the point of care: Reduced-cost, in situ training via a mobile cart. *Pediatric Critical Care Medicine, 10*(2), 176–181.
Wertsch, J. V. (1985). *Vygotsky and the social formation of mind*. Cambridge: Harvard University Press.
Wiggins, G. (1993a). *Assessing student performance. Exploring the purpose and limits of testing*. San Francisco: Jossey-Bass.
Wiggins, G. (1993b). Assessment: Authenticity, context, and validity. *Phi Delta Kappan, 75*(3), 200–214.
Williamon, A. (Ed.). (2004). *Musical excellence: Strategies and techniques to enhance performance*. Oxford: Oxford University Press.

Chapter 4
Researching Surgical Education

Heather Fry, Nick Sevdalis, and Roger Kneebone

4.1 Introduction

Chapter 1 has already referred to education being a composite of many fields and disciplines. Surgical and medical education research can be viewed, arguably, as specialised branches of social science/education research; this view is contested, see for example Gill and Griffin (2009). The context of the problems to be researched is different, but many of the issues are essentially similar to those in other forms of education, for example, how do learners acquire knowledge or learn a particular skill, is assessment reliable, does training teachers make any difference, what is the optimal strategy for teaching and learning knowledge or a particular skill, what motivates learners, etc. There are particular parallels with other areas of professional education. A good introduction to various types of social science-based medical education research, by leading international experts, can be found in Swanwick (2010). A major exception to reliance on social science research methods is that neuroscience is increasingly drawn on by some branches of education.

However, a number of differences exist between surgical education and other forms of educational research. An obvious one is that surgeons do not just depend on factual knowledge, nor do they use technical skills on an inanimate object, nor do they just develop highly expert and sophisticated analytical and synthesising skills.

H. Fry (✉)
Higher Education Funding Council for England (HEFCE), Bristol BS16 1QD, UK
e-mail: h.fry@hefce.ac.uk

N. Sevdalis
Division of Surgery and Centre for Patient Safety and Service Quality,
Imperial College London, London, UK
e-mail: n.sevdalis@imperial.ac.uk

R. Kneebone
Surgical Education, Imperial College London, London, UK
e-mail: r.kneebone@imperial.ac.uk

H. Fry and R. Kneebone (eds.), *Surgical Education: Theorising an Emerging Domain*,
Advances in Medical Education 2, DOI 10.1007/978-94-007-1682-7_4,

They learn all these and more. Moreover, the focus of surgical practice is the patient, and the patient therefore has to be considered as part of the learning context; this adds to the uncertainty and variability of the surgical context, making it an even richer and more complex field for research. The patient's interests and needs will predominate over a focus on learning and training; the critical nature of surgical practice means the need to safeguard the patient and their health throughout the learning process is dominant. Patients, also, may act as part tutor; some patients' behaviours may distract the learner; some patients will have more complex problems to treat than others and the flow or the symptoms of the presenting patients cannot be controlled for educational purposes. A second difference is that the trainee surgeon or physician more often than not works and learns as part of a team, unlike the lone university student taking a mathematics examination. However, it could be argued that the 'patient, team and safety factors' are little different in essence from, say, the client and product team building a bridge in engineering, or from the client and barrister in practice of law – in other words the context of surgical practice is not similar in its essential nature from the context in which other professional education occurs.

The research tradition that surgical education draws on is more that of education and related social sciences, and less that of traditional surgical science. This means that lab-based testing, for example, is not something that can be used straightforwardly in surgical education. It also means that biomedical traditions of, for example, clinical trials can rarely be used because the component parts of the research can rarely be sufficiently controlled or isolated to render such an approach valid – and even if they can be, the conditions created are then far from the ones usually prevailing 'in reality', which will themselves be varied. A characteristic of surgical education research is therefore one in which, even when quantitative methods are used, the human factor and the difficulty of controlling variables are never far away. Another distinctive feature of social science research is its use of theory, for example, drawing on disciplinary knowledge to ensure that research problems contribute to the evolution of a field and forming theoretically informed research questions (Albert and Reeves 2010 and Teunissen 2010).

This chapter explores the two main paradigms used in surgical education research; they are often used together in mixed methods studies. The chapter is not sufficiently detailed to act as a manual of such methods. Its primary purpose is to introduce the non-social scientist to surgical educational research techniques, to tease out some key premises and features and to act as a useful backdrop to understanding some of the research studies that are developed/referred to in subsequent chapters.

4.2 The Quantitative and Qualitative Educational Research Paradigms Compared and Contrasted

Quantitative research relies heavily upon deductive reasoning, where a hypothesis is formulated and then tested statistically. This type of approach to education research will be immediately recognisable to surgeons in that it may use similar sampling techniques and statistical approaches to some biomedical research. Research investigations are designed which allow for a systematic approach, aiming for results that are generalisable beyond the limits of an individual investigation. Here attention is paid to random or representative sampling from large populations, adequate experimental control of extraneous variables, use of validated metrics, minimisation of investigator bias and other similar notions. But even here, a social science use of statistics is more likely to be in relation to something such as questionnaire responses or assessment scores rather than outcomes from randomised controlled trials. Such quantitative methods are extremely powerful, but there are limits to the kinds of questions they can address. This type of research tends to be published in the form of relatively short journal articles, with a consistent and highly formalised structure. The ordered sequence of Introduction, Methods, Results, and Discussion (IMRaD) provides a familiar framework, allowing key information to be conveyed quickly and compared with other articles. Critical appraisal involves being able to judge the quality of research design and methodological rigour, analyse statistical methods and weigh up the validity of conclusions.

Qualitative research tends to focus on capturing the perspectives of individuals, using methods such as interviewing and observation. Such methods make no claim to produce generalisable results, but instead aim to shed light on the area being investigated – often opinions, behaviour, interactions and processes. Qualitative research relies much more upon inductive than deductive reasoning. Understanding evolves through a process of observation and analysis, which looks to see what is there, without having a preconceived hypothesis. What is needed is a detailed description of what individuals think, feel or do. Research of this kind is likely to acknowledge that there may be many 'truths', and that each person's experience may be as valid as anyone else's. This kind of research tends to be published in the form of books or much longer articles, using a different set of conventions where the author often appears as a person, and his or her responses to the research are acknowledged as a factor. The research itself is framed within an extensive discussion of what has been written by other authors, and the findings are often interwoven with a critical discussion of what is already known. The criteria for assessing the quality of the research outcomes are very different from those of quantitative research, often depending on the transparency, thoroughness and suitability of the process, rather than an 'objective' evaluation of an impersonal method, and on how far findings are recognised by those in similar situations. 'Authenticity' is strived for. The results of this kind of work can rarely be exactly reproduced because every person observed or interviewed has a unique perspective, but the process by which the researcher has reached his or her conclusions must be laid open for scrutiny and critique.

Table 4.1 aims to capture some of the key differences between the two research paradigms, being a schematic representation of two broad approaches to research.

As mentioned above, in practice, educational research often uses a mixed method approach and none of the methods may be at the purest or most extreme end of either research paradigm.

Table 4.1 Characteristics of qualitative and quantitative research to illustrate their different approaches and emphasis

Qualitative research	Quantitative research
Acknowledges a degree of subjectivity and reflexivity	Claims objectivity
Focuses on individuals or groups	Focuses on populations
Exploration	Trends
Usually starts from an open question	Usually starts from a hypothesis
Inductive reasoning	Deductive reasoning
Analysis of text	Statistical techniques
Purposive sampling	Preference for random, or appropriately stratified sampling
Asks about why and how	Asks how many, in what proportion and is it significant
Findings often not transferable	Findings may be transferable
Rarely generalisable	Usually generalisable
Takes place in the real world, often uses observation, opinion and perception	Based on codified observations or responses
Analysis may start alongside on-going data collection, conclusions may start to emerge as data is being collected and influence subsequent data collection and analysis	Analysis will happen after all data has been collected
Both methods may generate models and theories	

4.3 Quantitative Surgical Education Research

As highlighted above, quantitative research approaches in the context of surgical education share numerous facets with similar approaches across the entire breath of biomedical and clinical sciences – from laboratory-based science to translational research aiming to take scientific and technological advances to the bedside and evaluate their impact on patient care. These approaches are also common in some social science disciplines. A key aspect of this type of research, which sometimes differentiates it from more qualitative approaches, is that decisions about *all* aspects of research have to be made at the early stages of the research and strictly adhered to whilst the research is being carried out. Such decisions include choice of research designs, endpoints and other metrics to be collected, and analytical (statistical) approaches. The stages of data collection and analysis are kept separate. In the light of this, adequate piloting of the scientific techniques, tools, and materials to be used is a key aspect of this type of research, which ensures feasibility and quality of the entire research endeavour.

In the remainder of this section, we consider the way quantitative research questions and hypotheses are set, the range of quantitative research methods used and the range of analytical tools that are available in the context of surgical education. These aspects of quantitative educational research will be highlighted in order for comparison with qualitative approaches to become apparent; it does not provide a comprehensive overview. Numerous research methods textbooks are available to surgical education researchers, which should be consulted for in-depth coverage of the issues discussed below (Blalock 1979; Cohen et al. 2007; Shadish et al. 2002; Zeller and Carmines 1980).

4.3.1 Research Questions and Hypotheses

Quantitative research in surgical education is typically driven by well-defined questions and hypotheses set prior to the commencement of the research. Research questions tend to be broad in nature. Recent examples of research questions tackled within the quantitative research paradigm include 'what is the impact of stress on surgeons' performance in the operating theatre?' (Arora et al. 2010a) and 'can behavioral and cognitive skills of surgeons be captured reliably and validly in the operating theatre?' (Sevdalis et al. 2009). These questions are in effect open-ended: there is no preconceived direction in the possible answer that will emerge from the data. Research hypotheses tend to be narrower than questions, typically specifying a direction in the anticipated research outcomes. For instance, the research question about surgeons' stress could be 'translated' into a research hypothesis as follows: 'Stress impairs surgeons' performance in the operating theatre'. Analysis of the data that the researcher collects should subsequently be able to determine whether the research hypothesis is supported or not, and how strongly.

Because of the specific, pre-specified nature of research questions and, particularly, research hypotheses, successful quantitative research in surgical education tends to be theory or evidence driven. Research questions and hypotheses do not arise in a vacuum; rather, they emerge as the 'where next' questions of empirical research that has already been carried out. Previous research within a certain topic thus drives quantitative approaches, so that forthcoming research builds onto the empirical evidence already accumulated and takes it to the next scientifically logical step. For example, research on the efficacy of surgical simulators as training and education tools for technical skills in novice surgeons started with providing evidence that such simulators can differentiate between novice and expert performance, went on to ask whether trainees' skills improve over time following simulator-based training, followed this up by asking whether the skills acquired on a simulator transfer to performance in the real environment of an operating theatre, and is now addressing the question why skills under certain conditions show transferability to real-life performance, whereas under other conditions they do not (for relevant reviews, see Issenberg et al. 2005; Lynagh et al. 2007; Sutherland et al. 2006; Sturm et al. 2008). Adequate reviews and/or meta-analyses of past research findings within the domain of interest are invaluable in shaping the direction of quantitative educational research and the specific content of the questions asked and hypotheses tested.

4.3.2 Research Methods

A key aim of quantitative educational research is robustness and generalisability of findings. The key idea here is that all tested participants are sampled from more or less similar populations. By collecting quantitative data and submitting these data to statistical analyses, quantitative researchers use the data they collect from their samples to make robust inferences about the populations from which the samples have been drawn. A key aspect of this process is that in order for an inference to be accurate, the sample that is being tested should be as similar as possible to the target population. For instance, if a researcher is interested in teaching and learning opportunities in Emergency Departments (EDs), a range of EDs need to be sampled to ensure that factors like whether the ED belongs to teaching or non-teaching hospital, staffing levels (low or high), and volumes of patients seen by ED personnel (low or high) are taken into account. Deciding which factors should be taken into account is driven by the existing evidence base, which reveals whether some factors are likely to affect the measure(s) of interest. Sampling considerations are therefore of critical importance in quantitative research and care should be taken in choosing a sampling strategy.

For our purposes here, it is important to highlight the relevance of random sampling and stratified sampling for quantitative research. In the former, all members of a population are equally likely to be drawn into a researcher's sample; in the latter, the sample is constructed in such a way that important population strata (e.g., gender, age and level of expertise) are accurately represented in the sample. True random sampling is often difficult to achieve in surgical education research. Instead, evidence-driven stratification is a viable alternative, which ensures that potentially confounding variables are built into the design of the research – and therefore can be taken into account when the data are being analysed.

Once the sampling strategy has been decided, quantitative educational researchers are faced with a range of approaches to the design of the research. A number of options are available here, with the 'true experiment' (randomised controlled study) being thought to offer the highest level of unbiased empirical evidence. Such studies offer truly random allocation of research participants (individual subjects, clinical units or entire institutions) to the various conditions of the researcher's design and include a control group, in which no educational intervention/treatment is carried out. In addition, ideally both the research and the participants should be blinded regarding which condition a participant has been allocated to, to prevent bias from the research as well as from the participant. For practical reasons, however, such studies are often not feasible in educational research: for example, it is not feasible for a researcher to be blinded to the treatment condition of a group of participants, if s/he is the one to deliver the training intervention to them (a problem often encountered in clinical surgical research too). Apart from true experimental studies, other design possibilities include quasi-experiments, with pre- and post-intervention treatment groups, or even only post-intervention studies, when a pre-intervention baseline is not available.

It is important to stress here that, because surgical education research is typically carried out with busy clinicians, often in highly pressurised environments, researchers often find themselves having to make informed trade-offs between what would be scientifically desirable versus what is practically achievable. Practical considerations should be taken into account early on in educational research designs, as they are often important determinants of how many participants will be available and when, how much time is available for an intervention to be delivered, whether the same participants will be traceable for a post-interventions assessment, and similar considerations. Whereas a laboratory scientist exerts adequate control over such issues, surgical education researchers often have to 'make do' within the constraints of service and education delivery as they currently stand. Although this does not mean that the research will be of a lower standard, practical considerations very often feature in the relevant 'Methods' sections of educational research articles.

The final step in the research method process is the choice of outcomes, or endpoints and the tools that will be used to capture them. As in all quantitative research, in surgical education too measures should be reliable (i.e. they should be measuring educational and learning constructs consistently) and valid (i.e. they should capture the constructs they purport to capture). A significant body of quantitative educational research in surgery focuses on the development and validation of assessment tools, which can then be used in further studies. Recent examples of such research include the development of tools to capture stress experienced by surgeons in real time in the operating theatre (Arora et al. 2010b), and tools to capture the quality of team working behaviours exhibited by surgeons (Sevdalis et al. 2008, 2009). Once such tools have been developed and evidence exists on their reliability and validity, they can be used to capture factors that affect learning outcomes (e.g. the impact of stress on the transfer of skill from simulation-based training to real operating theatre) or to assess directly the efficacy of training modules for surgical trainees (e.g., to capture improvements in team skills and behaviours following simulation-based team training).

Regarding types of data collection tools used in surgical education research, tools tend to capture research participants' knowledge, their attitudes/views, and their skills/behaviours. Paper and pencil, or electronically administered knowledge tests are typically used to capture knowledge. Attitudes or perceptions are typically assessed via self-report questionnaires, ideally validated (i.e. that have been shown to adequately capture the attitudes, beliefs and perceptions of interest in a manner that allows scores derived from such questionnaires to be correlated with other measures). Such tools offer robust measurement of participants' subjective views. Finally, skills and behaviours can be captured via a variety of more objective metrics, which are typically obtained from direct observation of research participants and scoring of relevant scales. Observation can be carried out in real time, or retrospectively using audiovisual recording equipment and video/audio analysis. In recent years, with the advent of simulators and virtual reality technologies into surgical education, simulator-derived metrics are also used to capture technical or procedural skills. Finally, in the last 5 years or so, there has been a significant expansion of the evidence base on observational tools to capture behaviour in surgical contexts – with validated tools such as the Observational Teamwork Assessment for Surgery (OTAS) (Sevdalis et al. 2009; Undre et al. 2007a) and Non-Technical Skills for Surgeons (NOTSS) (Yule et al. 2008) being increasingly used in research.

4.3.3 *Quantitative Approaches to Data Analysis*

Quantitative research typically utilises quantitative endpoints (see previous section), which therefore require quantitative handling and analyses. Descriptive statistics are typically used to summarise findings across groups, or interventions in this type of research. These statistics provide numerical information for the central tendency of the responses (e.g. mean, median and mode), as well as the dispersion or 'noise' in the collected data (e.g. variance and range). Graphical representations of such findings (including frequency plots, box plots, bar graphs, and scatterplots, amongst other options) often accompany numerical indices to visually illustrate findings. Statistical description is typically followed by statistical inference, in which statistical tests are applied to the data to discover quantitative patterns and trends in them and to determine whether such patterns are likely to hold for the populations from which the samples have been drawn (i.e. whether they are 'statistically significant'), or can be attributed to chance (i.e., random, non-systematic variations). Well known and widely used such tests include the following:

- *t*-test: a parametric test used to compare two independent or paired groups of subjects, or observations (parametric test make assumptions that may or may not be met by the data to hand)
- Analysis of variance: a parametric test used to compare three of more groups of subjects or observations, independent or paired
- Wilcoxon's test: a non-parametric equivalent to the paired samples *t*-test (non-parametric texts attempt to relax the assumptions about data and therefore have wider validity in dubious cases)
- Mann–Whitney test: a non-parametric equivalent to the independent samples *t*-test
- Correlation coefficients and regression analysis: a range of tests (Pearson *r* or Spearman's rho coefficients, simple or multiple regression, linear or logistic regression, etc.) that allow the researcher to establish whether there are significant relationships between different variables or measures of interest.

It is important to stress here that in quantitative research, statistical handling of the data and the relevant analyses should be thought through and specified at the early stages of a research project – with the design of the research. The choice of endpoints and outcome measures (e.g. multiple choice knowledge tests, standardised validated surveys or quantitative observation protocols) predetermines to a large extent the range of statistical analyses that can be used once the data have been collected.

4.4 Qualitative Surgical Education Research

Often a study may be designed from the outset to use both qualitative methods and statistical approaches – for different types of data related to the same phenomena. Qualitative research is also often thought of as being used in the preliminary stages of research, for example, to interview a group of trainee surgeons to seek opinion about the usefulness of the lecture teaching method for learning. The findings could help inform the topics and nature of questions to ask on a questionnaire. Alternatively, interviews can be used to explore the reasons and perceptions behind a finding from quantitative data. But qualitative approaches are also often used in their own right, simply to generate better understanding of phenomena that are suited to their approach (see Sect. 4.5.2).

Qualitative research is often lengthy in all its stages. Determining how to best collect the data and how to analyse it is vital. As with quantitatively based approaches, failure to consider these aspects at the start will often limit the type of analysis that can be conducted later. Collecting data can be time consuming, as can processing it. The amount of data generated is often enormous. Analysis is complex and can rarely rely so much upon a computer as is the case for statistics. Such research often requires comparatively lengthy writing up to ensure methods, analytical processes and how conclusions have been derived, are transparent; and as findings are usually discussed alongside preceding relevant literature, length is again likely. Discussions will tend to be quite discursive.

4.4.1 Key Approaches in Qualitative Research

Table 4.1 has already indicated many of the key characteristics of qualitative research. There are probably three major types of activity for which it is best used: the understanding of processes (e.g. how a trainee learns to make a particular type of flap, which might use observation and the interviewing of all parties involved, this might lead to improvements in training); exploring people's reactions, perceptions and opinions (e.g. 'what in your experience are the biggest challenges that learning minimally invasive techniques pose?', with a view to minimising these in training) and analysing documents (e.g. a report on future training requirements for surgeons, for example such a study might take a historical approach to such documents, tracing policy and practice shifts). Other key areas for qualitative research are as follows: evaluation studies that have an emphasis which qualitative research can address, and which typically draw conclusions about the impact of something; in depth comparative write-ups of circumstances/contexts (case studies); and action research in which the researcher investigates their own practice, usually through cycles of evaluation and amendment to practice. Words and what is seen are the focus of qualitative research, not numbers or precise measurement. There are innumerable general works that consider in some detail the main methods and approaches to qualitative research in education and the social sciences (e.g. Cohen et al. 2007;

Miles and Huberman 1994; Pope and Mays 2006; Robson 2002; Seale et al. 2006; Somekh and Lewin 2005); Kneebone and Fry (2009) consider how these methods may be used in surgical research and have a useful glossary explanation of key concepts in qualitative research.

Setting aside the analysis of documents, people, their actions and opinions are usually at the centre of qualitative research. For this reason, qualitative research has a strong consideration of ethical factors, including obtaining appropriate ethical permission to start the study, obtaining individual consent to take part, and with clear agreement about anonymity (or otherwise) and how data will be used, stored and published.

Rigour in qualitative research in best achieved and demonstrated by careful and appropriate selection of methods and modes of analysis; declaration of the position/possible influence on outcome of the researcher; triangulation of methods and findings by the use of multi-methods and perspectives; detailed description of the use of methods and analytical techniques; critical analysis of the strengths and weaknesses of the study design; the drawing together of ideas and conclusions into a model or theory with explanatory power that others recognise as an appropriate abstraction that also represents and aids the understanding of what was being researched.

4.4.2 Design and Methods

Selection of subjects or episodes for study is a tricky part of qualitative research. As with quantitative research, rarely can all examples of something be researched. Moreover it can be extremely difficult to create a truly random or representative sample, not least because such a sample might be too large for most qualitative studies to tackle; sometimes an opportunistic sample is all that can be achieved, in this case its likely representativeness or otherwise will typically be commented on when the researchers discuss the strengths and weaknesses of their study design. Some might even argue that it is pointless to try to create or hold up as desirable a representative sample, as all teachers and learners are different, patients and contexts also vary and trying to control for factors such as age, sex or length of training in one group of subjects, or interviewing every tenth trainee or trainer will not address the multiple layers of sampling issues. For many qualitative researchers, true sampling is therefore anathema; to undertake it is to misunderstand the strengths of what qualitative research can offer, and seeking to ape the quantitative paradigm risks losing the power, consistency and authenticity of the approach in use. However, many qualitative researchers do undertake purposive sampling, that is, they will seek out persons and situations so as to intentionally include a wide spectrum of types or likely variation across a range of parameters, based on previous literature and studies or personal knowledge of context.

Although there is probably wide recognition that face-to-face or telephone interviewing is the most commonly used method in qualitative research, there is less recognition of the variety of types of interview that can be conducted. These may be not only individual or group but also tightly structured or much more free flowing. This means that there could be a set of fixed questions used consistently with all subjects or there could be questions that are little more than general starting points and which are followed up as seems sensible depending upon the responses, to try and elicit very detailed and thoughtful answers. Although questions should always be open and non-leading, more 'free' approaches will likely lead to more complex and less focused data – with obvious benefits and drawbacks. (Free response questions on questionnaires also produce qualitative data and in some cases may be little different from other types of interview – but they lack the opportunity for further exploration and follow up. Comment below about analysing qualitative data also applies to free response sections of questionnaires.) In this book, Chaps. 6, 10 and 12 especially draw substantially on interview techniques.

Interview data recorded as notes loses much that makes for the strengths of interviews – it loses complexity and much of the actual wording used, and may be less useful than written answers on a questionnaire, even when these are of limited length. Most qualitative researchers will wish if at all possible to record and transcribe interviews for these reasons, perhaps keeping notes as well about matters such as the body language of the interviewee. Transcription enables close study and coding of the text into themes, which can be recorded and ordered using proprietary software. Transcription will also seek to note hesitancy, tone of voice, etc. to capture as much as possible of the nuance of the response. Audio or video recording of interviews or other situations that may be observed, such as consultations, is often considered intrusive, and much is written about the possible impact this has on detracting from the 'naturalness' of the situation. Such intrusion always has to be commented on when the research is written up.

There are various specific techniques for eliciting opinion about carefully defined topics, which are quite different from the interview. The term focus group is often used as if it were synonymous with interviewing a group of people, this is not so. The focus group usually considers a single topic or issue and is heavily structured to reduce the influence of any dominant voices; moreover, its aim is to gradually sort and reduce views towards a single consensus output by means of a staged process that controls against the view emerging being that of the strongest personalities present (Moore 1987). The nominal group technique is a similar method but does not seek a consensus view from the group. The Delphi technique (conducted through written iterations that downplay minority views and rewrite statements in forms that seem to reflect a more consensual view) is a comparable technique that is not conducted face to face. Its purpose is to determine some form of majority view among the participants. This process has, for example, been used as a method of drawing together experts who are geographically dispersed to develop curricula (Paterson Davenport et al. 2004). Again it is a structured process that, for example, a video conference meeting would not replicate.

Observation studies can use both quantitative and qualitative methods, and many use both side by side. Qualitative approaches to observation are less widely recognised than interviews, but have much to contribute to the understanding of process. They may also be followed up with interviews that seek further elucidation of what appear to be key incidents that occurred during the observation. They can be very time consuming, yield much data and pose particular challenges for analysis. Again, where something can be well recorded or filmed, the data may be particularly rich and can be studied many times over and in great depth; however, filming is not always possible for reasons of cost and ethics – and it may not actually capture all the nuances seen by a trained observer with a full view of everything (e.g. in a teaching episode on whom should the camera focus?). Participant observation may yield greater nuance and understanding, and more data. Human observers typically take free flowing notes or focus on particular features that are thought to be most pertinent to the study. All types of observation research run the risk of 'normal' behaviour being altered by the intrusion of the observer's eye, lens or microphone. Attempts to mitigate this with a camera usually take the form of making the instrument as unobtrusive as possible and with participant observation of greater immersion, not less, of the researcher in the context, so that they become almost an accepted part of the situation. A case in point here would be the famous 'boys in white' study of medical students (Becker 1976) or a more recent example from surgery (Bosk 2003). The methodology of observation studies draws heavily on ethnography.

The analysis of written documents and of discourse more generally is another area that might be described as a qualitative method (see Gill and Griffin 2010, for example), in that issues of interpretation cannot be ignored. There is overlap with how interview data (for example) is approached. Textual analysis can be undertaken in a range of ways that are reflective of some of the dilemmas and divisions at the heart of being a qualitative researcher (e.g. how far one imposes an external structure on written data and how far one seeks to have that structure emerge from the data itself). Other considerations that arise are similar to those that historians need to consider, for example, the bias of the writer. Some of these issues are explored further in the section below.

As with quantitative studies, piloting is usually a vital part of qualitative research and will be another feature that critical readers of such research will look for. Piloting, for example, would include trying out interview questions on two or three subjects and seeing if questions are clear, unambiguous, yield the complexity and depth of data required etc. It would also be checked that the proposed approach to analysis will work. A pilot also enables a check that appropriate subjects are being targeted. Adjustments will be made before the study resumes. This process helps to ensure the research is as effective as possible and resources are not committed to larger scale activity before it is warranted.

4.4.3 Analysis

There are many possible approaches to analysing qualitative data, but most fall into one of two camps. Taking a grounded theory approach (Glaser and Strauss 1967) means that no preconceived concepts, fields or themes are imposed on the data. Instead the data is read and re-read closely, and emerging themes and concepts (ones that are 'grounded' in the data, not, for example in previously published studies) are noted. As more data is read and provisionally analysed, such emerging themes are refined and altered. The text is marked up or coded with these emergent categories in an iterative process. At the extreme of this approach, the signal to end data collection arises when no new categories or concepts are emerging from the data – when saturation is reached. Thus, in grounded theories, categorisations of ideas and actions emerge from the data through careful analysis.

An alternative approach is to come to the data with preconceived ideas of themes or categories and look for these in the data. Both approaches can have strengths and weaknesses and be used better and less well. The grounded approach generally requires more time. Both approaches can use software, or be conducted in more old fashioned ways using highlighter pens of different colours for each 'code' or literal cut and paste of transcribed text. It is partly because of the fundamental difference between a pre- and post-imposition of categorisation that careful description of methods is vital in qualitative research. The more inductive the approach the more vital it is to be able to return to the actual words and actions used to show how these verify one's research. Notes of interviews do not enable the same close analysis as recording and transcription.

However, analysis into major themes should not be the end of research. The hallmark of fully analysed data is the emergence of models and theories about the phenomena being researched. These will be abstractions, but are intended to be the embodiment of the context or situation being studied and will be based on the themes analysed out of the data. They are not models or theories that actors in the situation/process would themselves readily articulate, but should subsequently be recognisable as 'true' to that situation by participants. They usually offer insight. Sections 4.5.1 and 4.5.2 illustrate this feature of qualitative research. Qualitative research may or may not be able to make suggestions about how research findings can be used (and often has not had this aim), but may nonetheless yield pointers for further investigation and consideration.

4.4.4 Writing Up

It will be apparent that when using qualitative methods the influence of the researcher cannot be completely nullified (although neither can it in quantitative research, in that the researcher in both instances has made choices about methods and analysis that influence the output). The researcher sets the questions, does the coding, selects the extracts, may be present during data collection and affect the context etc. Qualitative research compensates for this usually through using different forms of triangulation, that is, through the use of multi-methods, multiple researchers comparing their analysis of the same data, checking findings and conclusion with study participants for 'recognition', etc.

Transparency is vital, in the sense of absolute clarity as to methods and modes of analysis. Being able to present depth and complexity is another necessary feature. Educational qualitative research is typically written up with reference to and use of existing research and theory that is pertinent; results and conclusions are not necessarily separated – nor is any of this necessarily separated from theory and already published research. This is quite unlike the approach taken in science papers. Qualitative research aims to generate insight and understanding. As has been mentioned, this is typically presented as themes, or ideally developed into models to present a representation of reality that participants will recognise, but would not have been conscious of themselves before the research (e.g. Stewart 2008). As has been noted, a critique of the research is also usually expected from the authors, pointing to strengths and limitations of the work.

4.5 Case Studies of Educational Research

The purpose of this section is to briefly describe a few pieces of educational research so as to 'put flesh' on the bones of methods and approaches described above.

4.5.1 Case Study 1: The Qualitative Paradigm

Meyer and Land are the authors of Chap. 6 of this book. They have developed a theory of learning that, to simplify, suggests that in each (sub) discipline area, there is a key concept that is crucial to understanding that subject but which often poses challenges for learners such that some learners can never get beyond it – a threshold concept. Meyer, Land and others have conducted further studies to investigate what these threshold concepts might be for a number of disciplines. In this book, Meyer and Land present their first attempt to explore threshold concepts in surgical education. They developed their ideas through a series of interviews with consultant and trainees surgeons. Through asking pertinent questions, analysing respondents' replies and 'applying' their theory they emerged with a suggestion for a threshold concept in surgery. They quote from their interviews in showing how this concept emerged; it is akin to the development of a model or theory as referred to above.

4.5.2 Case Study 2: The Qualitative Paradigm

Jane Stewart adopted a grounded theory approach to the data she collected about how junior doctors make decisions about calling out a senior (Stewart 2008). She used purposive sampling, semi-structured interviews and group presentation and 32 hours of direct observation. From these she constructed a complex model that attempted to capture the criteria that governed their decisions 'to call or not to call'. The importance of the research is that it elucidated not only the actual practice in these situations but also that the researcher was then able to draw out suggestions about how junior doctors hone their skills and decision-making capacity and the implications this has for education and training.

4.5.3 Case Study 3: The Quantitative Paradigm

Simulation-based training for health-care teams (especially in interventional specialties such as surgery, obstetrics and anaesthesia) has been highlighted in the surgical education literature as a key learning environment for trainee as well as expert clinicians to hone their skills in crisis management, as well as communication, leadership and other 'nontechnical' factors (Issenberg et al. 2005; Lynagh et al. 2007; Sutherland et al. 2006; Sturm et al. 2008). Working independently, a number of research teams across the world piloted simulation-based training modules for individual clinicians and entire teams (e.g. operating theatre teams or maternity care teams) and assessed their efficacy using participants' attitudes to safety, and also validated, quantitative metrics of performance (Ellis et al. 2008; Moorthy et al. 2006; Paige et al. 2009; Robertson et al. 2009; Undre et al. 2007b). Following initial studies, prospective cross-sectional studies were subsequently carried out, with randomised controlled studies being increasingly reported in the international literature across a variety of specialities (Thomas et al. 2010). Learning outcomes are increasingly paired with clinical outcomes in such studies, aiming to demonstrate direct, quantitative translation of education and training into improved care processes, and ultimately, patient outcomes (Haller et al. 2008; Nielsen et al. 2007).

4.5.4 Case Study 4: Using Mixed Methods

In a recent series of interrelated studies, Arora and her colleagues have explored the impact of stress on the performance of surgeons, and how best to educate and train them to enable them to better cope with it in their clinical practice. This work started with reviewing the relevant evidence base, to determine what is known about the topic (Arora et al. 2010c). It then proceeded with a qualitative assessment, having conducted semi-structured interviews, of what surgeons feel about stressors in their environment, and what they would like a training and educational intervention to consist of (Arora et al. 2009). This work delivered a very rich context for an intervention to be delivered, with both senior and junior surgeons highlighting the role of systematic feedback on their performance as a key driver to learning and better coping with stress. The role of high-fidelity simulation environments also emerged as safe environments for learning and rehearsal of cognitive strategies to manage stress. These findings led to the subsequent development and validation of a mental practice protocol for surgeons to mentally rehearse their responses to stressors (Arora et al. 2010a; Arora 2010d). This was done by developing the protocol, administering it to expert and novice surgeons (two independent groups design), and comparing statistically the quality of their self-reported mental imagery pre- and post-exposure to the protocol. Once the protocol was shown to improve both novice and expert surgeons' imagery, it was deployed within a context of full immersion simulation (two independent groups design again), in which surgeons had to deal with a range of stressors in their theatre environment. One group of surgeons was exposed to the protocol (intervention group) whereas a second group of surgeons was not (control group). Findings of this study showed that surgeons' imagery did improve as a result of the protocol, and so did their response to stress and their performance in the simulation – all measured using standardised, validated scales (Arora 2010d).

4.6 Conclusion

This chapter has set out some of the key features of the two main paradigms used in surgical education research. It has used examples and case studies to exemplify the use of these varied approaches. It has also attempted, very superficially, to indicate the differing philosophical underpinnings of these paradigms, their differing starting points and intents. The purpose of the chapter has been to provide a sufficient account of the techniques of educational research for readers unfamiliar with this area to appreciate the research and approaches referred to in this book.

References

Albert, M., & Reeves, S. (2010). Setting some new standards in medical education research. *Medical Education, 44*(7), 638–639.

Arora, S. (2010d). Stress, safety and surgical performance. Unpublished Doctoral Dissertation, Imperial College, London.

Arora, S., Sevdalis, N., Nestel, D., Tierney, T., Woloshynowych, M., & Kneebone, R. (2009). Managing intra-operative stress: What do surgeons want from a crisis training programme? *American Journal of Surgery, 197*, 537–543.

Arora, S., Sevdalis, N., Aggarwal, R., Sirimanna, P., Darzi, A., & Kneebone, R. (2010a). Stress impairs psychomotor performance in novice laparoscopic surgeons. *Surgical Endoscopy, 24*, 2588–2593.

Arora, S., Tierney, T., Sevdalis, N., Aggarwal, R., Nestel, D., Woloshynowych, M., Darzi, A., & Kneebone, R. L. (2010b). The Imperial Stress Assessment Tool (ISAT): A feasible, reliable and valid approach to measuring stress in the operating room. *World Journal of Surgery, 34*, 1756–1763.

Arora, S., Sevdalis, N., Nestel, D., Woloshynowych, M., Darzi, A., & Kneebone, R. L. (2010c). The impact of stress on surgical performance: A systematic review of the literature. *Surgery, 147*, 318–330.

Becker, H. S. (1976). *Boys in white*. New Brunswick: Transaction Publishers.
Blalock, HM, Jr. (1979). *Social statistics* (Revised 2nd edn). New York: McGraw-Hill.
Bosk, C. L. (2003). *Forgive and remember. Managing medical failure*. Chicago: University of Chicago Press.
Cohen, L., Manion, L., & Morrison, K. (2007). *Research methods in education* (6th ed.). London: Routledge Falmer.
Ellis, D., Crofts, J. F., Hunt, L. P., Read, M., Fox, R., & James, M. (2008). Hospital, simulation center, and teamwork training for eclampsia management: A randomized controlled trial. *Obstetrics and Gynecology, 111*, 723–731.
Gill, D., & Griffin, A. (2009). Reframing medical education research: Let's make the publishable meaningful and the meaningful publishable. *Medical Education, 43*(10), 929–1024.
Gill, D., & Griffin, A. (2010). Good medical practice: What are we trying to say? Textual analysis using tag clouds. *Medical Education, 44*(3), 316–322.
Glaser, B., & Strauss, A. (1967). *The discovery of grounded theory*. Chicago: Aldine.
Haller, G., Garnerin, P., Morales, M. A., Pfister, R., Berner, M., Irion, O., Clergue, F., & Kern, C. (2008). Effect of crew resource management training in a multidisciplinary obstetrical setting. *International Journal for Quality in Health Care, 20*, 254–263.
Issenberg, S. B., McGaghie, W. C., Petrusa, E. R., Gordon, D. L., & Scalese, R. J. (2005). Features and uses of high-fidelity medical simulations that lead to effective learning: A BEME systematic review. *Medical Teacher, 27*, 10–28.
Kneebone, R., & Fry, H. (2009). Principles and methods in qualitative research. In T. Athanasiou, H. Debas, & A. Darzi (Eds.), *Key topics in surgical research and methodology* (pp. 243–254). Heidelberg: Springer. chapter 20.
Lynagh, M., Burton, R., & Sanson-Fisher, R. (2007). A systematic review of medical skills laboratory training: Where to from here? *Medical Education, 41*, 879–887.
Miles, M. B., & Huberman, M. (1994). *Qualitative data analysis* (2nd ed.). Thousand Oaks: Sage.
Moore, C. M. (1987). *Group techniques for idea building*. Newbury Park: Sage.
Moorthy, K., Munz, Y., Forrest, D., Pandey, V., Undre, S., Vincent, C., & Darzi, A. (2006). Surgical crisis management skills training and assessment: A simulation-based approach to enhancing operating room performance. *Annals of Surgery, 244*, 139–147.
Nielsen, P. E., Goldman, M. B., Mann, S., Shapiro, D. E., Marcus, R. G., Pratt, S. D., Greenberg, P., McNamee, P., Salisbury, M., Birnbach, D. J., Gluck, P. A., Pearlman, M. D., King, H., Tornberg, D. N., & Sachs, B. P. (2007). Effects of teamwork training on adverse outcomes and process of care in labor and delivery: A randomized controlled trial. *Obstetrics and Gynecology, 109*, 48–55.
Paige, J. T., Kozmenko, V., Yang, T., Paragi Gururaja, R., Hilton, C. W., Cohn, I., Jr., & Chauvin, S. W. (2009). High-fidelity, simulation-based, interdisciplinary operating room team training at the point of care. *Surgery, 145*, 138–146.
Paterson Davenport, L. A., Hesketh, E. A., Macpherson, S. G., & Harden, R. M. (2004). Exit outcomes for the PRHO year: An evidence base for informed discussion. *Medical Education, 38*(1), 67–80.
Pope, C., & Mays, N. (2006). *Qualitative research in health care* (3rd ed.). London: BMJ Books/Blackwell Publishing.
Robertson, B., Schumacher, L., Gosman, G., Kanfer, R., Kelley, M., & DeVita, M. (2009). Simulation-based crisis team training for multidisciplinary obstetric providers. *Simulation in Healthcare, 4*, 77–83.
Robson, C. (2002). *Real world research* (2nd ed.). Oxford: Blackwell.
Seale, C., Gobo, G., Gubrium, J., & Silverman, D. (Eds.). (2006). *Qualitative research practice*. Thousand Oaks: Sage.
Sevdalis, N., Davis, R. E., Koutantji, M., Undre, S., Darzi, A., & Vincent, C. A. (2008). Reliability of a revised NOTECHS scale for use in surgical teams. *American Journal of Surgery, 196*, 184–190.

Sevdalis, N., Lyons, M., Healey, A. N., Undre, S., Darzi, A., & Vincent, C. A. (2009). Observational teamwork assessment for surgery: Construct validation with expert vs. novice raters. *Annals of Surgery, 249*, 1047–1051.

Shadish, W. R., Cook, T. D., & Cambell, D. T. (2002). *Experimental and quasi experimental design for generalized causal inference*. Boston: Houghton-Mifflin.

Somekh, B., & Lewin, C. (Eds.). (2005). *Research methods in the social sciences*. Thousand Oaks: Sage.

Stewart, J. (2008). To call or not to call: A judgement of risk by pre-registration house officers. *Medical Education, 42*(9), 938–944.

Sturm, L. P., Windsor, J. A., Cosman, P. H., Cregan, P., Hewett, P. J., & Maddern, G. J. (2008). A systematic review of skills transfer after surgical simulation training. *Annals of Surgery, 248*, 166–179.

Sutherland, L. M., Middleton, P. F., Anthony, A., Hamdorf, J., Cregan, P., Scott, D., & Maddern, G. J. (2006). Surgical simulation: A systematic review. *Annals of Surgery, 243*, 291–300.

Swanwick, T. (Ed.). (2010). *Understanding medical education: Evidence, theory and practice*. Oxford: Wiley-Blackwell.

Teunissen, P. W. (2010). On the transfer of theory to the practice of research and education. *Medical Education, 44*(6), 534–535.

Thomas, E. J., Williams, A. L., Reichman, E. F., Lasky, R. E., Crandell, S., & Taggart, W. R. (2010). Team training in the neonatal resuscitation program for interns: Teamwork and quality of resuscitations. *Pediatrics, 125*, 539–546.

Undre, S., Sevdalis, N., Healey, A. N., & Vincent, C. A. (2007a). The Observational Teamwork Assessment for Surgery (OTAS): Refinement and application in urological surgery. *World Journal of Surgery, 3*, 1373–1381.

Undre, S., Koutantji, M., Sevdalis, N., Selvapatt, N., Williams, S., Gautama, S., McCulloch, P., Darzi, A., & Vincent, C. A. (2007b). Multi-disciplinary crisis simulations: The way forward for training surgical teams. *World Journal of Surgery, 3*, 1843–1853.

Yule, S., Flin, R., Maran, N., Rowley, D., Youngson, G., & Paterson-Brown, S. (2008). Surgeons' non-technical skills in the operating room: Reliability testing of the NOTSS behaviour rating system. *World Journal of Surgery, 32*, 548–556.

Zeller, R. A., & Carmines, E. G. (1980). *Measurement in the social sciences: The link between theory and data*. Cambridge: Cambridge University Press.

Part II

Chapter 5
Conceptualising Surgical Education Assessment

Lambert W.T. Schuwirth and Cees P.M. van der Vleuten

5.1 Introduction

Assessment of surgical competence is conceptually not much different from assessment of competence in other medical domains. Of course, the types of patients and consultations and the specific needs for dexterity all may slightly differ between surgery and medical disciplines, but this does not necessarily mean that the principles underlying assessment must differ. The way these principles are translated into real assessment practices, however, may and does vary considerably from discipline to discipline. The balance of purposes for assessing may also differ.

In this chapter, we address the concepts underlying the current approaches to assessment. We first discuss the main purposes assessment can and probably should serve, the main aspects determining the quality of assessment and the current methods in practice-based assessment, as these are especially important in surgical training. Then, we will present the most popular instruments and how to combine the results of the various assessments. We conclude by summarising some of the most important lessons about assessment.

5.2 Purposes of Assessment

The most frequently mentioned purpose of assessment is to distinguish between those who are competent and those who are not. This is logical because in all educational settings we need to be able to take the responsibility for the quality of graduates and specialists. Both society and teachers do not want to invest in

L.W.T. Schuwirth (✉) • C.P.M. van der Vleuten
Department of Educational Development and Research, Maastricht University, PO Box 616, 6200 MD Maastricht, The Netherlands
e-mail: l.schuwirth@maastrichtuniversity.nl

H. Fry and R. Kneebone (eds.), *Surgical Education: Theorising an Emerging Domain*, Advances in Medical Education 2, DOI 10.1007/978-94-007-1682-7_5,

incompetent students or trainees. The importance of this goal sometimes leads us to forget that there are other purposes also. The results of larger groups of candidates, for example, can provide valuable information as to the quality of the educational programme. If a large proportion of candidates fail, it is very likely that the course was not taught well or the test did not really assess the subject matter well.

A purpose most often forgotten is using assessment to drive learning in the desired direction. Most learners are strongly focused on the assessment and will adapt their learning to it.

5.3 General Issues Concerning Assessment

An important question is of course what determines the quality of an assessment procedure. Shared opinion on this question is that the quality of a procedure is always a trade-off between various criteria. Typically, criteria such as reliability, validity, educational impact, cost efficiency and stakeholder acceptability are included (Van der Vleuten 1996). The first three are briefly considered below.

5.3.1 Reliability

Reliability of an assessment pertains to the reproducibility of the results. This can be approached at two different levels. If an examination tries to establish whether the candidate scores above a certain level, in other words whether the candidate scores above an absolute threshold, reliability determines whether the candidate would obtain the *same* score on a so-called parallel test. A parallel test is a hypothetical test with different questions on the same topics and of equal difficulty. So, suppose a candidate scores 58% on a test on surgical knowledge, then the question arises whether he would score the same percentage again if he were presented with another test of equal difficulty on the same topics.

An assessment can also be used to determine the relative position of candidates in the rank ordering. In this case, reliability determines to what extent the candidate would obtain the same position in the rank ordering on a parallel test.

Good reliability in assessment is important because it supports the individual decisions made about progression and remediation of candidates. In addition, it may be important to realise that unreliability works both ways; it leads not only to competent candidates failing the test (a sort of false negative) but also to incompetent candidates passing the test (false positives).

The most important threat to reliability is poor sampling (Van der Vleuten et al. 1991). For this, it must be realised that every assessment should be seen as a sample from the almost infinite domain of possible questions, assignments, tasks, and techniques. Therefore, short tests, for example, a test using only one patient case/operation, cannot be reliable, simply because the sample is too small.

In general, therefore, high-stakes decisions must not be made on small samples but only on the collection and collation of extensive information.

A second source of unreliability is measurement error. Many factors contribute to this, for example, poorly constructed items on a multiple-choice test, poorly defined model answers in open-ended questions, judgement biases in orals or practice-based assessment. The two best known judgement biases are halo and primacy effects. In the former, the assessors can be influenced by non-relevant characteristics, for example, judge the competency of a candidate higher because he or she is well dressed or handsome. The latter means that the first impression dominates the assessment. So, a candidate whose first answers, actions or behaviours are spot-on will be judged more favourably on all subsequent questions than if the first answer had been incorrect.

Although it is often believed that to make an assessment reliable it should be objective, this is not correct. Objectivity is not equal to reliability nor is subjectivity equal to unreliability (Van der Vleuten et al. 1991). To achieve high reliability, the following measures are most helpful:

- Increase sample size. The most important source of unreliability is the content sample size (items, stations, cases, operations, etc), the solution is simple. Never rely on small samples for high-stakes decisions.
- Sample through all possible confounding factors. An Objective Structured Clinical Examination (OSCE, a station-based skills examination) is a good example (Harden and Gleeson 1979). In an OSCE, the candidate rotates through various rooms (stations) and in each room there is a new assignment (e.g. perform a resuscitation), a new examiner with a rating scale or checklist and a new manikin or simulated patient. This way, the final judgement is based not only on the impression of one examiner but also on the aggregated judgement of many. Some may be hawks and others doves (stringent or more lenient markers), but basically, for all students, a large sample of examiners is used. The same applies to the simulated patients.
- Provide examiners with some global criteria. It is important not to overdo it. Too detailed checklists (trying to make it as objective as possible) tend to trivialise the assessment. Some global criteria ensure that all candidates are judged roughly equally but leave room for the examiner to use his/her expertise in the assessment. Suppose in an observation-based assessment intubation is assessed and the examiner is an experienced anaesthetist, he or she does not need 30 yes/no items to determine whether the candidate demonstrates sufficient skill in the procedure. Instead the examiner needs to judge whether the procedure was performed with sufficient skill, whether complications were managed, whether sufficient care was taken for the patient, etc. For this, a more-point rating scale can be used. Again, it needs to be stressed here that no tick list will eliminate the difference between hawks and doves, but only sampling will.
- Train the examiners. Especially in workplace-based assessment, examiners need to be trained in using the assessment instruments and in the provision of feedback.

5.3.2 Validity

Where reliability is a rather straightforward concept, validity is more nebulous. Basically, validity indicates to what extent the test actually measures what it purports to measure. This is not easy to define. Many different types of validity have been described in the literature, but all can be subdivided in two mainstreams (Cronbach 1983; Ebel 1983). One – the so-called indirect validity – starts from the assumption that all that we test is a personal characteristic that we cannot observe directly (a so-called latent trait), much like intelligence or blood pressure. The validity of the test must, therefore, be inferred from the scores, for example, by demonstrating that experts outperform lesser experts or novices (Cronbach 1983).

The other starting point is that a test is a collection of directly relevant assignments or questions. As such (direct) validity can and must be built into a test, by careful item construction and review, a good blue print by which the distribution of topics within the test is determined, comparison with the curriculum or intended learning and careful consideration of the pass–fail scores (Ebel 1983).

Setting a pass–fail score is not an easy task, however. The literature describes more than 30 different standard setting methods. The logical conclusion from this is that there is no single superior method (Cusimano 1996). Every method has its inherent pros and cons, a careful consideration of which is the best basis for any decision in this matter. Some methods are so-called criterion referenced, which indicates that a judgement on the difficulty of the content is made by experts, and by this, the pass–fail score is determined. A second group of standard setting methods is the so-called norm-referenced procedures. In this, the performance of the candidates as a group is used to determine the pass–fail score (e.g. the mean score minus one standard deviation). No matter which method is used, it is always based on the *careful* collection of judgements and/or opinions, giving rise to the well-known aphorism that standard setting may always be arbitrary but may never be capricious.

5.3.3 Educational Impact

Often, assessment is part of a training programme. Although, in such a context, an important purpose of assessment is to determine whether the competence of the candidate is sufficient to progress to the next training phase or to graduate, this is not the only goal. Often in surgical training, it is intended that each assessment is part of the on-going education and training, the cumulative performance is what is important and the immediate educational impact is as much to receive feedback on performance as it is to demonstrate the current level of ability. As there is shared opinion that assessment is a powerful driving force for the learning behaviour of trainees, it is important to design the assessment programme as such that it stimulates desired learning behaviour (Frederiksen 1984; Newble and Jaeger 1983). In this respect, the two most obvious factors are the content and the format of the assessment. Additional aspects, however, are regulations and scheduling. The former relates to how scores on different assessment parts are combined (e.g. compensation or conjunction, which will be discussed later), weighting of different parts and resit possibilities. To ensure an optimal educational impact, it is advisable to evaluate the consequences of assessment on the learning regularly and make the necessary modifications.

5.4 Developments in Practice-Based Assessment

The notion of practice-based assessment is not new; for centuries, observations in practice have been part of assessment. Our understanding of reliable practice-based assessment, however, has improved. In recent decades much research and development has focused on making assessment more objective. The OSCE is a typical example of these developments. In OSCE research, however, an important finding was that the structuring did not really contribute much to reliability, but the use of multiple independent raters across stations and multiple different tasks was more important (Petrusa 2002). In other words, it was found that the 'objectivity' of the assessment was not essential, but careful sampling was. It was this robust finding that led to the design of the in-practice assessment procedures we are using today. This was a positive development because it enabled us to take the assessment of practical performance back to where it belongs, authentic practice. This has important implications for the design of a practice-based assessment programme.

5.4.1 Careful Sampling is Essential

One single observation is never enough to come to a decision about a candidate's competence. Typically, an assessor may be convinced after a short observation that he or she knows enough to reach a conclusion, but such an individual judgement is proven to be unreliable. In order to reach a sufficiently reliable conclusion typically 7–10 observations are the minimum (Williams et al. 2003).

5.4.2 Sampling Through Various Error Sources Is Needed

A typical error source is the assessor. Some are more stringent and others are more lenient; at various occasions, assessors may be more or less tired or inattentive and different settings (outpatient clinic, the operating theatre) may influence the candidate's performance (Van der Vleuten and Swanson 1990). Here, it must be stressed again that unreliability works in two ways and that insufficient reliability may not only lead to competent candidates failing the assessment but also to incompetent candidates passing.

5.4.3 Some Criteria are Important, too Detailed Checklists Lose Ground

It must be clear what the criteria for the observation of performance are, but the criteria must be set in such a way that the expertise of the observer is acknowledged. Typically, current practice-based instruments have a limited set of global criteria and a rating scale, with some explanation as to how to use the criteria (Pangaro and Holmboe 2008; Regehr et al. 1998). In general, good teacher/assessor training is a more important means to improve the quality of the assessment procedure than making the criteria more structured.

5.4.4 Assessment in the Framework of Training Requires Feedback

While the typical primary purpose of examinations was to optimally decide whether a candidate is a pass or a fail, in-training assessment aims to give more detailed information. Typically, every observation is followed by a brief feedback session in which it is determined what went well and what did not, what the specific learning goals or practice points are and how they are going to be met. Essential here is not per se to be soft and gentle to the trainee, but to analyse carefully how he or she can improve. Feedback, therefore, has to be concrete, constructive and combined with specific advice about improvement (Pendleton et al. 1984). In an in-training assessment programme a follow-up of the learning goals must be integral and failure to achieve successfully a learning goal (by the trainee) must have consequences (Carr 2006).

5.4.5 In-Training Assessment must be feasible

The life of a practising surgeon is busy; supervising trainees is often the work that comes on top of the rest. Designing a wonderful but unrealistic programme is not efficient. Even if the staff are of good will and dedicated to putting in maximum effort, any assessment programme will eventually be watered down if it turns out to be incompatible with everyday practice. Therefore, a careful consideration of what is manageable in the long run is necessary. This is not a plea for a minimalistic approach, but for pragmatism. If 5 min/day per trainee is doable, a system of 5 min/day each day is better than 1 h/month. To reiterate the issue of sampling, many observations of 5 min each draw a better general picture than one or only a few observations of 1 h.

This is not to say that it should always be short observations. Often, in the operating theatre, the consultant and the trainee jointly perform an operation.

Here there is ample room for a longer observation and the provision of feedback (as well as short observations). The only extra effort here is to document briefly the observations and the feedback. The bottom line is still to find ways to incorporate the work-based assessment in the daily routine as well as possible.

5.5 Instruments for Practice-Based Assessment

There are many different instruments available for practice-based assessment, and many of them have been adapted from the original form to fit better the local/speciality training situation. In light of the previous paragraphs, we would certainly advocate this; if slight adaptations make the assessment more practical and doable they should be made. We discuss the most important instruments and their use here. For each instrument, we describe what it is and how it is best used. Some are based directly in practice, others simulate practice.

5.5.1 Mini-Clinical Evaluation Exercise

Mini-Clinical Evaluation Exercise (mini-CEX) is an observation-based assessment instrument. John Norcini and colleagues developed it in the mid-1990s at the American Board of Internal Medicine (Norcini et al. 1995). Typically, it is used to assess the practical performance of a trainee or registrar in daily practice. In surgery, it spurred the developments to assess longer periods of practice and has been given various names.

Administratively, a mini-CEX consists of a form with a small number of criteria. Each criterion has a rating scale. Originally, this was a 9-point rating scale, but, as said, several adaptations have been made and used since. Examples of such criteria are as follows:

- Medical interviewing skills
- Physical examination skills
- Humanistic qualities/professionalism
- Clinical judgement
- Counselling skills
- Organisation/efficiency
- Overall clinical competency

There is also some room for meta-data, like time needed for observation and to provide oral and/or written feedback.

A mini-CEX is completed after a direct observation of a clinical patient encounter. The observer is instructed to complete only those items on which a judgement could be made. As said before, observations can be kept brief. When used properly mini-CEX combines summative (decision making) and formative (to inform the candidate about his/her performance) values of assessment. For these purposes, qualitative remarks and a short verbal feedback session are as essential to the use of mini-CEX as is the rating.

It is important to instruct the observer that the purpose of a single observation and completed mini-CEX is not to give a judgement of the overall competence of the registrar or his suitability for the discipline, but only to provide a judgement as to what has been observed directly. More general judgements or inferences can only be made reliably when sufficient independent mini-CEX results are obtained.

The literature shows that in general 7–10 *independent* observations suffice for higher stakes decisions (Wilkinson et al. 2008; Williams et al. 2003). For summative assessment purposes, the ideal is that 7–10 different examiners should have each observed and judged an encounter. Since the mini-CEX was developed for the clinical-patient encounter and not so much for the assessment of procedural skills, it may be clear that its place is not the operating theatre, but rather the outpatient clinic or the wards. For procedural skills and operations, other instruments (e.g. DOPS (Direct Observation of Procedural Skills) discussed below) are more useful.

If the same assessor judges all the encounters, a confirmation bias will influence the reproducibility of the results. This means that during the early encounters, the examiner has formed an opinion that is not very likely to change during subsequent encounters.

For formative purposes, it is essential that the learning goals arising from one feedback session are followed up during the next feedback session, to see whether they have been met or not. This again poses problems for practice-based learning in surgery.

5.5.2 Multi-source Feedback (360° Feedback, Multi-rater Feedback)

Multisource feedback is a tool that was originally used in Human Resource Management (Ward 1997). It is an assessment based on the judgement of colleagues, peers, etc. from various viewpoints. The purpose is not to provide information about the average performance of the assessee, but more to provide insight into specific strengths and weaknesses as seen from various angles. Because different rater groups (including the assessee himself/herself) are used, a more complete or balanced picture about the assessee's abilities can be obtained.

In surgery, the various judges should not only be drawn from peers and supervisors, but also from paramedical staff, nurses and administrative staff – patients can also provide valuable information. Of course, every judge can evaluate only what he or she is 'expert' in. Patients, for example, cannot comment on the technical competence of the assessee, but they can evaluate the professionalism, communication, empathy, etc. It is therefore important to brief the respondents about the purposes and limitations of the method. Typically the rating form contains several (30–60) items with a so-called Likert scale. Likert scales are the type used in many questionnaires; each possible response is shown as four or five tick boxes, ranging, for example, from 'completely disagree' to 'completely agree'.

In its normal use, the assessees complete the questionnaires evaluating themselves and then the other forms are distributed amongst the various stakeholder groups. Although some early research showed that it does not matter whether the respondents are selected by the assessee or chosen at random (Ramsey et al. 1993), it is best advised to at least select half of the judges at random. In many surgery training settings, it may be difficult to randomly select in certain rater groups (like fellow registrars), but it is possible to select randomly in other groups (i.e. patients). Ideally the distribution and collection is done by someone else than the assessee (administrative personnel), and the results are collated first and then fed back to the assessee (e.g. in an appraisal session). Technology can be useful to collect, collate and redistribute scores.

5.5.3 Key-Feature Approach Case-Based Testing and Extended-Matching Items

One of the robust research findings in the expertise literature is that central to expertise and problem-solving ability is the possession of well-organised knowledge (see also Chap. 10). Therefore, the 1970s mantra, 'You don't have to know it as long as you know where to find it', has been disproven to a large extent. In order to find relevant knowledge and to appraise new knowledge critically, you have to have sufficient knowledge already (Chi et al. 1982; Posner 1988). This being said, it is also quite clearly demonstrated that the possession of irrelevant knowledge and wrongly structured knowledge (e.g. by learning lists by rote) is not very useful for successful problem solving. Knowledge is best learnt and applied if it happens in the context of a realistic case. In assessment, this has led to the development of long-branched patient simulations for the assessment of medical problem solving. Due to various psychometric problems, this approach has been abandoned by all major testing bodies. The most striking problem was that long simulations take a long time to complete and therefore extremely long testing times would be needed for sufficient reliability. Instead, both the key-feature approach to assessment (developed by Bordage and Page for the Medical Council of Canada (Page et al. 1995) and extended-matching items (developed for the National Board of Medical Examiners in the USA; Case and Swanson 1993) have in common that they are based on short cases with questions asking for decisions to be made in each specific case. They do not try to test general medical knowledge, but instead focus on medical decision making or clinical reasoning.

The biggest advantage of the key-feature approach is that a large number (roughly 30) short cases can be asked per hour of testing time. Thus, the sampling is broad.

Each case presents a patient problem, the setting in which the patient is seen and the role of the assessee ('You are a registrar in surgery. At the emergency you see

Mr. Johnson ...'). The presentation also describes pertinent elements from history taking and physical examination, and other possible diagnostics. The number of questions per case is restricted to the essential decisions that have to be made; decisions that determine whether each case is managed successfully or not. The question format is not prescribed, and preferably it is decided based on the content – or more specifically the number of realistic options – of the question.

In extended-matching items, a panel of options is given first (varying from 15 to 26 options) and then a collection of short case presentations (vignettes). The assessee now has to choose the most likely correct option from the panel of options. Some options are not applicable to any of the vignettes and some options can be the correct answer in more than one vignette.

5.5.4 Objective Structured Assessment of Technical Skills

Objective structured assessment of technical skills (OSATS) is a method of assessing technical skills (Bodle et al. 2008). It is an OSCE type of assessment where the assessees move around through different rooms with different assignments, examiners and manikins or simulated patients, but each station usually lasts for a longer time than in an OSCE. It is therefore better suited to more experienced doctors.

The examiner has two forms – one is a checklist on the specific procedure to be tested in that station. This form is specifically designed for the task of the particular station and the criteria on the checklist are tailored to the specific technical skill to be assessed, for example, haemorrhage control and repair of a traumatically ruptured big vessel. The second form is more generic and contains criteria such as respect for tissue, time and motion, instrument handling, knowledge of instruments, use of assistants, flow of operation and forward planning, and knowledge of specific procedure. This can be used in all stations. Further discussion of simulation in learning and assessing can be found in Chaps. 3, 8 and 9.

5.5.5 Direct Observation of Procedural Skills (DOPS)

Directly observed procedural skills was developed in the UK (Davies et al. 2005). It is based on the direct observation of procedural skills (e.g. intubation and inserting a central line) and a generic rating scale to be completed by the examiner. It is similar to the mini-CEX approach the only difference being the criteria on which to rate the procedure. These are tailored more specifically to surgical procedures. Typically, these criteria are as follows:

- Demonstrates understanding of indications, relevant anatomy, technique of procedure
- Obtains informed consent

- Demonstrates appropriate preparation pre-procedure
- Appropriate analgesia or safe sedation
- Technical ability
- Aseptic technique
- Seeks help where appropriate
- Post-procedure management
- Communication skills
- Considerations of patient/professionalism
- Overall ability to perform procedure

The rating form also has space for some qualitative feedback.

Similar to the mini-CEX, the basis for DOPS is a direct observation of the performance of the procedure. Observations can be kept brief; there is little usefulness in observing a registrar or trainee longer than 15–20 min, and the examiner completes only those items on which a judgement could be made. In DOPS, summative and formative aspects of assessment are combined: on the one hand, a judgement as to whether a certain standard has been reached, on the other hand giving feedback which is required for learning purposes. The guidelines and tips for use in practice are the same as for the mini-CEX.

5.5.6 Case-Based Orals/Chart Stimulated Recall

Case-based orals (in the North American literature: Chart stimulated recall; in the UK: case-based discussion) are designed to assess the process of clinical judgement, decision making and the application of medical knowledge in the context of practical patient care. It should be based on those patient cases the trainee has been directly responsible for.

As with all other instruments, some structure in the form of a criteria list is embedded in the method. The oral element is a discussion between the assessor and the trainee on what has happened during a consultation and what the reasons for actions were or what the relevant background knowledge of the trainee is. Apart from the medical-technical content, ethical and medico-legal issues with respect to the case may be discussed.

The (typical) criteria on the form are:

- Medical record keeping
- Clinical assessment
- Investigation and referrals
- Treatment
- Follow-up and future planning
- Professionalism
- Overall clinical judgement

The assessment should normally take no more than 15–20 min and a subsequent feedback session of roughly 3–5 min. Ideally, there is a safe learning environment in which the trainee can use the feedback to improve most effectively, so that he or she feels free to select more challenging cases and not to use routine cases.

5.5.7 Portfolio

Portfolios come in many forms and shapes. They have become very popular in a short time span, leading some authors to call them a hype. Indeed, a simple internet search reveals over 194,000,000 hits (search performed September 2009). Some see a portfolio as an instrument to teach and assess reflection, perhaps especially in pre-registration education, but others use them as a dossier with a self-reflection on strengths and weaknesses. For the training of registrars in surgery, the latter seems more appropriate. In this case, the portfolio is not so much another instrument to assess a certain aspect of competence, but it is the instrument in which all results, both quantitative and qualitative and formal assessment results, as well as informal feedback can be collected and collated – often with an element of reflection on these being expected.

Recent reviews confirm that portfolios used in such a way effectively assess day-to-day performance (Driessen et al. 2007). A comprehensive range of information, collated in this way, will produce a well-founded summative judgement, which is discussed later. At the same time, however, it provides a good basis for trainees to formatively analyse their own performance. In this way, they can reflect on and improve their practice and set realistic objectives for further learning.

When a portfolio is used in this way, it can be seen as analogous to a patient chart. This normally contains a dossier with a report of all the symptoms and findings, a section with the doctor's notes on working diagnosis, further diagnostic and therapeutic actions and possible impact on the prognosis. We suggest the portfolio of surgical trainees contain:

- A dossier in which the evidence or underpinning for the competencies of the candidates are stored (e.g. min-CEX forms, DOPS, 360°, results of knowledge and knowledge application assessment on the one hand and informal observations and deliberations on the other hand),
- A documentation of procedures and operations conducted,
- A part in which the trainee produces a SWOT, self-reflection if you will (an analysis of strengths, weaknesses, opportunities and threats), an analysis of his/her competencies with learning goals and
- Short minutes of meetings between the fellow/registrar and his/her supervisor.

First, good mentoring is the single most decisive success factor (Driessen et al. 2007). Second, the portfolio must be smart and lean. Portfolios should never become piles of paper or the digital equivalent of this; it should be trimmed down to essential information. The principle of 'enough is enough' should really be adhered to in portfolios, otherwise they become unmanageable. So, both trainees and their supervisors should sift the relevant information from the irrelevant. Another important aspect is that the SWOT analysis is always supported by concrete evidence from the dossier. So the analysis must be traceable to the individual trainee. Careful implementation is crucial. A strong resistance to the portfolio can be unleashed when learners are forced to stick to a rigidly prescribed format.

5.6 How to Combine the Results of Various Sources

In the previous sections, we have talked about some general issues and specific characteristics of individual assessment methods. But on coming to high-stakes decisions about whether or not a trainee can progress to a next phase, the information from various assessment instruments needs to be combined in a fair and defensible way. There are different ways of combining results, each of which has its own advantages and disadvantages.

Probably the most well-known approach is the so-called conjunctive method. Simply put, this means that a candidate is deemed to be competent only if all the assessments were satisfactory. In most assessment programmes, conjunction is used between assessment methods. Various royal college membership examinations consist of multiple parts, all of which must have been passed in order to become a member. This is a typical example of a conjunctive structure.

The opposite is a compensatory structure. This is typically the case *within* an assessment part. In a case-based written assessment, for example, a registrar who completes case 1 correctly and case 2 incorrectly will receive half of the total credits. The same applies, however, for the registrar who completes case 2 correctly and case 1 incorrectly. So, there is total compensation between parts within an examination.

Of course, a fully conjunctive model is more stringent; it will minimise the number of false positives (registrars passing without sufficient competence) but at the cost of producing larger numbers of false negatives. Of course, the dangers of false positives are quite obvious; letting an incompetent surgeon loose on the public is dangerous. But, the opposite should not be neglected either, that is, unjustified denial of the chance to earn a (higher) salary and withholding from society of a competent surgeon. So, in either way the stakes are high.

A compensatory model may then seem to be more useful, but here too there are caveats to consider. First is the negative influence it may have on the learning behaviour of the registrars. Especially in those cases in which the early performances were very good, it may lead to complacency as even with low marks on the later examination parts the compensatory mark will still be sufficient (e.g. someone who scored 9/10 on a first test may not be inclined to study hard for the second as a 3/10 would still lead to a satisfactory mark).

In many situations where examination results are combined quantitatively, limited compensation can be used. Limited compensation is simply based on an extra rule that compensation is only possible if none of the individual marks is too far below the pass mark. In the example previously given, one could add the rule that if one of the individual results is lower than 5, the final decision is always 'fail'.

Compensation and conjunction are easy to understand when the results of all assessment parts are quantitative. Numbers can easily be averaged. But nowadays more qualitative judgements are incorporated in assessment programmes. It may go without saying that converting qualitative data into numbers (e.g. 'good' = 8, 'satisfactory' = 6, 'unsatisfactory' = 4) is not the ideal route to take. Many assessment-based decisions are simply too important to be based on poor statistics.

How then, one may ask, can we combine meaningfully the results from both quantitative and qualitative sources? We would argue that much can be learnt from clinical practice. It is the bread and butter of a clinician's daily work. In many consultations, numerical lab values, qualitative interpretations (history taking, physical examination) and opinions of expert third parties (pathologist, radiologist) are combined. Factors that ensure that judgements based on such information are fair and defensible are found in careful documentation, note taking, second opinion, inter-collegial consultations, etc. In assessment programmes, where a variety of information is collected about the progress and competency of the trainee, there is certainly room for individual judgement even for high-stakes decisions as long as the same careful procedures are adhered to as in normal patient care. In such cases, a portfolio appears to be the best suitable instrument, not for the assessment of reflection, but as the assessment analogy of a patient chart.

5.7 Epilogue, What is the Use of all this?

A question often asked, and rightfully so, is whether this really produces better surgeons, as it certainly produces more supervisory work. The answer is a clear 'yes', but requires some elaboration. If the question is whether there has ever been a large randomised controlled trial conducted comparing the old assessment approaches to the new ones the answer must be clearly 'no'. This is much the same as there being no randomised control trial to demonstrate that the use of imaging techniques in medical diagnostics has improved the health care of the population of the UK or that medical education with anatomy teaching or learning leads to better doctors than medical education without anatomy. Yet there is overwhelming evidence that imaging techniques in health care are beneficial and apparently to the extent that we are willing to spend time and resources on them. It is the same with innovations in medical education and assessment; there is good research underpinning all kinds of decisions about assessment methods and how to use them in a plethora of international peer reviewed journals. The evidence on what influences reliability and validity of assessment methods, what constitutes medical/surgical expertise, how trainees learn more effectively and the value of specific, timely and concrete feedback is robust enough to support the descriptions and suggestions made in this chapter. We hope that our descriptions and suggestions have also been clear enough to help the reader in his or her roles as teacher, examiner and supervisor.

References

Bodle, J. F., Kaufmann, S. J., Bisson, D., Nathanson, B., & Binney, D. M. (2008). Value and face validity of objective structured assessment of technical skills (osats) for work based assessment of surgical skills in obstetrics and gynaecology. *Medical Teacher, 30*, 212–216.

Carr, S. (2006). The foundation programme assessment tools: An opportunity to enhance feedback to trainees? *Postgraduate Medical Journal, 82*, 576–579.

Case, S. M., & Swanson, D. B. (1993). Extended-matching items: A practical alternative to free response questions. *Teaching and Learning in Medicine, 5*, 107–115.

Chi, M. T. H., Glaser, R., & Rees, E. (1982). Expertise in problem solving. In R. J. Sternberg (Ed.), *Advances in the psychology of human intelligence* (pp. 7–76). Hillsdale: Lawrence Erlbaum Associates.

Cronbach, L. J. (1983). What price simplicity? *Educational Measurement: Issues and Practice, 2*, 11–12.

Cusimano, M. D. (1996). Standard setting in medical education. *Academic Medicine, 71*, 112–120.

Davies, H., Archer, J., Heard, S., & Wouthgate, L. (2005). Assessment tools for foundation programmes – A practical guide. *British Medical Journal, 330*, 195–196.

Driessen, E., Van Tartwijk, J., Van der Vleuten, C., & Wass, V. (2007). Portfolios in medical education: Why do they meet with mixed success? A systematic review. *Medical Education, 41*(12), 1224–1233.

Ebel, R. L. (1983). The practical validation of tests of ability. *Educational Measurement: Issues and Practice, 2*, 7–10.

Frederiksen, N. (1984). The real test bias: Influences of testing on teaching and learning. *The American Psychologist, 39*, 193–202.

Harden, R. M., & Gleeson, F. A. (1979). Assessment of clinical competence using an objective structured clinical examination (OSCE). *Medical Education, 13*, 41–54.

Newble, D. I., & Jaeger, K. (1983). The effect of assessments and examinations on the learning of medical students. *Medical Education, 17*, 165–171.

Norcini, J., Blank, L. L., Arnold, G. K., & Kimball, H. R. (1995). The mini-CEX (clinical evaluate on exercise); A preliminary investigation. *Annals of Internal Medicine, 123*, 795–799.

Page, G., Bordage, G., & Allen, T. (1995). Developing key-feature problems and examinations to assess clinical decision-making skills. *Academic Medicine, 70*, 194–201.

Pangaro, L. N., & Holmboe, E. S. (2008). Evaluation forms and global rating scales. In E. S. H. R. E. Hawkins (Ed.), *Practical guide to the evaluation of clinical competence*. Philadelphia: Mosby Elsevier.

Pendleton, D., Schofield, T., & Tate, D. (1984). A method for giving feedback. In *The consultation: An approach to learning and teaching*. Oxford: Oxford University Press.

Petrusa, E. R. (2002). Clinical performance assessments. In G. R. Norman, C. P. M. van der Vleuten, & D. I. Newble (Eds.), *International handbook of research in medical education*. Dordrecht: Kluwer Academic Publishers.

Posner, M. I. (1988). What is it to be an expert? In M. T. Chi, R. Glaser, & M. J. Farr (Eds.), *The nature of expertise* (pp. xxix–xxxvi). Hillsdale: Lawrence Erlbaum Associates, inc.

Ramsey, P. G., Wenrich, M. D., Carline, J. D., Inui, T. S., Larson, E. B., & Logerfo, J. P. (1993). Use of peer ratings to evaluate physician performance. *Journal of the American Medical Association, 269*, 1655–1660.

Regehr, G., Macrae, H., Reznick, R., & Szalay, D. (1998). Comparing the psychometric properties of checklists and global rating scales for assessing performance on an osce-format examination. *Academic Medicine, 73*, 993–997.

Van der Vleuten, C. P. M. (1996). The assessment of professional competence: Developments, research and practical implications. *Advances in Health Sciences Education, 1*, 41–67.

Van der Vleuten, C. P. M., & Swanson, D. (1990). Assessment of clinical skills with standardized patients: State of the art. *Teaching and Learning in Medicine, 2*, 58–76.

Van der Vleuten, C. P. M., Norman, G. R., & De Graaf, E. (1991). Pitfalls in the pursuit of objectivity: Issues of reliability. *Medical Education, 25*, 110–118.

Ward, P. (1997). *360-degree feedback*. London: CIPD.

Wilkinson, J. R., Crossley, J. G., Wragg, A., Mills, P., Cowan, G., & Wade, W. (2008). Implementing workplace-based assessment across the medical specialties in the united kingdom. *Medical Education, 42*, 364–373.

Williams, M., Klamen, D., & McGaghie, W. (2003). Cognitive, social and environmental sources of bias in clinical performance ratings. *Teaching and Learning in Medicine, 15*, 270–292.

Chapter 6
The Scalpel and the 'Mask': Threshold Concepts and Surgical Education

Ray Land and Jan H.F. Meyer

6.1 Introduction

Surgery is an unusual and distinctive practice and the education of new entrants to this profession is a particularly complex affair. An important consideration in the analysis of any form of learning, and this applies equally to forms of professional training such as surgical education, is the particular lens through which the process of development, and the learning environment in which it takes place, are viewed. In this study, the conceptual framework of 'Threshold Concepts and Troublesome Knowledge' is employed (Meyer and Land 2003, 2005; Land et al. 2005). Within all disciplinary areas there seem to be particular concepts that can be considered as akin to a portal, opening up a new and previously inaccessible way of thinking about something. A threshold concept represents a transformed way of understanding, or interpreting, or viewing something without which the learner cannot progress. As a consequence of comprehending a threshold concept, there may thus be a transformed internal view of the subject landscape, of practice or even world view, and the student can move on.

6.2 Threshold Concepts and Troublesome Knowledge

In attempting to characterise such conceptual gateways, we have suggested in earlier work (Meyer and Land 2003) that they are *transformative* (occasioning a significant shift in the perception of a subject), *integrative* (exposing the previously hidden

R. Land (✉)
Learning Enhancement, University of Strathclyde, Glasgow, UK
e-mail: ray.land@strath.ac.uk

J.H.F. Meyer
The University of Queensland, Australia

H. Fry and R. Kneebone (eds.), *Surgical Education: Theorising an Emerging Domain*, Advances in Medical Education 2, DOI 10.1007/978-94-007-1682-7_6,

interrelatedness of something) and likely to be, in varying degrees, *irreversible* (unlikely to be forgotten, or unlearned only through considerable effort). They also entail a shift in the learner's sense of self, what we might term their subjectivity. For example, they may feel, in some particular respect, that they are now thinking and practising a little more like a surgeon. Thresholds also invariably entail a changed (usually more sophisticated) use of the specialised language (discourse) of the discipline or profession. These learning thresholds are often the points at which students experience difficulty. The transformation may be sudden or it may be protracted over a considerable period of time, with the transition to understanding often involving *troublesome knowledge*. Depending on discipline and context, knowledge might be troublesome because it is ritualised, inert, conceptually difficult, alien or tacit, because it requires adopting an unfamiliar discourse, or perhaps because the learner remains 'defended' and does not wish to change or let go of their customary way of seeing things.

Having to cope with a threshold concept as an integral aspect of surgical practice, may leave the new entrant in a state of 'liminality', a suspended state of partial understanding, or 'stuck place', in which understanding approximates to a kind of 'mimicry' or lack of authenticity. Insights gained by new entrants as they encounter thresholds can be exhilarating but might also be unsettling, requiring an uncomfortable shift in identity, or, paradoxically, a sense of loss. A further complication might be the operation of an 'underlying game', which requires the learner to comprehend the often tacit games of enquiry or ways of thinking and practising inherent within specific disciplinary knowledge practices. In this sense, we might wish to talk of 'threshold practices' or 'learning thresholds', which are necessary for the learner's development.

6.3 Ontological Shift

There is now a substantial body of writing (Meyer and Land 2006, 2010; Land et al. 2008) which furthers our understanding of the *ontological* transformations – the changes in being, identity or awareness of self that are necessarily occasioned by significant learning. These learning thresholds, as we might term them, might not be strictly conceptual, but are concerned with shifts in identity and subjectivity, with procedural knowledge, or the ways of thinking and practising customary to a given disciplinary or professional community such as surgical practice. This has significant implications for the analysis and design of learning environments.

> ..the stuck places encountered by students ... can have an ontological dimension ... This obviously renders problematic any simplistic schematic attempt to overcome troublesome knowledge by technicist redesign of curricula alone, and challenges easy assumptions that if the learning environment is suitably ordered and constructively aligned then the intended transformations will ensue. (Meyer and Land 2005, p. 378)

Furthermore, running throughout this transformational process, there is often the 'underlying game', mentioned above, in which ways of thinking and practising that are often left tacit come to be recognised, grappled with and gradually understood. This underlying game is a common feature of the processes of entry, meaning-making and identity formation typically required for entry to a given community of practice (see Chaps. 2 and 11).

> ... in some instances students may grasp concepts but the barrier to their learning appears to lie at a deeper level of understanding, where the student finds difficulty in appreciating what David Perkins ... has termed 'the underlying game', or an 'epistemic game'. He defines an episteme as 'a system of ideas or way of understanding that allows us to establish knowledge'. It might also be seen as a 'way of knowing'. Epistemes are 'manners of justifying, explaining, solving problems, conducting inquiries, and designing and validating various kinds of products or outcomes.' (Meyer and Land 2006, p. xvi)

Entry to the community of practising surgeons offers an illustration of the ontological transformations that are frequently mentioned in the literature on threshold concepts. These 'learning thresholds', conceptual or otherwise, seem necessarily occasioned by significant learning and are more concerned with shifts in identity and subjectivity, with procedural knowledge, or the ways of thinking and practising customary to a given disciplinary or professional community. An underlying implication here is that there is always some form of self-relational trajectory to the discipline being learned (Cousin 2009). One might be, for example, a student and practitioner of music *in order to become* a performing pianist. Being and knowing are inextricably linked. We are what we know, and we become what we learn. As Davies (2006) has pointed out, an act of learning is an act of identity formation.

Kegan (1982) claims that individuals experience such 'shifts of consciousness' through recurring patterns or phases of stability and change during their lives. Timmermans (2010) points to the elusiveness and inherent difficulty of examining these transitional phases.

> It is these periods of change, these transitions that characterise the learning process, which I find most intriguing. These transitions remain nebulous; however, understanding them is crucial. Cross (1999) notes that 'in developmental theory, the periods of greatest personal growth are thought to lie in the unnamed and poorly-defined periods *between* stages' (p. 262; emphasis in original). We might therefore imagine that the most significant aspect of learning lies not in the *outcomes* of learning, but in the *process* of learning. Understanding this process and how best to facilitate it is thus essential to our work as educators. (Timmermans 2010, p. 3)

6.4 Attitudes of Perfection: The Needle

To gain some understanding of the process of surgical education, a series of individual face-to-face interviews was conducted in London with a small sample of surgeons. The group can by no means be regarded as representative but contained surgeons from both sexes, of different ages and nationalities, and ranging in level of professional experience from relatively new entrants to those with considerable experience, and, in one case, of world renown.

Regarding conceptual knowledge and possible candidates for threshold-like points of transformation in the process of professional training, considerable emphasis was placed on how to appreciate the anatomy and how to handle tissue. A particular concern and priority was the capacity to navigate and make sense of strange anatomical terrain in cases when the patient had undergone previous surgery that had led to alterations in anatomy. The more normal representations of organs and tissue in the textbook become less recognisable in such situations. But a number of respondents commented on the difference they found generally when encountering anatomy in surgical contexts compared with what they had learned as medical students from textbooks.

> I'm a general surgeon. One of the most common elective operations in general surgery is Inguinal hernia repair ... so that's a growing hernia repair and I learned the anatomy to quite a large extent in medical school but never really... I thought I understood it but then when it came to actually doing the operation I really did find it quite difficult. It was a competence and confidence issue with me there, because I thought it was just me that didn't understand it. And I had spent hours... I had a very traditional medical school basic science course with a lot of anatomy, so I had really spent hours poring over this anatomy and I felt very frustrated that when it came to actually doing it on the patient I really didn't 'get it'.
>
> [Interviewer: What was it that you didn't get?]
>
> The different layers. And how they interact. Yeah. And there's also ... because obesity's quite a problem now ... the levels ... there's a layer of fat that isn't in the anatomy books.

One significant realisation is that surgical learning often involves a 'letting go' of the dependence on formal textbook learning.

> I was trying to find out what was important in the operative thing. Some of the planes – the layers – you just have to put your finger in and sweep round. You can't really explain that in a book very much. There's two different kinds of hernia – one is where it pushes through ... the wall is quite weak ... you actually have to feel that yourself to see how weak it is and how much of the flap you have to take up and you can't learn that from a picture. And in the book what's called pre-peritoneal fat. The peritoneum is when you're *right* inside the abdomen, so that's when you're guggling around for the appendix. And just before you get through that last thin layer there's a layer of fat that is definitely not in my anatomy text books and you think 'Oh my god! I'm really in the wrong area here!' You know? 'I've gone through the wrong layer! Am I *in* the abdomen? Why is there this fat?' And then, you know, it makes clear ... but it can be very scary when you're on your own in the middle of the night and you're trying to get your confidence up, and suddenly it really doesn't look like in the books! [*laughs*]

Respondents tended to feel that three-dimensional medical computer simulations held promise for better future preparation for surgeons (see also Chaps. 3 and 8), but there was a general concern that conventional two-dimensional anatomical drawings were often unhelpful, and occasionally misleading.

Another realisation is that others have also faced this difficulty and that a problem shared is often halved:

> But then I did find – it was a female surgeon actually – who was visiting from overseas and I said to her 'I don't really get this,' and she said 'Ooh! It's very difficult! You know *I* found it very difficult.' And suddenly the light went on and I thought 'Gosh! It's not just me!' She

> became quite a good friend. So we sat down at home one day and went through the anatomy in the books, which didn't completely solve the problem, but it certainly went quite a long way to building up my confidence, so when I was in there[*the operating theatre*] it certainly helped a lot.

Such professional frankness, it was acknowledged, was sometimes troublesome in a culture where, often 'To be wrong is to be weak'.

Technical precision, neatness and accuracy in stitching were taken as a foundational skill. An eye surgeon, a fairly recent entrant to the profession who was still undergoing training, commented:

> Precision and control are essential. 'Cos it's quite an alien skill. For instance, just moving an instrument inside the eye – the whole diameter of what you're dealing with is a just a few millimetres. So it's dexterity and confidence and calm. Fine dexterity. Sometimes the level of proficiency requires a certain slickness. It's being able to do very fine movements, with deftness. Surgeons are cool people. They have to be.

Of course eye surgery is particularly a fine work, so this emphasis is especially likely in this context, but we are reminded here of McLuhan's (1994) observation of 'technology as an extension of the human body'. Surgical technical dexterity exemplifies his claim that an extension of our body and senses occurs when we can extend the reach of our embodied mind beyond our natural limited means. Surgical use of high technology and microscopy offers a dramatic illustration of this extension of vision.

However, though the initial experience of opening the skin and performance stitching was recognised as stressful, this was considered to be a practice that was relatively quickly routinised and normalised. More challenging and demanding, the more senior surgeons emphasised, was the essential capacity for *decision making*. This occurs pre-operatively, when deciding whether or not to operate on the patient, during operational procedure as complications or unforeseen factors arise, and post-operatively in terms of the provision of appropriate post-operative care. The impact of such decisions can of course be quite profound and both the process and the consequences of the decision making are relatively public. One experienced surgeon commented:

> Surgical skill is not technical skills only. Technical skill is part of surgery but decision-making is crucial for surgery and is more important than technical skills. A surgeon needs good decision-making, needs attitudes of perfection. We need precision. The patient might get post-operative complications. There can be no short cuts. And we need high standards of post-operative care. Everything has a set of skills but they are of different intensity.

The difference in intensity relates to the risk involved. Another senior surgeon, as part of the novice surgeon's process of learning, observed that:

> You can divide the operation into components. I divide the operation into high risk and tolerant risk. For example high risk is near a critical site, a vein or artery, as opposed to opening the skin. The new surgeon doesn't assist the whole operation but will do the components that they can do well.

There is inevitably variation in the rate of progression between new entrants and also in the contexts in which they will operate. 'A good surgeon', one respondent commented, 'should be a good physician plus the technical aspect of what he does'. This surgeon had worked with an ergonomist and had learned to appreciate the need for task analysis, to break process down into components. Surgeons require a capacity for deconstructive thinking, to disassemble the procedures of their own practice. At the novitiate level there is little room for personal flair in this highly procedural approach, with checklists and protocol-driven tasks. The personal is to a great degree reduced through the routine nature of common place tasks. However, the same surgeon adds:

> It's a technical craft. You should rationalise and standardise. But to convert a surgeon to a technician just doesn't make sense. Surgery is an art. When you are working in theatre with highly experienced people it is wonderful to watch.

The surgeons interviewed often found it difficult to articulate the experience and process of gaining surgical expertise (see Chap. 7). In the light of earlier observations about the nature of troublesome knowledge, this is possibly owing to the tacit (because routinised and suppressed) nature of expert practice. But the proficient surgeon has to be able to deconstruct the whole operative practice and procedure into parts, techniques and rules that can be orchestrated with high efficiency. They have to become proficient in a range of component skill sets, like islands of expertise, and gradually integrate these. They need to achieve what one leading surgeon termed a 'proficiency–gain curve', a kind of threshold proficiency. Such task analysis is crucial for error reduction. And the new surgeon is then encouraged to move in stages from one component to another of greater complexity, challenge, uncertainty and risk.

So new surgeons need to be exposed to the widest possible set of clinical situations in order to gain a repertoire of skills that are drawn on judiciously and appropriately much in the manner, to draw an analogy with a very different kind of real-time skilled performance, in which the jazz musician improvises around an emerging theme. To gain the requisite degree of precision and confidence, a highly experienced surgeon considered that, in his own specialist area, performing an operation or large parts of it 50–60 times would probably be required. 'But less for operating on an appendix'.

As Timmermans noted earlier '[t]hese transitions remain nebulous; however, understanding them is crucial' and as Cross (1999, p. 262) observed, 'in developmental theory, the periods of greatest personal growth are thought to lie in the unnamed and poorly defined periods *between* stages'. The new surgeon moves through stages from a novice state of being supervised to a state of proficiency characterised by the consultant's expertise. There is difficulty in moving from one stage to another and the duty to the patients is paramount. In the light of the latter, the criterion required by one experienced mentor was 'I let people do things if they can do it as good as me'. It is better for the surgeon to be excellent in the components that they can do well'. It was also observed that not all surgeons perform consistently well across all components, across all skill sets, and this gives rise to questions of future practice.

6.5 Uncertainty – 'The Untravelled World'

> I am a part of all that I have met;
> Yet all experience is an arch wherethro'
> Gleams that untravell'd world whose margin fades
> For ever and for ever when I move.
> (Alfred Lord Tennyson 1842)

Nevertheless assembly is not integration. The 'proficiency–gain curve' involves more than the efficient sequencing of component skill sets, manoeuvres and rules. It is in the time of uncertainty, and the moment of unpredictability, that the error reduction mentioned above no longer applies to the same extent. Minimisation of risk implies that other things will remain constant. Indeed, though the appreciation of anatomy and the handling of tissue are core epistemic areas, it is *uncertainty* that emerges as a predominant threshold concept. The emphasis noted earlier on precision ('attitudes of perfection') decision making and error reduction are all forms of minimising the risk that comes from operating under conditions of high uncertainty, complexity, volatility and speed – for there is the accompanying temporal urgency of dealing with the uncertainty in real time. In this regard, decision making in surgery is different in nature than that in medicine. The surgeon makes decisions *continuously* with significant consequence. There is a need for continual reading of the situation (see also Chap. 10). Things come into play and recede continually, with different factors being foregrounded and issues that were formerly on the periphery suddenly staring one in the face with alarming urgency. There is a powerful dynamic about this kind of decision making against uncertainty and instability. There is variation in the inherent risk.

> I remember a situation when [A], a colleague] was operating on an elderly gentleman. It wasn't envisaged as being a very complicated procedure but when the patient was opened up they found that the quality ... the state of his arteries ... the walls of the arteries ... was so poor that they just started disintegrating and they just couldn't stitch the walls and couldn't stem the bleeding. The patient just bled to death very rapidly. And there was nothing they could do in theatre in time. They hadn't expected anything like that. [A] met the patient's wife afterwards in the hospital corridor. She was devastated and said 'But he trusted you ...' That's very hard to live with afterwards.

There are different ways in which the uncertainty of surgical procedure can manifest itself. There is the uncertainty characterised by the unpredictability and volatility of events, as above. This might also take the form of uncertainty of technical knowledge, where routine scenarios do not conform to what is in the surgical text book, as in this instance:

> I had to perform what I thought was to be a routine appendix removal and everything started off as normal. What I didn't expect to happen was that I couldn't find the appendix! It got to where I was thinking can I cut another four inches with the scalpel through this layer of fat here, which is getting very near to the liver? I decided I had to call the consultant in, for what is normally considered a very routine operation. I remember sitting waiting for him to arrive feeling useless. I was thinking 'I'm totally useless'. And then I remember feeling great for the next hour and a half whilst the consultant couldn't find it either! [*laughs*]

There is also the uncertainty of recognition, where, through trauma or post-operative 'joins', organs or tissue might be swollen and distended or cavities filled with pus or blood so that they cease to be recognisable through touch.

There is a risk inherent in the process which can be either attenuated or increased potentially in terms of what the surgeon does. He or she can turn a low-risk situation into a high-risk procedure very quickly through, for example, contact with an artery. In this way, uncertainty acts as an example of a 'provoked liminality'. This can happen to quite experienced surgeons who find themselves plunged into an unanticipated liminal state of troublesome knowledge and transformational learning.

> If I make a mistake, I have to have the confidence and knowledge to fix it – and you often are the only one to fix it. I have to know what to do when something goes wrong. If something unforeseen happens you have to deal with it. And a new form of uncertainty is, if one of your trainees makes a mistake, you've got to be able to fix it.

The experience of an eye surgeon, relatively new to practice, succinctly captures these tensions:

> There is the idea of 'complication'. You have to predict the consequence of what you do. There's a difference between a routine situation and a complication. You have to apply your knowledge a lot more. There's the unpredictability of the situation – you may be totally unprepared for it. Something very minor that you do that you weren't expecting, for instance the patients lens is weak. There's a thing about having to deal with uncertainty everywhere you look. (And the patient is conscious. In eye surgery pre-operative care continues into the operating theatre). There's a recipe, a pathway that you follow, but if something goes wrong – it can go wrong in any sort of way. It might be any bit of the eye – the patient might be fidgety. You're dealing with a finite object that's always in view, but sometimes you can lose the view of what you're seeing – sometimes the cornea that you're looking through can go hazy or there can be bleeding that obscures the view.

6.6 Surgical Ontologies: The Scalpel

The operating theatre can be an unforgiving place. The surgical community might be a tolerant society in some regards but attitudes of perfection are required and there is little tolerance of imperfection, though this is often complicated by time pressures and the need for swiftness. Many of the respondents interviewed spoke of their anxiety, whether it be at three o'clock in the morning in the operating theatre wondering, when an unforeseen complexity has arisen, if they might have to call out the consultant from her bed 60 miles away, or whether the theatre sister might take that initiative upon herself. Or 'lying awake all night thinking about the list that I'll be responsible for on my own the next day.' This is both a psychological and a social process.

> You're dealing with uncertainty – and accepting that you will have to deal with risk, despite all the procedures. The risk ... it's always there ...

This ties with the perspective within threshold concept theory that in the liminal phase an *ontological shift* or *change in subjectivity* accompanies change in cognitive understanding, often as part of a recognition that such shifts are necessary and appropriate for entry into and subsequent membership of a given community of practice, in this case the surgical community. In the thresholds framework, the process is also recognised as troublesome and occasionally incurring resistance. The theory also contends that such shifts are also irreversible. This is a point also noted within transformational learning theory, for example, by O'Sullivan and colleagues:

> Transformative learning involves experiencing a deep, structural shift in the basic premises of thought, feelings, and actions. It is a shift of consciousness that dramatically and irreversibly alters our way of being in the world. (O'Sullivan et al. 2002, p. 11)

To enter the transformative liminal space leading to the community of surgical practice requires a very particular set of ontological credentials. 'To achieve well in surgery', one respondent commented, 'you have to see surgery in a certain way'. Pre-eminent amongst these ontological credentials are a resilience, confidence and coolness under pressure, a tolerance of uncertainty and an unflappability in the face of the unpredictable.

> You have to get used to very fine movement and looking down a microscope. Sometimes they [*novice surgeons*] don't have the temperament. You have to be calm. Because the patients are awake. Our interactions with the patients carry on into the operating theatre. People recover more quickly if they remain awake. It's better for the patient. Patients prefer it too. They don't feel groggy waking up.

Layered on to this, moreover, is an ethical dimension with a long Hippocratic provenance. In the words of a very experienced consultant:

> A surgeon needs to be a good human being, honest, credible, respectful, straightforward. Doesn't say anything bad. No politics. Empathetic, straight, honest person who cares about the patient. Does things perfectly. Takes his time. No short cuts. Cares about the patient against pressures of time. You judge yourself by your own standards, which have to be high. It has to be interdisciplinary – you can't do it single handed. You need to be multidisciplinary. You need good communication skills. You don't need anaesthetic technical knowledge, but the surgeon needs to know whether the patient would be fit enough for the anaesthesia. You need to be able to make a risk analysis for the other disciplines. You need to know how to interact with them and what sort of information they need to make a decision. For example with obesity, you're working with a psychiatrist and a nutritionist, and you're the one to decide on the best option for the patient.

This is a challenging set of demands. But the following account from a fairly newly qualified consultant is worth quoting at length for its demonstration of the previous (experienced) respondent's emphasis on *Does things perfectly. Takes his time. No short cuts. Cares about the patient against pressures of time*.

> I did a below knee amputation about six months ago on a youngish man, and he already had a below knee amputation on the other side. So there was a real pressure because if he's going to walk on a prosthesis it has to be the right shape and, because he's got another stump, you want it to be fairly symmetrical and you didn't want him to have any problems with healing because he had all sorts of vascular problems ... I felt terribly pressurised doing it, because it's an operation which I've only done a couple of times before, never on

> my own. It can be difficult to do to get right. ... I could have made the operation shorter. But I didn't. I kept reshaping the flap. ... A whole number of people are working round you, and they've all got different priorities. The nurses often want to have a break. It's night time and what they want is someone who can do it quickly. And the anaesthetists don't like their patient to be on the table for too long.

In thresholds parlance, this pressure can sometimes lead to a form of 'mimicry'. Mimicry is the posturing of the behaviours of an imagined postliminal state whilst remaining in a liminal or even preliminal state. It is however often a temporary coping strategy, a means of buying time or taking measure of the situation until the liminal state can be successfully negotiated. It might be argued that every time surgical procedure is undertaken, the degree of uncertainty renders the journey different. In this respect, surgeons, in a similar fashion to that reported by both artists and engineers, do not ever permanently escape liminal space.

The interview data suggests that, although it is learned, there is a 'self-selecting element' to the achievement of surgical modes of reasoning and practising.

> I'm involved in Interviews now for people wanting to come into surgery. Looking at the people wanting to be trainees, there's definitely an element of self-selection going on.

There is what might be termed an *ontological predisposition*, that is, an ontological shift that has taken place even whilst, in developmental terms, the learner is still firmly in the preliminal mode. Whilst many medical students are petrified by the thought of surgical practice, another surgeon amongst our respondents remarked that: 'Even in the first year of the medical school I always liked to be a surgeon – I don't know why'.

6.7 Performing Identities in the 'Theatre': The 'Mask'

The acquisition of surgical identity, the required change in subjectivity, seems partly owing to the ontological predisposition discussed earlier. It is also formed through medical study and the shift in subjectivity which, according to threshold theory (Meyer and Land 2005), accompanies any significant cognitive shift in learning. With any discipline, there is always a self-relational attitude towards that discipline like, 'I am studying this in order to become this particular kind of practitioner.' In the case of surgery, however, it seems also strongly developed by the contingencies that arise in the sociocultural relations within the community of practice.

> Circumstances often put you in a situation that you hadn't quite prepared for. It's what other people ask you to do that makes you step into that role.

Situations arise that, in a quasi-peristaltic fashion, push the novice surgeon into the next (higher) stage of their professional practice, with an accompanying ontological shift in confidence, self-status (or anxiety). A respondent quoted earlier had commented:

> And I did that at night, when I was having a bit of pressure from the people around me, and not much support. And I felt that that had moved me forward. I was glad that I had completed that operation. I felt that it had been a difficult couple of hours but I felt that I'd done the right thing.

This social intervention is, in effect, an endorsement, and, though it often arises from contingent factors, a manifestation of the confidence that the community now has in the new entrant. It is a bestowal of a gradually more centralised status within the community of practice.

> Part of it is how other people treat you. One senior colleague says to another 'We're short of a surgeon. Sarah *[not her real name]* can do it'.

The conferring of status can take apparently casual forms:

> One time [the senior surgeon] just said 'OK I'm going on holiday. You can have the list this week'. What they are saying is 'You are one of us. We trust you'.

Reference to the list occurs frequently in the interview data. It seems to serve as shorthand for trust, and for acknowledgment of membership of the community of practice, somewhat in the manner of handing over the keys of your house as a mark of trust. These reported events characterise recognition of emergence into a postliminal state of transformation, into fledgling membership of the profession. They are transitional moments:

> There comes one day when you think 'I'm a surgeon'. I'm doing it. For example you might be in theatre when a complication arises, and you think 'I can do this myself'. The consultant might be there but you can say to yourself 'I'm OK; I'm going to carry on'.

This self-assurance, however, may have to be gained operation by operation. Asked when they first felt they had achieved the ontological status of being a surgeon respondents provided the following observations:

> It's when you do it on your own with no-one supervising you.
>
> It's when someone junior rings you up for advice – that doesn't happen to you when *you're* junior. One day you're the one phoning for advice and the next you're the one being phoned and that's an external thing that's imposed upon you.

Factors in the transition to the new identity seem to involve autonomy, independence from consultation and supervision and speed of performance.

> Is there a change of identity? Yeah, I agree with that. It's the circumstances that bring about those changes. It's things about when you start to feel that you've done the list as fast as the consultant would have done. Or you've done the whole clinic and you've not had to ask anyone's advice.

Ascension to new levels of proficiency, and the accompanying shifts in ontology, can be affected through changed levels of signification, particularly regarding official status:

> My competence didn't change, but my status changed and people's expectations of you change. It's not necessarily a bonus that you can now perform that particular thing but people expect you to do that. It's what your status is expected to signal.

But in the responses of some respondents, there were still indications of oscillative behaviour, indicating a continuing state of liminality:

> Sometimes you think you're doing OK but then the consultant swoops in and finishes the operation for you.

Power relations can add to the troublesomeness:

> And that was another complication with this operation that I found quite difficult . . . This was when I was a junior surgeon, in the operating theatre, scrubbed up, with my boss showing me how to do it. And the other thing is you're usually at the opposite side of the patient so you're seeing it back to front – so that doesn't help. And also having quite a didactic boss, I found it very difficult to say 'No, actually I don't get that'. So that's quite difficult – a real power imbalance.

And it is common, with different operations and with new situations in much used operations, for even quite experienced surgeons to find themselves entering liminal states, experiencing ontological insecurity and oscillation.

> To be quite frank, I've been practising now for over ten years but there are often days when I think, do I want to carry on doing this? Do I still *want* to do it? Can I carry on being *able* to do it?

A further significant, potentially stressful, dimension of surgical practice is its performed and visible nature, always open to scrutiny.

> It's a public act – you're being watched. The theatre sister and the other theatre staff are judging your confidence.
>
> [Interviewer: So does it feel like a performance?]
>
> For sure, surgery is like a performance. Yeah, definitely. I feel like I'm on display for the senior surgeon (if there is one), the junior surgeons (if they're there), the medical students (if they're in theatre) and the patients and the nurses. And we know they talk behind your backs.

The following is a particularly graphic account of the pressure that sometimes needs to be resisted and the resilience that has to be achieved:

> And they put pressure on you, and people look over your shoulder and, you see, it does sometimes happen that other people will call the consultant. That decision will be taken out of your hands. That you'll find that somebody's rung them...
>
> [Interviewer: Without you knowing about it?]
> Without you knowing about it.
>
> [Interviewer: And who does that? The anaesthetist or the..?]
>
> It's usually the nurse! [*laughs*] It's usually a senior nurse. It's very unnerving because it calls your judgement into question...Sometimes you don't feel much team spirit behind you. [*laughs*] You feel like you're on your own.

Surgical identities, similarly, seem performed. Some of the respondents, who were amateur musicians themselves, drew comparisons with the demands of public concert performance where accuracy and concentration are paramount, and proficiency is, similarly, under scrutiny. One respondent commented:

> It's a bit of a ritual. A ritual performance. I'm a musician too and I started to get stage fright about it when I was relatively junior. It's the same stage fright as for a musical performance. I can't sleep the night before doing the list. If I drink too much tea I start getting affected. When I was a SHO some other younger colleagues would say 'I'm not going to have a drink the night before'. I would think 'Big cissies!' And then there's a shift when you think, mmm... I'd better not stay up late. There's a need for self-regulation. I don't go skiing or ice skating any more, in case of injury falling on my hands. I'm learning the bass guitar but I'm worried about getting calluses that might affect delicacy of touch.

Sometimes the performance is explicitly judged.

> You know you're being judged. A patient might say afterwards. 'Hmm. You took a long time over the operation, doctor'. Or they might say, 'You're very gentle doctor, but, ooh, that hurt a bit!' So they do make judgements.

Like actors or musicians there is a sense of (literal and metaphorical) theatricality.

> Another colleague of mine used to say 'They don't call it theatre for nothing!'
> Going into theatre I still sometimes get very nervous. With the nerves you just have to say 'I've got to get through this'.

In relation to the question of the development of professional identity or a surgical ontology one experienced surgeon pondered:

> Hmm. Do disciplines change people? Or do they attract people who want to be surgeons. Or is it to do with the way we follow the line that we have laid out, the path we have drawn... that you follow into this profession.

What emerges from the data is an indication that the adoption of, or the transformation into, a sense of 'surgeonhood', of professional identity is strongly influenced by the entrance into the procedural formality and pattern of surgical practice. In these highly pressured settings, in the midst of uncertainty and potential complexity, and beset by unpredictability, there is a strapping on not just of the literal surgical mask, but, *metaphorically*, a simultaneous donning of the surgical identity, much like an ancient Greek actor fitting a theatrical mask. This too might be seen as a warding off of the forces of uncertainty and the unpredictable, and a gaining of a certain assurance and security from the 'perfected' procedure discussed earlier.

> Through surgery you build up, and build up, and build up your own internal set of references and judgements to help you decide what to do. You have to take circumstances into account. You have to integrate the whole thing. And there is this sense in surgery that you have to be a little bit tough. You have to listen to them as well, but you have to weigh it up and see what you think is in the patient's interest. But always, as trainees, in the back of our mind, we're thinking, what's in my interest as a trainee? That's not our first priority but it's something we're always aware of.

Masks have been used in nearly all cultures, throughout the centuries, for protection, disguise, luck, gratitude and therapy. They serve complex psychological functions. Caillois (1965, p. 4) argued that: 'There is no tool, no invention, no belief, no custom nor institution that to that same degree accomplishes and manifests the unity of mankind as does the wearing of masks'. Janzing (1998, p. 151) suggests that they serve a mediating purpose:

> Originally an object of ritual ... the mask creates contact with an inaccessible world. It is a mediator. For the duration of a ritual, it transmits to those who wear it the strength of that which it represents and it allows the wearers to transcend their everyday identity... Within all cultures, the mask has never been a mundane object. This mask, which hides at the same time as it proclaims, which conceals while it reveals ...

Janzing cites Landy (1986, p. 45), who observes that in work with theatrical actors, 'as for the Greeks, the mask transformed the human head into the godhead, the particular and mundane into the universal and sublime' and the theatre producer Peter Brook, who in his book *The Shifting Point* (1988), reports that the mask permits actors to overcome their 'natural human limitations'. Janzing draws on the work of a range of commentators – from the fields of anthropology, theatre and therapy – who variously report uses of the mask that foster expressiveness, 'greater awareness, choice and control in physical expression', self-discovery, 'the testing out and adoption of new roles', disinhibitory effects and experimentation with new attitudes and behaviours. Further reported effects of this rather strange simultaneously camouflaging/revelatory device, which is both mediator and container, include perceptual heightening, concentration, precision and accuracy. Janzing sounds a cautionary note as to the power it bestows:

> To wear a mask with this kind of power is not, evidently, given to everyone. Depending on the culture, the right to this privilege is bestowed according to age, lineage or the spiritual experience of the individual (Raabe 1992). As a rule, it seems that the mask wearer has to demonstrate a certain maturity and particular precautions are necessary to avert the danger associated with the use of this instrument of metamorphosis. (Janzing 1998, p. 155)

Weiss (1992) similarly, warns against the risk of 'superidentification' with the mask. No more is suggested here, however, than that the assumption of the surgical role and its accompanying (somewhat mask-like) *persona*, in the context of the different but equally performative and public *theatre* of the operating room, may play a strong part in the powerful ontological shift and change in subjectivity required for effective surgical practice.

6.8 Conclusion

We have indicated here that a dominant threshold concept for surgical education seems to be uncertainty, and this chapter has focused mainly on the analysis of that concept. It is of course highly unlikely that one learning threshold would be adequate to account for such a complex field as surgery, and further work could productively investigate such other thresholds. For example, all surgeons first train as doctors following the same preregistration curriculum as all other doctors and at some point there is a requirement to establish and indeed 'practise' a certain 'distance'. This was beginning to emerge in the section on the 'mask'.

The importance of speed in surgical practice would also merit further investigation. In terms of troublesome knowledge, the degree of complexity with which surgeons continually have to deal would be worth exploring.

There are interesting implications of the foregoing arguments for surgical training and continuing professional development. We have argued that uncertainty as a learning threshold requires coping with (and on occasion even embracing) uncertainty, and that this is as much ontological in nature as epistemological. There then arises the problematic issue of how the capacity to cope with uncertainty can be adequately assessed. Also, there is a question of how one can communicate an ontological shift, which is not yet apprehended, to those for whom it is beyond their ontological horizon (Land and Meyer 2010). In this regard, surgical education is making increasing use of technological simulation to enhance the teaching and learning of surgical procedures. There are interesting initiatives also underway to simulate conditions of uncertainty through the use of professional scenarios, and it will be interesting to see how educational practice develops in this respect in the near future, as well as in relation to new forms of reflective assessment being developed that seek to render visible and capture personal professional development where this is not easily observable. Other implications for the future of surgical training are suggested elsewhere in this volume, including being picked up by Heather Fry and Roger Kneebone in the Afterword.

Acknowledgments The authors are deeply indebted to the surgeons who took part in these interviews for the generous way in which they gave their time despite busy schedules and for the thoughtful and frank observations that they contributed concerning their practice and experience. We are also grateful to the Oxford Centre for Staff and Learning Development for their kind permission to adapt material originally published as Meyer, J. H. F. and Land, R. (2003) below.

References

Brook, P. (1988). *The shifting point: Theatre, film, opera 1946–1987*. London: Methuen Drama.

Caillois, R. (1965). Preface. In M. Guimet (Ed.), *Masques* (pp. 3–8). Paris: Olivier Perrin.

Cousin, G. (2009) *Threshold concepts*. Video webcast, Central Queensland University. http://onlinemedia.cqu.edu.au/media_request.htm?file=cqu/staff/asdu/interview/2009_g_cousin&formats=3

Cross, P. (1999). What do we know about students' learning and how do we know it? *Innovative Higher Education, 23*(4), 255–270.

Davies, P. (2006). Threshold concepts: How can we recognize them? In J. H. F. Meyer & R. Land (Eds.), *Overcoming barriers to student understanding: Threshold concepts and troublesome knowledge*. London/New York: Routledge.

Janzing, H. (1998). The use of the mask in psychotherapy. *The Arts in Psychotherapy, 25*, 151–157.

Kegan, R. (1982). *The evolving self: Problem and process in human development*. Cambridge: Harvard University Press.

Land, R., & Jan Meyer, H. F. (2010). Threshold concepts and troublesome knowledge (5): Dynamics of assessment. In J. H. F. Meyer, R. Land, & C. Baillie (Eds.), *Threshold concepts and transformational learning*. Rotterdam: Sense Publishers.

Land, R., Cousin, G., Meyer, J. H. F., & Davies, P. (2005). Threshold concepts and troublesome knowledge (3): Implications for course design and evaluation. In C. Rust (Ed.), *Improving student learning 12 – Diversity and inclusivity* (pp. 53–64). Oxford: Oxford Brookes University.

Land, R., Meyer, J. H. F., & Smith, J. (Eds.). (2008). *Threshold concepts within the disciplines*. Rotterdam: Sense Publishers.

Landy, R. (1986). *Drama therapy*. Springfield: Charles C Thomas.

McLuhan, M. (1994). *Understanding media: The extensions of man*. Cambridge: MIT Press.

Meyer, J. H. F., & Land, R. (2003). Threshold concepts and troublesome knowledge (I): Linkages to ways of thinking and practising. In C. Rust (Ed.), *Improving student learning – Ten years on*. Oxford: OCSLD.

Meyer, J. H. F., & Land, R. (2005). Threshold concepts and troublesome knowledge (2): Epistemological considerations and a conceptual framework for teaching and learning. *Higher Education, 49*, 373–388.

Meyer, J. H. F., & Land, R. (Eds.). (2006). *Overcoming barriers to student understanding: Threshold concepts and troublesome knowledge*. London/New York: Routledge.

O'Sullivan, E. V., Morrell, A., & O'Connor, M. A. (2002). *Expanding the boundaries of transformative learning: Essays on theory and praxis*. New York: Palgrave.

Raabe, E. C. (1992). Mythos maske. Frankfurt: Museum für Völkerkunde. Tennyson, A. L. (1842) Ulysses. Reprinted in Trilling, L. & Bloom, H. (1973) *Victorian prose and poetry* (pp. 416–418). New York/Oxford/Toronto: Oxford University Press.

Timmermans, J. (2010). Changing our minds: The developmental potential of threshold concepts. In J. H. F. Meyer, R. Land, & C. Baillie (Eds.), *Threshold concepts and transformational learning*. Rotterdam: Sense Publishers.

Weiss, B. (1992). Maske und Therapie im integrativen Ansatz der Arbeit mit kreativen Medien und der Kunsttherapie: Ein Überblick. In H. Petzold & I. Orth (Eds.), *Die neuen Kreativitätstherapien II* (pp. 777–805). Paderborn: Junfermann Verlag.

Chapter 7
The Surgeon's Expertise

K. Anders Ericsson

7.1 Surgical Expertise: A Perspective from the Expert-Performance Approach

The emphasis on general education, problem-based training, and professional experience for the acquisition of skill, expertise, and professional achievement has varied during the history of training of professionals, such as engineers and medical doctors. As knowledge in the corresponding professional domain increased, it became clear that students had to attain a general education, such as a pre-medicine college education for doctors, before beginning their studies at their respective professional school. Following this primarily theoretical training, graduates were trained as apprentices and interns under the supervision of experienced practitioners for several years until they could earn the credentials to practice independently.

Traditional models of skill and expertise (Dreyfus and Dreyfus 1986; Fitts and Posner 1967) distinguish different phases of development of performance that are consistent with the distinction between general theoretical knowledge and professional skill. The first phase of the beginner, such as a medical student, involves reasoning from basic principles and then following instructions by teachers for applying step-by-step procedures. During this phase, gross errors occur and are noticed by the teacher, or even the student, and are corrected, and subsequently decrease in frequency. With increasing opportunities for performing similar tasks, the student becomes more able to generate better outcomes faster, more smoothly and with less effort. Some researchers of expertise (Dreyfus and Dreyfus 1986) consider individuals after extensive experience in the domain to become experts, who are able to respond rapidly and intuitively. Some domains, such as driving a car, are simple and "almost all novices [beginners] can eventually reach the level

K.A. Ericsson (✉)
Florida State University, Tallahassee, FL, USA
e-mail: ericsson@psy.fsu.edu

H. Fry and R. Kneebone (eds.), *Surgical Education: Theorising an Emerging Domain*, Advances in Medical Education 2, DOI 10.1007/978-94-007-1682-7_7,

we call expert" (Dreyfus and Dreyfus 1986, p. 21). In other more complex domains, such as telegraphy and chess, they argue that it may take over a decade to reach the highest levels (Simon and Chase 1973). The pioneering research on expertise by Herbert Simon and Bill Chase (1973) emphasized the improvements in performance associated with further experience in the domain and how increasingly complex patterns (or chunks) are acquired and stored in memory, providing the basis for pattern recognition to mediate rapid retrieval of appropriate actions from memory. Numerous studies in the late 1970s and early 1980s compared the performance of beginners with experts (Chi 2006; Feltovich et al. 2006). In these studies, it was common to identify experts by using peer-nomination procedures among highly experienced professionals (Elstein et al. 1978).

In the latter part of the 1980s, the conception was that accumulated knowledge of a domain, followed by an extended period of professional experience, would inevitably lead to expertise and superior performance, and peer nominations became increasingly criticized (see Chap. 1). Early studies of medical diagnosis were unable to establish superior accuracy of peer-nominated best general physicians compared to a group of undistinguished physicians (Elstein et al. 1978). Similar findings were subsequently obtained for clinical psychologists, where more advanced training and longer professional experience was unrelated to their success in treating patients' problems. Reviews show that there is a surprisingly weak relation between the length of professional experience and objective performance in a wide range of domains (Ericsson 2006a; Ericsson and Lehmann 1996). For example, the accuracy of heart sound diagnosis and many types of measurable activities of nurses and general physicians do not improve as a function of professional experience, and sometimes the performance even gradually decreases as a function of years since graduation from training (Choudhry et al. 2005; Ericsson 2004; Ericsson et al. 2007).

It is important to note that in the majority of these domains, there is very little immediate feedback on the success or failure of a diagnosis. Many doctors never see the final diagnosis for a patient whom they try to diagnose, and if they do eventually see the diagnosis, their memory for their initial diagnostic process is too fragmentary to help assess what they overlooked or should have done. This situation is different in surgery, where mistakes, problems, and successful outcomes are often perceived during surgery, within hours of the completed surgery, or at least the next day, so accurate timely feedback is frequently available to help surgeons to learn and improve their skills. Consequently, as one of the exceptions from this general lack of learning from experience in professional domains, surgeons with more experience (larger number of completed surgical procedures of a given type) often have been found to have significantly superior outcomes for their patients (Ericsson 2004).

In response to this dissociation between superior performance and professional experience, Ericsson and Smith (1991) proposed that researchers should redirect research from studying socially recognized experts to studying reproducibly superior performance in a given domain.

7.2 The Scientific Study of Expert Performance and its Acquisition

The establishment of any science, including the study of expert performance, starts with accumulation of a body of reproducible empirical phenomena such as superior performance (Ericsson 2006a, b). Unless it is possible to reproduce such phenomena consistently, under standardized and experimental conditions, it will not be possible to analyze them with experimental methods.

The most successful efforts to demonstrate reproducibly superior performance under standardized conditions are found in sports. Athletic competitions in ancient Greece have a long history of attempting to design standardized situations that would allow fair competition between athletes. For example, they built straight and flat running tracks that were the same for all runners and devised methods to allow runners to start at the same time and then to cross the same finishing line—to make it easier to determine who got there first. More recently, competitions in music, dance, and chess, have been designed to evaluate the best performance with reliable and often objective methods for scoring. In all of these traditional domains, elite individuals reliably perform better than less accomplished individuals, when given technically difficult tasks.

There have also been efforts to measure performance in professional domains. In many of these domains, large numbers of professionals encounter and perform similar tasks on a daily basis. For example, professional investors on the stock market have essentially equal opportunities to purchase and sell stocks in companies; medical professionals, especially in emergency rooms of larger cities, treat patients with similar symptoms; and psychotherapists treat patients with similar reported problems. The number of encountered patients with the same type of challenging problems will be very small for a given professional, even if one were to aggregate their experience over a month or a year. There are, however, exceptions involving specialists, who are approached by people from a large area for help with particular procedures, such as specialized surgery. However, simply knowing that a surgeon has had better outcomes than other surgeons for some 50–100 patients (following surgical procedures that last around 4 h) makes it difficult to identify the nature and locus of the differences.

There is a similar problem in understanding what distinguishes chess masters from weaker players, when the games last several hours. In his pioneering research on chess expertise, de Groot (1946/1978) developed a methodology of selecting critical events. He extracted critical situations in games between chess masters and then set up a controlled laboratory situation where he could present the associated positions one at a time to an individual chess player (see Fig. 7.1). This method focuses on that part of a chess game where the masters' ability to select the best move in complex challenging situations is paramount to success. This excludes any differences in the beginning of a chess game, since these are typically simple and routine and are based on shared knowledge of openings. De Groot's method thus focuses on complex and challenging situations, where routines and prior experience will not lead to the best approach and actions.

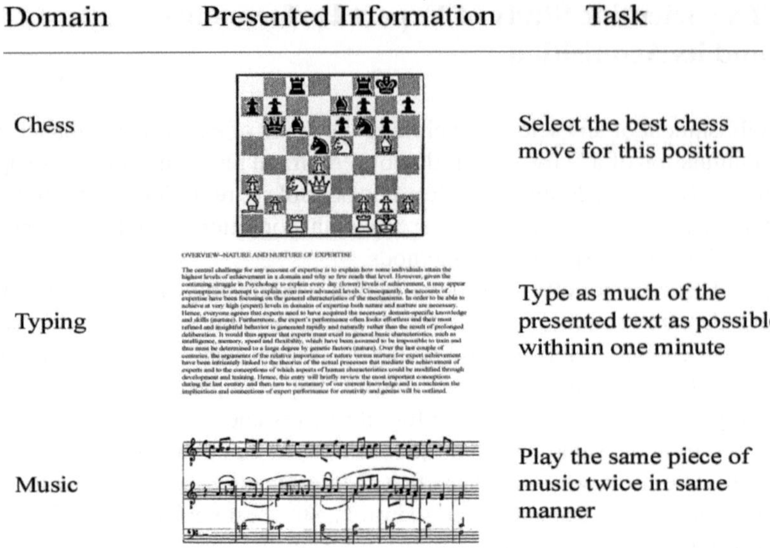

Fig. 7.1 Three examples of laboratory tasks that capture the consistently superior performance of domain experts in chess, typing, and music (From "Expertise," by Ericsson and Lehmann 1999)

For other types of tasks, the difficulty of selecting the correct actions may not be as important as the speed to complete typical tasks. Expertise in typing should be generalized to any type of material to be transcribed, so that one can present all typists with the same text material and ask them to type it accurately as fast as possible for a fixed time period. The final example given in Fig. 7.1 illustrates the skill of musical sight reading, where an accompanist would be presented with a sheet of music and asked to accompany a singer without having a chance to prepare the performance in advance. The ability to accurately play as many of the written notes as possible in a musically pleasing fashion is one characteristic that differentiates skilled accompanists from other pianists (Lehmann and Ericsson 1993). It is important to note that the speed of accurate sight reading is not an end in itself, but it demonstrates the musicians' ability or capacity for performance, which in turn allows them to musically express their pieces when they play at lower than maximal speed. Expert musicians are able to play a relatively simple piece twice in a row with a high degree of consistency, whereas novices are unable to reproduce the microstructure of their performance from trial to trial (Krampe and Ericsson 1996). Similarly, speed of surgeons' performance as well as their ability to reproduce their performance (displaying higher level of control) is likely to be correlated with surgical skill and surgical outcomes.

Over the last few decades, it has been possible to develop standardized test situations, where performance on these representative situations can be assessed in around an hour, yet are highly correlated to real-world performance. Examples include tournament performance in chess, golf, and Scrabble, performance in music competitions, and medical diagnosis (Ericsson 2006a, b). These findings are consistent with the hypothesis that there is an underlying factor of attained expertise in a domain, where the majority of the tasks can be ordered on a continuum of difficulty. In many domains, there is a rank ordering of difficulty for mastery of different tasks. For example, in diving competitions each dive is assigned a difficulty score, while in music, pieces are rated by the number of years of study recommended before attempted mastery. In addition, gymnastics and martial arts have a clear progression of levels defined by mastery of increasingly difficult tasks, and a similar progression of mastery is found in mathematics and many of the sciences.

7.2.1 *Applying the Expert-Performance Approach to Surgery*

The central question for the expert-performance approach when applied to surgery concerns if, and under what circumstances, it is possible to identify surgeons who have consistently superior outcomes for their patients—although it may sometimes be difficult to separate the effects of the individual surgeon from the contributions of their team members and the influence of post-surgery care. Superior data on patient outcomes is the most compelling for procedures with stable individual differences in objective outcomes, such as mortality and morbidity. Recently, Vickers et al. (2007) reported large differences in mortality as a function of the number of procedures of that same type previously completed by the surgeon—patients whose surgeon had performed less than ten procedures were almost twice as likely to have a recurrence of the cancer as patients whose surgeons had performed more than 250 procedures. The biochemical recurrence following this particular procedure (removal of the prostate) is claimed by Vickers et al. (2007, p. 1171) to be a particularly good measure on surgical performance "because adjuvant therapy is not commonly given for prostate cancer and recurrence is not substantially affected by other aspects of postoperative care." With statistical control for severity of the patients' cancer condition, it is possible to determine that these differences in outcome are due to acquired skill. In fact, Vickers et al. (2007) compared the same surgeons' outcomes for their first 10 procedures and after 250 procedures and observed the same significant improvement. In a subsequent study, Vickers et al. (2008) discovered that when cancers that were confined to an organ, the recurrence of cancer was monotonically reduced with increased surgeons' experience for the first 1,500–2,000 procedures to a point at which recurrence of cancer was essentially eliminated. In a different analysis of outcomes of laparoscopic procedures, Vickers et al. (2009) found that decreases in recurrence of cancer were seen for the first 1,000 procedures, whereas with open surgery a stable plateau was attained after 250 procedures. More generally, individual differences in outcomes for practicing board-certified surgeons are often found for the more complex procedures with the highest mortality rates. For example, Prystowsky (2005) found no differences for mortality as a function of number of procedures for simple cases of alimentary tract surgery (ATS), but only for complex ATSs. He reviews seven other studies demonstrating a higher mortality or complication rate for the first 15–50 cases of complex procedures by certified surgeons. Recent reviews of this research demonstrate that surgical performance minimizing mortality and morbidity requires procedure-extended specific experience and training, and that general surgeons require considerable training in laparoscopic techniques to overcome the steep learning curve (Kumar and Gill 2006; Prystowsky 2005; Vickers et al. 2009).

Several successful approaches can be adopted for identifying superior (expert) performance. For example, it is possible to study surgical teams which differ in their associated risk-adjusted mortality rates, then have all teams adopt the procedures of best-performing teams. This adoption of expert methods with frequent monitoring of units' outcomes has led to significant improvements in system-wide mortality outcomes (Nugent 2005).

It is much more difficult to analyze the infrequent instances leading to mortality that measure and give immediate feedback on the performance of individual surgeons. For example, recurrence of some types of cancers will happen up to 1–5 years after the operation, thus precluding immediate feedback after surgery. It is, however, possible to monitor the detailed processes of a given operation by video recording or even having a surgeon "think aloud" while performing the operation. Frequently, the surgeons discover mistakes themselves or other staff notice problems during or after surgery. In addition, it is possible to gain additional feedback about the surgical outcome using special tests. For example, following radical prostatectomy, Atug et al. (2006) analyzed the tissue removed during surgery to assess whether the edges included cancerous tissue or whether the cancerous tissue was completely contained within the removed tissue. They found that with increased surgical experience, the number of collected samples with cancerous tissue decreased by a factor of 4. Similarly, Bacha et al. (2008) describe how the outcomes of congenital heart surgery can be evaluated almost immediately after the surgery by post-procedure echocardiographic testing that assesses the repaired heart's function. By developing similar auxiliary tests, conducted for the primary purpose of giving feedback on outcomes within hours or days after the completed surgery, the continued learning and improvement of surgeons would be facilitated.

The most promising approach to studying individual differences in surgical performance and its relation to surgical experience involve videotaping actual surgeries operations, followed by blind assessment of the surgeons' performance. There are few studies that have compared live operations performed by highly experienced surgeons who have completed training (internship and residency). In a pioneering study, Sarker et al. (2006) compared video tapes from laparoscopic cholecystectomies by four less-experienced registrar/resident surgeons with those by five experienced consultant/attending surgeons, and found significantly faster and higher ratings for general and specific performance for the more experienced experts. In a more recent study, Murphy et al. (2008) completed a task analysis to identify serious errors, such as organ perforations and tissue tearings. They then assessed the error rates for novices (interns and junior registrars) and experts (senior specialist registrars and consultants) and found significantly lower rates for the more expert group. These findings should permit better targeted training on the development of control of the movements with one's instrument, and inform the design of training activities outside the operating theater that would permit repeated attempts with immediate feedback to develop that control.

There has not been any research requiring surgeons to "think aloud" during a particular surgery or to give a retrospective report immediately after the surgery in order to link individual differences in thinking to superior surgical outcomes. One of the few "think-aloud" studies was conducted by Abernathy and Hamm (1994), who asked a master surgeon to "think aloud" about how to treat sick patients in different scenarios. The focus, however, was not on the planning or execution of surgery but on general diagnosis and treatment (see Ericsson 2004, 2007, for discussions of diagnosis of patient vignettes and simulated patients). The methodology that most closely resembles an application of the expert-performance approach to surgery is illustrated in a recent study by Sarker et al. (2009). They relied on a library of videotapes of over 100 operations to identify situations requiring a decision, where two highly experience laparoscopic surgeons agreed on the correct decision. These situations were presented to experts and intermediate surgeons, and the expert group made significantly better surgical decisions.

Another interesting approach involves inviting experienced surgeons to perform simple tasks used for training surgical students, to provide reference points for mastery of six laparoscopic tasks. An established simulator is the Minimally Invasive Surgical Trainer-Virtual Reality (MIST-VR), a device simulating laparoscopic surgery by using realistic instruments to perform geometrical tasks on computed visual images. Van Sickle et al. (2007) tested over 40 experienced surgeons (who had an average of over 1,000 laparoscopic procedures) on the MIST-VR after a single training trial for each laparoscopic task. Completion time and errors were recorded for each task, but showed no significant correlations with years of laparoscopic experience or number of previous laparoscopic procedures. The lack of correlation with experience was not due to any ceiling effects, as the surgeons' previous experience with the particular simulator MIST-VR was associated with superior performance.

In sum, it is possible to identify individuals whose performance is consistently superior to that of other individuals in the same domain. In particular, in the domain of surgery, the number of times a particular surgeon has completed a given procedure is a potent predictor of surgical outcome for complex and challenging procedures. In the following sections, I will discuss how we can learn from the expert performers and their developmental path to superior performance.

7.3 The Acquisition of Superior Reproducible (Expert) Performance

In most of the traditional domains of expertise, such as chess, sports, and music, it has been possible to describe the time course of development that generalizes across different domains of expertise (Ericsson 2006a, b; Ericsson and Lehmann 1996).

Unlike surgery, most international level performers in the traditional domains start their training and practice as children, often around 7–8 years of age but sometimes as early as 3–4 years. Even though surgical training starts two decades later, similar characteristics are observed.

When we are using the same objective standards to measure performance, such as chess-ratings, time to complete running events, and risk-adjusted mortality rates for surgical outcomes, there is no evidence for abrupt increases in performance, and learning curves show gradual smooth improvement. While analyses of performance in sport and chess tend to show that the age at which experts typically reach their peak career is in the 30s and 40s, analyses of surgical performance show a pattern similar to music (Krampe and Ericsson 1996) with no reliable decline for active professionals (Waljee et al. 2006). Finally, in other domains (including sports, sciences, and arts), researchers have found that all performers, even the most "talented," need around 10 years of intense involvement before they reach an international level (Ericsson et al. 1993; Simon and Chase 1973), and most elite individuals take considerably longer. In sports and even music there are regional, national, and international competitions to assess when someone is able to win at a given level of competition. In surgery, by contrast, there are no established competitions and associated measures of performance, so the most relevant evidence would be found in data on how long it takes to reach the lowest mortality rates for surgeries with high base rates for mortality, such as advanced forms of cancer. Consistent with the need for up to a decade of required engagement in domain-related activities, the best surgical performance is attained after 1,500–2,000 operations (Vickers et al. 2008) or over 7 years of experience in the emergency department (McKenney et al. 2009). Surgical skill is not a stable entity and is constantly in flux, with technical innovations and the new surgical techniques being constantly introduced. Today's surgeons need to acquire an ability to keep learning new methods and techniques during their professional careers.

7.3.1 The Acquisition of Surgical Expertise

The primary challenge for surgical training has been to handle the steep initial learning curve. Traditionally, surgical trainees were allowed to perform increasingly complex aspects of a surgical procedure under the direct supervision of a trained surgeon. The experienced surgeon would step in and handle any problems or difficult parts of the surgery until the trainee had acquired a proficient performance. Research has shown that trainees performing surgeries under the supervision of surgeons experienced in that procedure have mortality rates similar to surgeries performed by experienced surgeons (Stoica et al. 2008). This is the general method of apprenticeship training that has dominated surgical education until quite recently, when the weekly hours of surgical service by residents have been markedly reduced.

More recently introduced surgical techniques that differ radically from the traditional open operations, such as laparoscopic and robotic procedures, have led to a challenge. As reviewed earlier, when certified practising surgeons initially perform procedures for which they lack experience, there is a higher incidence of mortality and other postoperative complications, which is reduced after 30–100 completed operations. Consequently, surgeons need supervised training before they are able to independently complete operations at a proficient level. Given the diverse and large number of procedures and the need for lengthy supervised training for each procedure prior to the acquired proficiency, there has evolved a great interest in training in simulators that would allow skill acquisition outside the operating theater. Some recent research has suggested that expert performers in many domains, such as music, acting, and sports, have developed training methods that do not require the expert to be in front of an audience but allows the training to occur during rehearsal, instruction by a coach or teacher, and solitary practice.

In a review of research on skill acquisition in a wide range of domains, my colleagues and I (Ericsson et al. 1993) identified a set of conditions where practice had consistently led to increased performance. Individuals who were given a task with a well-defined goal were motivated to improve, were provided with feedback, and had ample opportunities for gradual refinements of their performance with repetition of the same or similar tasks, saw their performance improve significantly. Deliberate efforts to improve performance beyond its current level often require identification of those aspects of performance requiring improvement and finding better methods to perform the tasks. These activities demand full concentration, limiting daily duration (Ericsson 2006a, b).

Informal observation of learning of everyday skills, such as tennis, golf, typing on a computer, and using a mobile phone, shows that people initially figure out what to do slowly, but with more practice opportunities are able to reach a sufficient level in the target activity (such as sending e-mails or text messages or returning a tennis shot). Many people spontaneously adopt the most available strategies, such as hunt-and-peck in typing or idiosyncratic movement patterns in tennis. With further experience they become increasingly able to generate rapid adequate actions with less and less effort—consistent with the traditional theories of expertise and skill acquisition (Dreyfus and Dreyfus 1986; Fitts and Posner 1967) (Fig. 7.2, lower arm). When performance has reached a level of automaticity, additional experience will not improve the structure or accuracy of action selection, and consequently the amount of accumulated experience will not be related to attained level of performance.

In direct contrast, teachers help aspiring experts to adopt the best training methods and the appropriate fundamentals, gradually developing into expert performance without long periods of relearning poor fundamentals. By helping their students target weaker aspects of their performance with deliberate practice, improvements toward the expert performance is faster than if practice involves unstructured experience without explicit goals. In music and sports, most of the training is not completed during informal games, competitions and public performances, but takes place on the practice field or the practice room.

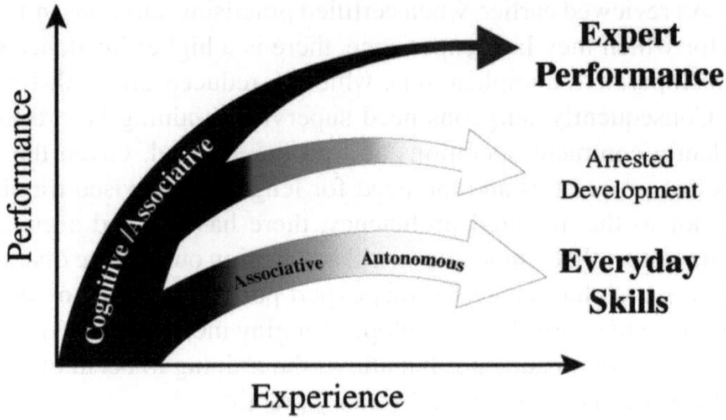

Fig. 7.2 An illustration of the qualitative difference between the course of improvement of expert performance and of everyday activities. The goal of everyday activities is to reach as rapidly as possible a satisfactory level that is stable and "autonomous." After individuals pass through the "cognitive" and "associative" phases they can generated their performance virtually automatically with a minimal amount of effort (see the *gray/white* plateau at the bottom of the graph). In contrast, expert performers counteract automaticity by developing increasingly complex mental representations to attain higher levels of control of their performance and will therefore remain within the "cognitive" and "associative" phases. Some experts will, at some point in their career, give up their commitment to seeking excellence and thus terminate regular engagement in deliberate practice to further improve performance, which results in premature automation of their performance (Adapted from "The scientific study of expert levels of performance: General implications for optimal learning and creativity" by Ericsson (1998). Copyright 1998 by European Council for High Ability)

7.3.2 *Simulation*

Simulation offers obvious potential here (see Chaps. 3 and 8). A recent review (Issenberg et al. 2005) has shown that the improvements in performance due to simulator training are primarily seen for training involving explicit performance goals with opportunities for feedback and repetitions until mastery (training activities satisfying the characteristics of deliberate practice). In a subsequent review, McGaghie et al. (2006) showed that the amount of deliberate practice showed a dose–response relation to performance. There has been a virtual explosion of research on the design of effective simulator training for surgical performance, especially for laparoscopic and robotic procedures. Recent comprehensive reviews (McGaghie 2008; Tsuda et al. 2009) note that education in simulators embraces the best methods, such as "distributed, structured, and deliberate practice with the appropriate mechanisms for feedback" (Tsuda et al. 2009, p. 336), with objective training goals based on experienced surgeons' performance in the simulator (c.f. Van Sickle et al.'s (2007) testing of expert surgeons in the simulators).

It is interesting to note that medical educators are adopting the characteristics of training (deliberate practice) originally observed among expert musicians (Ericsson et al. 1993). In music, the teacher identifies an aspect of the students' music performance that needs to be improved and then recommends particular training methods and techniques, where the targeted aspect can be gradually refined through repetition and refinement in response to feedback. The music student engages in the assigned practice activities until the goal is attained or the student is no longer able to engage in full concentration on their skill acquisition. The constraint on maintaining full concentration leads the students to limit training session to an hour and no more than 4–5 h of deliberate training each day.

There are now several impressive demonstrations of improvement in performance of surgical simulators as well as the transfer of simulator training to the operating room (Seymour 2007). For example, Ahlberg et al. (2007) showed a reliable decrease in errors for simulator-trained residents during their first ten laparoscopic cholecystectomies in the OR. In surgery and many other domains of traditional expertise, such as music, ballet, and sports, beginners need the help of teachers to identify appropriate aspects that are especially amenable to improvement. The teachers also are critical in helping students identify appropriate training techniques that lead to the desired goals within hours of training. Teachers are particularly important in evaluating and monitoring performance until the students eventually develop the skills to be able to monitor their own performance and become their own teacher.

In numerous domains, such as chess, music, and sports, aspiring experts acquire memory representations that allow them to rapidly encode situations and to evaluate and plan their future actions (Ericsson 2006a). Similarly, in surgery residents develop mental representations to support their ongoing evaluation and planning. For example, Bann et al. (2005) found a high correlation between residents' ability to detect errors in models and their ability to complete the same procedure in the operating room. In additional support for such representations, Wiegmann et al. (2007) found that residents discover most of their mistakes during surgery, but that interruptions of the operation by external factors, such as telephone calls, lead to increased probability of errors. Way et al. (2003) give examples of the challenges in identifying the anatomical structures during laparoscopic surgery and the associated skills allowing experienced surgeons to reduce the risks of injuring adjacent tissues, ducts, and vessels.

Once residents have completed their training and achieved their certification, they should remain motivated to continue improving and maintaining their skills. Unfortunately, some surgeons may develop automaticity during their practice (Fig. 7.2, middle arm). Consistent with such a development, Bann et al. (2005) argued that "senior surgeons are more prone to slips and lapses" (p. 414). Consequently, the key challenge for aspiring elite performers in any domain of expertise is to avoid the arrested development associated with automaticity. Individuals striving for excellence need actively to counteract tendencies toward automaticity (Fig. 7.2, upper arm). They do that by setting new and higher standards for their performance, requiring them to increase their speed, accuracy, and control over their action generation. For example, surgeons can assess their surgical margins (in cancer surgery), try to reduce redundant movements, and increase the safety and control of their movements by retrospective analysis of video tapes.

Experts deliberately construct and/or seek out training situations in which they can stretch themselves to attain desired goals that exceed their current level of reliable performance. They acquire and refine mechanisms that permit increased control and allow them to monitor performance in representative situations from the domain of expertise, so they can identify errors as well as improvable aspects (Ericsson 2006a, b).

There is compelling evidence for these complex cognitive mechanisms from studies in expert performance. For example, chess masters can select the best move for a chess position. When the chess position is removed, they are able to report their thoughts during the move selection and also recall the locations of all the pieces on the chess board virtually perfectly. Experts' superior incidental memory for relevant information for representative tasks has been demonstrated in a large number of domains, such as sports, music, ballet, and medicine (Ericsson and Kintsch 1995; Ericsson et al. 2000). When expert performers are given appropriately challenging tasks then they have to think, image, and reason. The most direct evidence for this type of thinking comes from asking the expert to "think aloud" during the procedure or to give a retrospective report on their thoughts immediately following the procedure (Ericsson 2006a).

7.4 Concluding Remarks

In this chapter, I have suggested parallels between findings on expert performance in surgery and those in other domains. From laboratory analyses of experts' superior performance in traditional domains, scientists have consistently found evidence for the acquired mediating mechanisms discussed above: very complex skills, highly refined representations, and extreme physiological adaptations to physical domains. In this chapter, I have tried to show how the acquisition of superior performance in surgery is closely related to the extent of engagement in practice with feedback during medical training and residency. I have also speculated that after the end of organized medical training, continued access to conditions for deliberate practice as well as feedback on daily medical practice might allow surgeons to keep improving their performance.

The complex integrated structure of expert performance raises many issues about how these structures can be gradually acquired and perfected over time. Medical students need to acquire representations that can support their planning, reasoning, and evaluation of the actual and intended performance to be able to make more appropriate adjustments to their complex skills (see Chaps. 3, 8, 10 and 12). This advantage becomes absolutely essential at higher levels of achievement. Given that deliberate practice involves mastering tasks that students could not initially attain, or only attain imperfectly or unreliably, successful students seem to acquire the ability to think, plan, and reason; this ability is further refined to allow them to solve problems and learn distinctions and consequences through planning and analysis.

In sum, I believe that the study of expert performance in surgery and other areas of medicine will provide unique insights for how to apply the expert performance framework to the study of many types of professional expertise. I anticipate that future research will show that the promising application of the expert-performance approach to medicine will advance our understanding of the development of professional expertise, and thus will yield measurable improvements in the performance of experts in many professional domains in our society.

References

Abernathy, C. M., & Hamm, R. M. (1994). *Surgical scripts: Master surgeons think aloud about 43 common surgical problems*. Philadelphia: Hanley & Belfus.

Ahlberg, G., Enochsson, L., Gallagher, A. G., Hedman, L., Hogman, C., McClusk, D. A., Ramel, S., Smith, C. D., & Arvidsson, D. (2007). Proficiency-based virtual reality training significantly reduces the error rate for residents during their first 10 laparoscopic cholecystectomies. *American Journal of Surgery, 193*, 797–804.

Atug, F., Castle, E. P., Srivastav, S. K., Burgess, S. V., Thomas, R., & Davis, R. (2006). Positive surgical margins in robotic-assisted radical prostatectomy: Impact of learning curve on oncologic outcomes. *European Urology, 49*, 866–871.

Bacha, E. A., Larrazabal, L. A., Pigula, F. A., Gauvreau, K., Jenkins, K. J., Colan, S. D., Fynn-Thompson, F., Mayer, J. E., Jr., & del Nido, P. J. (2008). Measurement of technical performance in surgery for congenital heart disease: The stage I Norwood procedure. *The Journal of Thoracic and Cardiovascular Surgery, 136*, 993–997.

Bann, S., Khan, M., Datta, V., & Darzi, A. (2005). Surgical skill is predicted by the ability to detect errors. *American Journal of Surgery, 189*, 412–415.

Chi, M. T. H. (2006). Two approaches to the study of experts' characteristics. In K. A. Ericsson, N. Charness, P. Feltovich, & R. R. Hoffman (Eds.), *Cambridge handbook of expertise and expert performance* (pp. 21–38). Cambridge: Cambridge University Press.

Choudhry, N. K., Fletcher, R. H., & Soumerai, S. B. (2005). Systematic review: The relationship between clinical experience and quality of health care. *Annals of Internal Medicine, 142*, 260–273.

de Groot, A. (1978). *Thought and choice in chess*. The Hague: Mouton (Original work published 1946).

Dreyfus, H., & Dreyfus, S. (1986). *Mind over machine: The power of human intuition and expertise in the era of the computer*. New York: Free Press.

Elstein, A. S., Shulman, L. S., & Sprafka, S. A. (1978). *Medical problem solving: An analysis of clinical reasoning*. Cambridge: Harvard University Press.

Ericsson, K. A. (1998). The scientific study of expert levels of performance: General implications for optimal learning and creativity. *High Ability Studies, 9(1)*, 75–100.

Ericsson, K. A. (2004). Deliberate practice and the acquisition and maintenance of expert performance in medicine and related domains. *Academic Medicine, 79*, S70–S81.

Ericsson, K. A. (2006a). The influence of experience and deliberate practice on the development of superior expert performance. In K. A. Ericsson, N. Charness, P. Feltovich, & R. R. Hoffman (Eds.), *Cambridge handbook of expertise and expert performance* (pp. 685–706). Cambridge: Cambridge University Press.

Ericsson, K. A. (2006b). Protocol analysis and expert thought: Concurrent verbalizations of thinking during experts' performance on representative task. In K. A. Ericsson, N. Charness, P. Feltovich, & R. R. Hoffman (Eds.), *Cambridge handbook of expertise and expert performance* (pp. 223–242). Cambridge: Cambridge University Press.

Ericsson, K. A. (2007). An expert-performance perspective on medical expertise: Study superior clinical performance rather than experienced clinicians! *Medical Education, 41*, 1124–1130.

Ericsson, K. A., & Kintsch, W. (1995). Long-term working memory. *Psychological Review, 102*, 211–245.

Ericsson, K. A., & Lehmann, A. C. (1996). Expert and exceptional performance: Evidence on maximal adaptations on task constraints. *Annual Review of Psychology, 47*, 273–305.

Ericsson, K. A., & Lehmann, A. C. (1999). *Encyclopedia of creativity*. San Diego: Academic Press.

Ericsson, K. A., & Smith, J. (1991). Prospects and limits in the empirical study of expertise: An introduction. In K. A. Ericsson & J. Smith (Eds.), *Toward a general theory of expertise: Prospects and limits* (pp. 1–38). Cambridge: Cambridge University Press.

Ericsson, K. A., Krampe, R. Th., & Tesch-Römer, C. (1993). The role of deliberate practice in the acquisition of expert performance. *Psychological Review, 100*, 363–406.

Ericsson, K. A., Patel, V. L., & Kintsch, W. (2000). How experts' adaptations to representative task demands account for the expertise effect in memory recall: Comment on Vicente and Wang (1998). *Psychological Review, 107*, 578–592.

Ericsson, K. A., Whyte, J., & Ward, P. (2007). Expert performance in nursing: Reviewing research on expertise in nursing within the framework of the expert-performance approach. *Advances in Nursing Science, 30*, E58–E71.

Feltovich, P., Prietula, M. J., & Ericsson, K. A. (2006). Studies of expertise from psychological perspectives. In K. A. Ericsson, N. Charness, P. Feltovich, & R. R. Hoffman (Eds.), *Cambridge handbook of expertise and expert performance* (pp. 41–67). Cambridge: Cambridge University Press.

Fitts, P., & Posner, M. I. (1967). *Human performance*. Belmont: Brooks/Cole.

Issenberg, S. B., McGaghie, W. C., Petrusa, E. R., & Scalese, R. J. (2005). Features and uses of high-fidelity medical simulations that lead to effective learning: A BEME systematic review. *Medical Teacher, 24*, 10–28.

Krampe, R. Th., & Ericsson, K. A. (1996). Maintaining excellence: Deliberate practice and elite performance in young and older pianists. *Journal of Experimental Psychology. General, 125*, 331–359.

Kumar, U., & Gill, I. S. (2006). Learning curve in human laparoscopic surgery. *Current Urology Reports, 7*, 120–124.

Lehmann, A. C., & Ericsson, K. A. (1993). Sight-reading ability of expert pianists in the context of piano accompanying. *Psychomusicology, 12*(2), 182–195.

McGaghie, W. C. (2008). Research opportunities in simulation-based medical education using deliberate practice. *Academic Emergency Medicine, 15*, 995–1001.

McGaghie, W. C., Issenberg, S. B., Petrusa, E. R., & Scalese, R. J. (2006). Effect of practice on standardised learning outcomes in simulation-based medical education. *Medical Education, 40*, 792–797.

McKenney, M. G., Livingstone, A. S., Schulman, C., Stahl, K., Lineen, E., Namias, N., et al. (2009). Trauma surgeon mortality rates correlate with surgeon time at institution. *Journal of the American College of Surgeons, 208*, 750–754.

Murphy, D., Doherty, G., & Luz, S. (2008). Differentiating between novices and expert surgeons based on errors derived from task analysis. *ECCE '08 Proceedings of the 15th European conference on Cognitive ergonomics: the ergonomics of cool interaction*. New York, NY, USA: Association for Computing Machinery.

Nugent, W. C. (2005). Building and supporting sustainable improvement in cardiac surgery: The Northern New England experience. *Seminars in Cardiothoracic and Vascular Anesthesia, 9*, 115–116.

Prystowsky, J. B. (2005). Are young surgeons competent to perform alimentary tract surgery? *Archives of Surgery, 140*, 495–502.

Sarker, S. K., Chang, A., Vincent, C., & Darzi, A. W. (2006). Development of assessing generic and specific technical skills in laparoscopic surgery. *American Journal of Surgery, 191*, 238–244.

Sarker, S. K., Rehman, S., Ladwa, M., Chang, A., & Vincent, C. (2009). A decision-making learning and assessment tool in laparoscopic cholecystectomy. *Surgical Endoscopy, 23*, 197–203.

Seymour, N. E. (2007). VR to OR: A review of the evidence that virtual reality simulation improves operating room performance. *World of Surgery, 32*, 182–188.

Simon, H. A., & Chase, W. G. (1973). Skill in chess. *American Scientist, 61*, 394–403.

Stoica, S. C., Kalavrouziotis, D., Martin, B.-J., Buth, K. J., Hirsch, G. M., Sullivan, J. A., et al. (2008). Long-term results of heart operations performed by surgeons-in-training. *Circulation, 118*, S1–S6.

Tsuda, S., Scott, D., Doyle, J., & Jones, D. B. (2009). Surgical skills training and simulation. *Current Problems in Surgery, 46*, 271–370.

Van Sickle, K. R., Ritter, E. M., McClusky, D. A., III, Lederman, A., Baghai, M., Gallagher, A. G., & Smith, C. D. (2007). Attempted establishment of proficiency levels for laparoscopic performance on a national scale using simulation: The results from the 2004 SAGES Minimally Invasive Surgical Trainer-Virtual Reality (MIST-VR) learning center study. *Surgical Endoscopy, 21*, 5–10.

Vickers, A. J., Bianco, F. J., Serio, A. M., Eastham, J. A., Schrag, D., Klein, E. A., et al. (2007). The surgical learning curve for prostate cancer control after radical Prostatectomy. *Journal of the National Cancer Institute, 99*, 1171–1177.

Vickers, A. J., Bianco, F. J., Gonen, M., Cronin, A. M., Eastham, J. A., Schrag, D., et al. (2008). Effects of pathologic state on the learning curve for radical prostatectomy: Evidence that recurrence in organ-confined cancer is large related to inadequate surgical technique. *European Urology, 53*, 960–966.

Vickers, A. J., Hruza, M., Koenig, P., Martinez-Pinero, L., Janetschenk, G., & Guillonneau, B. (2009). The surgical learning curve for laparoscopic radical prostatectomy: A retrospective cohort study. *The Lancet Oncology, 10*, 475–480.

Waljee, J. F., Greenfield, L. J., Dimick, J. B., & Birkmeyer, J. D. (2006). Surgeon age and operative mortality in the United States. *Annals of Surgery, 244*, 353–362.

Way, L. W., Stewart, L., Gantert, W., Liu, K., Lee, C. M., Whang, K., & Hunter, J. G. (2003). Causes and prevention of laparoscopic bile duct injuries. Analysis of 252 cases from a human factors and cognitive psychology perspective. *Annals of Surgery, 237*, 460–469.

Wiegmann, D. A., ElBardissi, A. W., Dearani, J. A., Daly, R. C., & Sundt, T. M. (2007). Disruptions in surgical flow and their relationship to surgical errors: An exploratory investigation. *Surgery, 142*, 658–665.

Chapter 8
Current and Future Simulation and Learning Technologies

Fernando Bello and Harry Brenton

8.1 Introduction

The last 20 years have seen great advances in the use of technological processes and resources to facilitate learning. Introduction of the personal computer into the classroom, data projectors, multimedia learning packages, virtual learning environments (VLEs), SmartBoards, online e-learning and, more recently, blogs, wikis and educational networking sites, have dramatically transformed the face of learning.

Similarly, simulation has established itself as a useful training tool, with a range of simulations and simulators[1] from simple benchtop models to highly sophisticated, computer-based multi-functional patient simulators being used across the mainstream surgical curriculum.

Whilst there have been clear educational benefits of such technological revolution, there are significant tensions between rapidly advancing technology and the slower pace of educational change. Not only new resources may need to be designed and distributed every so often but also the evolving nature of technology that may lead to it taking centre stage over the needs of learners and becoming an end, rather than a means to facilitate education goals. In addition, lack of proper training in the use of new learning technologies, inadequate integration of the technologies into

[1]We make a distinction between 'simulators', apparatus designed for practising specific surgical techniques across a range of complexity, and 'simulation', the wider universe within which simulators may be used.

F. Bello (✉)
Department of Surgery and Cancer, Surgical Graphics & Computing, Imperial College London, London, UK
e-mail: f.bello@imperial.ac.uk

H. Brenton
Department of Surgery and Cancer, Imperial College London, London, UK

H. Fry and R. Kneebone (eds.), *Surgical Education: Theorising an Emerging Domain*,
Advances in Medical Education 2, DOI 10.1007/978-94-007-1682-7_8,

the curriculum, or insufficient access to such technologies can all have a negative impact in the success and acceptability of a particular learning technology.

One of our aims in this chapter is to address these tensions by considering the complex relationship between learning technology (LT)[2] developments and actual educational needs, highlighting the importance of following a user-centred design and an iterative development cycle. We also argue that traditional LT resources such as multimedia (text, graphics, video clips, diagrams, etc.) and VLEs may be significantly enhanced by using different computer-based representations and interactions. Finally, we postulate that the educational value of simulation and LT changes as a surgeon progresses through his/her training.

This chapter starts by describing the broad context of simulation and learning technologies, defining its scope and introducing the concept of the 'Simulation Journey'. This is followed by a review of simulation and learning technologies, further detailed description and discussion of the Simulation Journey, and presentation of a case study. Finally, we highlight potential areas of future development and where these might lead.

8.2 Background and Scope

Simulation is widely acknowledged as offering a viable adjunct to the traditional apprenticeship model that has dominated surgical training in the past. Recently introduced limits in working hours have affected training opportunities, whilst increased political and public scrutiny demand more transparent and safer training practices. Economic and financial considerations have further affected on-the-job learning by pursuing ever increasingly optimal use of time and resources.

At the same time, the ubiquity and pervasiveness of computer technology, online connectivity and high-resolution three-dimensional (3D) graphics have put considerable pressure on educators to incorporate these technologies in their programmes, with students regularly demanding online access to high-quality multimedia resources, use of advanced software training packages, as well as engaging in training-related discussions through existing or tailored networking channels.

It seems obvious that novice surgeons should learn the basics of their specialty, including cognitive, technical and non-technical skills (e.g. communication, professionalism) before even being in contact with patients. Equally, surgeons in training should be able to continually refine their techniques, retain and advance their knowledge within a safe environment. Such learning and practising can be effectively supported throughout the undergraduate and postgraduate surgical curriculum, as well as in professional development opportunities, by a suitable combination of LT and simulation tools.

[2]Here we use the term Learning Technology as an equivalent of Educational Technology as per AECT's definition (Januszewski and Molenda 2008).

However, it is important to recognise that the educational value of simulation or a specific LT lies not on how technically advanced or sophisticated it is, but on how well it can support the learning outcomes of a particular educational encounter. Thus, educators need to have a good understanding of the affordances of a specific simulation or LT in order to be able to decide on its suitability and how best to incorporate it into specific section(s) of the curriculum.

In other words, the educational value of simulation and LT, and therefore the needs in terms of simulation and LT, change as a surgeon progresses through his/her training. Simple benchtop models that can effectively be used to learn and practise basic surgical skills at an undergraduate or foundation training level may not be adequate for higher surgical trainees. Equally, general anatomy multimedia resources suitable for the first years of undergraduate training would be unsuitable for learning more detailed surgical anatomy in preparation for performing a surgical intervention.

We refer to this trajectory of evolving simulation and LT requirements through the surgical curriculum as the 'Simulation Journey'. Acknowledging the close relationship between simulation and LT, and the need to coordinate and link such educational resources more explicitly, the Simulation Journey represents a purposely tailored continuum of different types of simulation and learning technologies, assembled together in an integrated manner to satisfy the learning needs of each individual student as he or she progresses through the curriculum, recognising that the success of an instructional strategy varies according to learner ability (Cronbach and Snow 1977).

This chapter looks at simulation and LT through this progression using a bottom-up, not prescriptive, approach, focusing on appropriate representations and interactions that address learner's needs, and highlighting the importance of a synchronised approach to the development of simulation and LT resources. Our particular emphasis is on computer-based representations, 3D modelling, hybrid and team simulations.

8.3 Technology Review: E-learning Technologies

Regarding Learning Technologies, we distinguish between *Equipment* used to facilitate learning such as SmartBoards (interactive whiteboard with touch control of computer applications), LCD projectors, digital video cameras, 3D displays, immersive Virtual Reality (VR) environments, tablet PCs, etc., and *E-learning* applications and processes that support learning and teaching. Here we concentrate on the latter and refer the reader to a recent review (Masters and Ellaway 2008), as well as to equipment providers for detailed descriptions of specific items of equipment (SMART 2010; i>clicker 2010).

The term 'E-learning' is widely used to indicate electronically supported learning and teaching; however, there are numerous different definitions available. For clarity, we adopt that proposed by Tavangarian et al. (2004):

"[E-learning comprises] all forms of electronic supported learning and teaching, which are procedural in character and aim to effect the construction of knowledge with reference to individual experience, practice and knowledge of the learner. [In E-learning] Information and communication systems, whether networked or not, serve as specific media to implement the learning process".

Key advantages of E-learning are improved learning delivery, simplification of course content standardisation and updating, and learning enhancement (Ruiz et al. 2006). Through E-learning, on-demand learning that eliminates the barriers of time and distance giving students greater autonomy regarding the point in time, the content and the method by which they learn becomes possible.

E-learning offers a new paradigm to educators capable of enhancing learning by allowing trainees to relate new learning to previous experiences, linking learning to specific needs and practically applying learning to real-life examples or case studies. Such enhancement permits greater interactivity and promotes efficiency, motivation, cognitive effectiveness and flexibility of learning style (Ruiz et al. 2006). A well-designed, interactive E-learning experience can motivate learners to become more engaged with the content, shifting the focus from a passive, trainer-centred model, to a more active, learner-centred one. Evidence suggests that E-learning is more efficient because learners gain knowledge, skills and attitudes faster than through traditional instructor-led methods (Clark 2002). This efficiency is likely to translate into improved motivation and performance, increased retention rates and better utilisation of content, resulting in better achievement of knowledge, skills and attitudes (Clark 2002). E-learning technologies may be grouped into offline and online.

8.3.1 Offline E-learning

Offline E-learning, also known as computer-assisted instruction, computer-based learning or computer-based training, uses computers to aid in the delivery of stand-alone multimedia packages on CD-ROMs or DVDs for learning and teaching (Ruiz et al. 2006; Ward et al. 2001). Multimedia refers to the use of two or more media (e.g. text, graphics, audio, video and animation) to produce more engaging content that learners and faculty can access through a computer. Whilst there exist a number of stand-alone computer-based learning packages dedicated to surgical education (Primal 2010; Toltech 2010; Reality Surgery 2010), there is an increasing trend towards online delivery facilitated by the availability of high-speed broadband and wireless connectivity.

8.3.2 Online E-learning

Online E-learning is also referred to as web-based Learning, online learning, distributed learning, Internet-based learning or distance learning. It uses information technologies to deliver instruction to learners who may be located at one or more remote locations from a central site. Several approaches can be used to develop and deliver online E-learning, ranging from replication of course materials online, to self-contained learning packages, to fully fledged Learning Management Systems (LMS) or virtual learning environments (VLEs)[3] integrating course material, interactive learning packages, assessment and support. However, based on the definition of E-learning adopted above, websites that are just repositories of knowledge, without links to learning, communication and assessment activities, are not learner-centred and thus cannot be regarded as true E-learning applications. Informational websites certainly have their uses, but a teaching site will be most effective if it stimulates active learning by supporting critical thinking, independent learning, evidence-based learning and providing constructive, timely and relevant feedback on the learner's progress.

Incorporating active learning in an educational website is not difficult, but it does require careful thought and planning (Minasian 2002). Developers need to combine established principles of curriculum development, adult learning and behavioural theory, along with principles of website design (Greenhalgh 2001). Cook and Dupras (2004) have outlined ten practical steps to effective web-based learning. Others have made recommendations on how to improve design and interactivity (De Rouck et al. 2008; Sisson et al. 2010).

Online E-learning applications for undergraduate and postgraduate surgical education are rich and varied. They cover both instruction and assessment (formative and summative), and include anatomy (Choi et al. 2008), problem-based learning (Corrigan et al. 2008), clinical examination (Criley et al. 2008), surgical internship (Meier et al. 2005), procedural skills (Chenkin et al. 2008), comprehensive course curricula (Kalet et al. 2007), real-time telementoring (Shimizu et al. 2007), life-support (Romero et al. 2006) and interprofessional education (Pulman et al. 2009). Offering different levels of interactivity, the degree of flexibility, engagement and learner-centredness of these applications varies considerably.

8.3.3 *E-learning 2.0*

The emergence of Web 2.0 as the next evolutionary stage of the World Wide Web has blurred the boundary between producers and consumers of content, shifting attention from access to information, towards access to other people. Web 2.0 applications facilitate interactive information sharing, interoperability, user-centred design and collaboration. New kinds of online resources (e.g. social networking sites, blogs, podcasts, wikis, RSS and virtual communities) have allowed people with common interests to meet, share ideas and collaborate in innovative ways.

[3]LMS is typically used in North America whilst VLE tends to be used in Europe. For consistency, we will use VLE throughout this chapter.

This new kind of participatory medium is ideal for supporting multiple modes of learning and has given rise to the term *E-learning 2.0*.

E-learning 2.0 refers to the second generation of online E-learning that makes use of Web 2.0 technologies such as collaborative authoring and social annotation in order to enhance online E-learning applications (Downes 2005). E-learning social networks resemble communities of practice capable of generating richer materials. Authors who belong to the same community can cooperate in providing more valuable E-learning content within the community, based on their different backgrounds and knowledge. Just as in Web 2.0 the boundary between producers and consumers of content is blurred, E-learning 2.0 involves both teachers and students in the content creation process, and thus the strict delimitations between tutors and students disappear.

This new online E-learning paradigm emphasises *Social Learning*, which is based on the premise that our understanding of content is socially constructed through conversations about that content and through grounded interactions with others around problems or actions (Brown and Adler 2008). Thus, the focus is not so much on what we are learning, but on how we are learning. This perspective shifts the focus of attention from the content to the learning activities and human interactions around which it is situated.

E-learning 2.0 is still an emerging field whose full potential is yet to be exploited. Early attempts to produce E-learning 2.0 authoring and delivery systems include those presented in (Ghali and Cristea 2009). Nevertheless, students have taken the lead in integrating social networking in their learning activities, medical schools and faculties already have a presence in all popular networking channels, and faculty members are increasingly participating in exchanges.

8.3.4 Virtual Learning Environments

The last decade has seen a rapid uptake of VLEs such as Moodle (Moodle 2010) and Blackboard (Blackboard 2010; Fig. 8.1). These are password-protected intranets with tools to support teaching and learning. For example, students can study course materials, take multiple-choice assessments, submit assignments and use discussion boards. VLEs provide a generic framework, which can be used across science and humanities subjects.

More specialised tools tailored towards medical education include the virtual patients (VPs) application tool (Fig. 8.2), which allows teachers to write clinical case studies that simulate a doctor–patient consultation. Students arrive at a working diagnosis by answering multiple-choice quizzes and are given textual feedback when a correct or incorrect answer is given.

Using different computer-based representations and interactions may significantly enhance conventional multimedia resources. For example, the VP in Fig. 8.2 is represented by text, photos and imaging scans. In contrast, the VPs in Fig. 8.3a, b

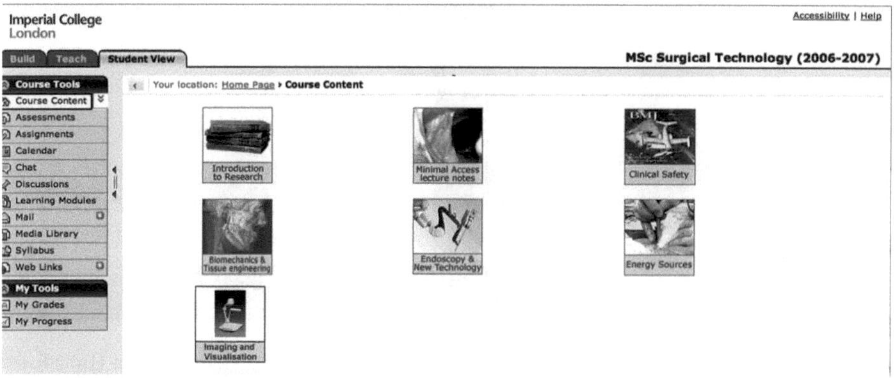

Fig. 8.1 Surgical Technology Blackboard course area at Imperial College London

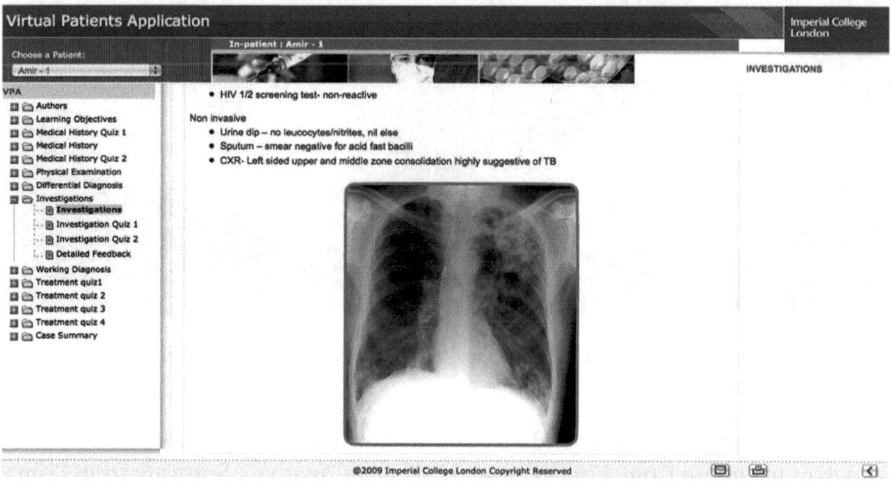

Fig. 8.2 The virtual patients application tool (Imperial College London) shows the X-ray results for a virtual patient suffering from tuberculosis

are embodied as animated 3D characters capable of supporting interaction through mouse clicks and text menus (Fig. 8.3b), or speech and body posture (Fig. 8.3a).

The use of 3D visualisation (Fig. 8.3a) through specialised stereoscopic display systems has been shown to improve recall of anatomical structures (Luursema 2008) and make it easier to locate a two-dimensional imaging scan within a 3D model (Gutierrez et al. 2007). Such enhanced spatial depiction of anatomical structures is one of the key justifications for using 3D virtual environments in medicine. Jurgaitis et al. (Jurgaitis et al. 2008) found that learners were significantly better at locating liver tumours using 3D anatomy than on equivalent 2D CT scans (Fig. 8.4).

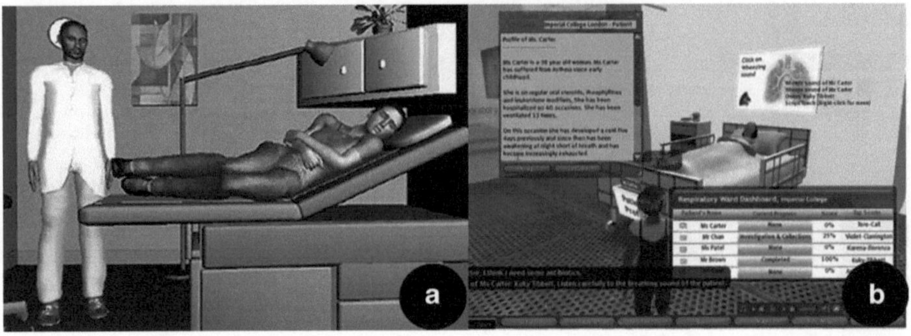

Fig. 8.3 3D virtual patients: (**a**) History taken from a patient with abdominal pain (Deladisma et al. 2008); (**b**) Respiratory ward in second life

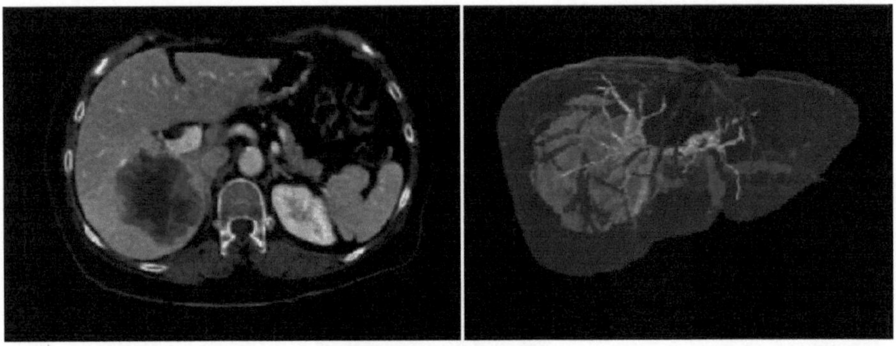

Fig. 8.4 Locating a tumour in an 3D model and an equivalent CT scan (Jurgaitis et al. 2008)

Medical students wishing to learn basic anatomy have a wide range of electronic resources to choose from. For example, 3D Human Anatomy Software from Primal Pictures (Primal 2010) allows a user to ‘strip’ between superficial and deep layers (Fig. 8.5) and rotate around multiple viewing angles (Fig. 8.6).

Some authors argue that this tractable demonstration of spatial information makes 3D graphics superior to 2D illustrations as it helps a learner to acquire ‘a fully plastic sense of the all-round shape of organs and how they fit together as a complex spatial puzzle’ (Kemp and Wallace 2000). Thus, 3D computer-generated anatomy may fulfil a valuable educational role for the many students who find it difficult to visualise in 3D (Heylings 2002). However, the educational value of rotating a 3D structure around multiple viewpoints is inconclusive. Garg et al. (2001) found that multiple viewpoints significantly improved spatial understanding of the carpal bones in the hand compared to looking at four ‘key’ views. But these results contradict two other studies by the same authors that found no significant difference between multiple and key views (Garg et al. 1999, 2002). Levinson et al. (Levinson et al. 2007) found that key views were significantly better than multiple views of

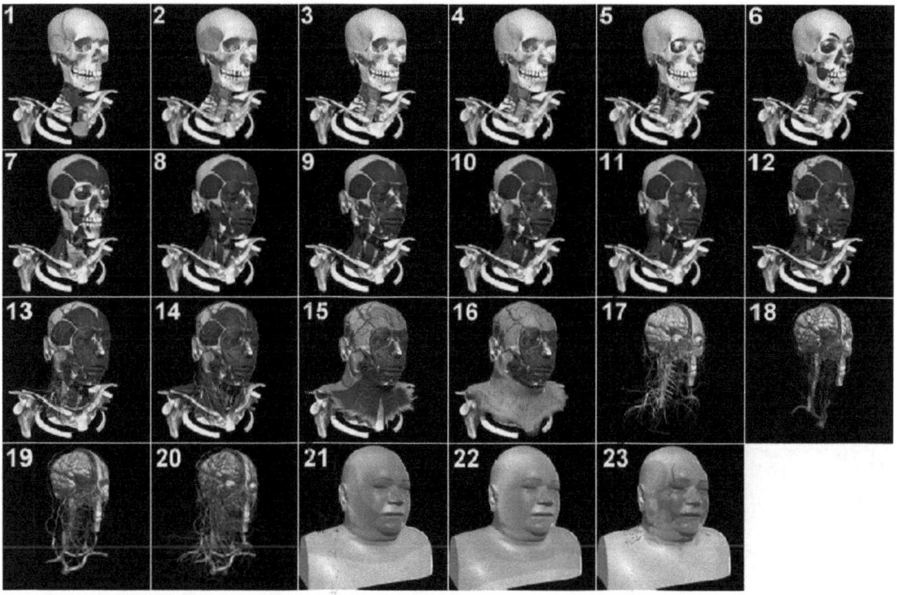

Fig. 8.5 'Stripping' interaction (Primal Pictures head and neck DVD ROM)

the abdomen when they were under the control of the learner, but no significant difference between key and multiple views presented in a sequence controlled by the computer.

Figures 8.5 and 8.6 are presented in an 'interactive encyclopaedia' format, which has become a de facto standard for anatomy interfaces (Temkin et al. 2006). Encyclopaedic interfaces are non-directive, presenting a large amount of information that can be accessed as the learner wishes. Figure 8.7 shows a more directive approach, which requires learners to snap muscles onto the correct area of a skeleton (Preim et al. 1999; Yip and Rajendran 2008). This 3D puzzle format imposes enough constraints upon construction to guide learners towards task completion, but enough freedom for them to make mistakes.

Thus, there is a wide variety of graphical representations in surgical/medical E-learning, ranging from static text and photographs (Fig. 8.2), to animated 3D characters (Fig. 8.3) and 3D anatomical models (Figs. 8.4–8.7). There are also several types of interaction: point and click (Fig. 8.2), speech and body posture (Fig. 8.3a), stripping (Fig. 8.5), rotation (Fig. 8.6) and snapping (Fig. 8.7).

The appropriateness of these representations and interactions changes during the course of surgical training. A medical student who has not yet decided to become a surgeon can acquire fundamental principles of patient management from a web browser (Fig. 8.2) and learn basic anatomy from DVD ROMs (Fig. 8.5) and 3D imaging (Fig. 8.4). Interfaces that impose constraints upon interaction can help novices 'unlock' concepts such as how muscles attach to limbs (Fig. 8.7). These

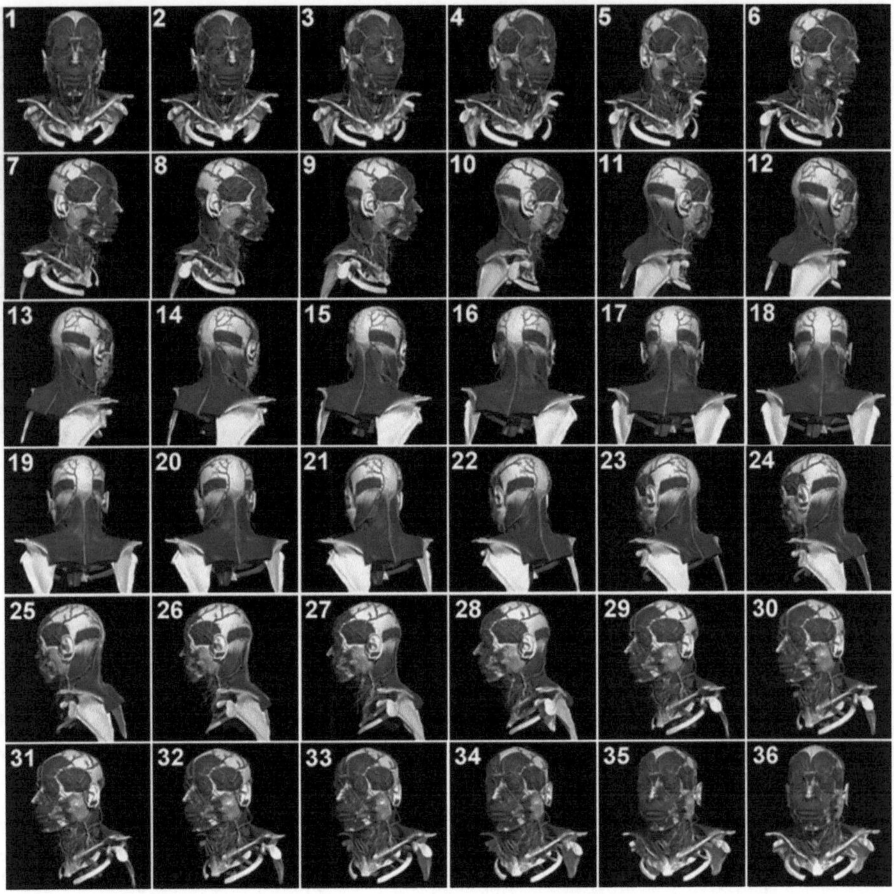

Fig. 8.6 Clockwise rotation (Primal Pictures head and neck CD-Rom)

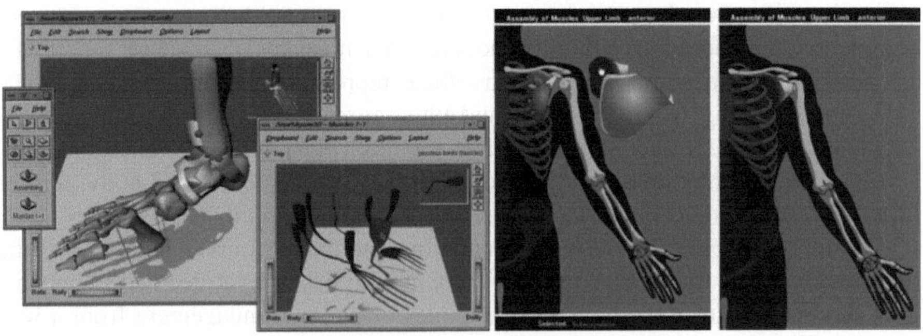

Fig. 8.7 Snapping interaction: (**a**) snap anatomy (Yip and Rajendran 2008); (**b**) 3D anatomy puzzle (Preim et al. 1999)

resources become redundant for a Senior House Officer (SHO) on a surgical rotation who requires surgically salient anatomy and an opportunity to practise technical and communication skills.

The educational value of learning technologies is contextual, so it behoves researchers to identify the circumstances under which they are most effective.

8.4 Simulation Technologies

We make a distinction between 'simulators', apparatus designed for practising specific surgical techniques across a range of complexity, and 'simulation', the wider universe within which simulators may be used.

Simulation has long been used as a tool for system modelling and analysis, performance optimisation, resource allocation and learning. Physical simulation makes use of real-life objects that are usually smaller, less complex and/or cheaper than the actual object or system being simulated. Computer simulation, on the other hand, uses computer software and mathematical formulations to model a real-life or hypothetical situation in order to study its behaviour and response to different stimuli. Both physical and computer simulations can be turned into interactive simulations with the intervention of human operators.

Simulator technology has benefited from advances in materials science, the realism of virtual reality computing and customised human–computer interfaces. For simplicity, we group simulators into three main types: physical models, virtual reality (VR) and hybrid simulators.

8.4.1 Physical Models

Physical or benchtop models (Limbs 2010; Gaumard 2010; Simulab 2010), also known as part-task trainers, are widely used at undergraduate and early postgraduate levels of surgical training (Bradley 2006). They are made from a variety of plastic, silicon and other materials that mimic the look and feel of real-life tissues and organs, and are available for a range of clinical procedures. They offer direct handling of instruments and interaction with real materials to show a range of tissue handling characteristics. Advances in materials technology have improved the realism of such models considerably (Kneebone et al. 2010). There is also increased interest and cross-fertilisation between film and television prosthetics experts, and medical/surgical benchtop models developers.

Box trainers allow laparoscopic and endoscopic procedures to be practised using real instruments. They are particularly helpful during the early stages of training since basic techniques such as camera handling, tissue dissection and endoscopic suturing can be rehearsed repeatedly. A dead animal and/or synthetic tissue may be used for practising more advanced procedures.

Whilst physical models are considerably cheaper than VR simulators, they exhibit fixed anatomy, are subject to considerable wear and tear and do not incorporate facilities for formative or summative assessment. Moreover, they tend to be separated from their clinical context and may lead to a reductionist approach to learning.

8.4.2 Virtual Reality

Virtual reality is best described as a concept of advanced human–computer interaction. VR enables humans to directly interact with computer-generated environments that simulate our physical world. VR applications vary greatly in their level of realism and user immersion. Voelter and Kraemer (Voelter and Kraemer 1995) group VR technology into four categories: immersive, desktop, pseudo and inverse. Immersive VR completely integrates the user into the world of the computer. Modern flight simulators are considered highly immersive. Pilots physically sit inside these simulators, and they are surrounded by realistic visual displays and sounds. Similar flight simulation programs available for personal computers are classified as desktop VR since they occur on a personal computer screen. Pseudo VR refers to programs with more limited computer–user interaction. These applications allow users to observe the virtual environment, but afford little ability to manipulate or affect it. As illustrated in the previous section, some VR anatomy programs allow users to adjust the orientation of 3D anatomic models, but cannot deform the models or virtually dissect them. Finally, inverse VR describes the integration of a computer into the user's world. An example would be the use of eye movements to control a computer that facilitates communication or other tasks in the real world. This type of VR has not yet played a role in medical education.

Augmented reality (AR) has been described as a fifth category of VR. In AR, virtual images are overlaid on the real world using see-through screens or head-mounted displays. Such technique has been successfully used in various surgical specialties to allow the surgeon to see 3D representations of internal anatomic structures (based on pre-operative radiographic studies) overlaid on the surface anatomy (Lamata et al. 2010). In effect, this allows the surgeon to 'virtually' see through the patient's skin.

Over the last 30 years, VR has proven to be a powerful teaching tool in several non-medical fields, including aviation, business, the nuclear power industry and the military (Krummel 1998). The aviation industry credits VR-based education as a major contributor to a nearly 50% reduction in the rate of human error-related airline crashes since the 1970s (Levin 2004).

The last decade has seen VR technology being used to recreate many surgical procedures with a high degree of realism, allowing learners to interact with a convincing computer-based environment. Minimal access procedures lend themselves especially to such simulations as manipulating objects with surgical instruments while watching a 2D screen reflects the reality of minimal access surgery. Such simulators consist of a suitable hardware interface (using instruments which resemble those used in surgical procedures), a screen to display the virtual environment and a computer to run the simulation. Learners choose procedures from a menu of varying levels of difficulty; performance metrics (e.g. time taken, economy of movement, bleeding and errors made) and the procedure itself can be recorded automatically. Feedback based on these metrics is normally provided after the procedure, with or without a tutor's input.

Several generations of VR simulators have been developed. The first generation focused on training basic skills by performing isolated tasks (e.g. pick and place, navigation) using abstract scenes and 3D representations of geometric solids (MIST 2010). The second generation focused also on basic skills, but attempted to achieve this by using more realistic procedural tasks, such as clipping blood vessels or intracorporeal knotting (LapSim 2010). The third generation allowed entire procedures (e.g. laparoscopic cholecystectomy) to be simulated, introducing anatomical variants to create a range of difficulty levels, moving beyond psychomotor skill and beginning to include decision making (LapMentor 2010). The current fourth generation aims to offer patient-specific simulation by using advanced image processing algorithms and 3D modelling techniques to combine scanned images of an individual patient's anatomy and pathology to generate individual simulations (PROcedure 2010). Such systems allow specialists to plan and rehearse challenging cases before an actual operation.

The more complex a simulation, the greater computing power it requires. This results in a trade-off between high visual and tactile fidelity, and the real-time response necessary for full interactivity. Another drawback of these simulators at present is their cost and their need for specialised support.

8.4.3 Hybrid Simulators

Hybrid simulators combine a physical model replicating the instruments as well as the anatomy interface, with a software program that creates interactive settings within which learning can take place. A key advantage of such technology is its potential for team training, for moving beyond the practice of isolated technical skills and for recreating the clinical context of practice.

Hybrid simulators include full-body automated mannequins designed to provide realistic tactile, auditory and visual stimuli (SimMan 2010; HPS 2010). They present a range of pathophysiological variables and can respond to the administration of drugs, as well as give immediate feedback to a range of interventions. Mannequins are well established within anaesthetic training and are becoming increasingly common in other domains (Bradley 2006; Grant et al. 2008). While full-body simulation exercises allow for basic procedural practice, immersive scenarios offer an opportunity to practise and reflect on critical diagnostic, management skills, communication, organisation and multitasking. As the field of simulation matures, mannequin simulators will develop increasingly realistic physical and procedural components to complement an already high level of situational realism.

By debriefing critical scenarios, crisis management skills can be identified and improved in conjunction with medical skills.

Other hybrid simulators such as endoscopy, endovascular or urological (Simbionix 2010) combine an authentic interface (the endoscope, catheters/guidewires, cystoscope, etc.) with realistic VR displays as seen by the operator. They simulate a range of diagnostic and therapeutic procedures, with a collection of virtual patient cases offering different levels of difficulty, allowing novice and intermediate learners to gain the basics of manipulative skill through repeated practice. The decision-making process is enhanced during the simulation by the display of vital signs, haemodynamic wave tracings and patient responses that appropriately reflect relevant physiology. Performance metrics are captured by the software and presented to the learner after each procedure. A range of pathological conditions and technical challenge levels is offered.

8.4.4 Virtual Worlds

Virtual worlds are a genre of web-based or online community where actors create their own world and interact with others within a computer-simulated environment that usually takes the form of an interactive 3D environment. Examples of virtual worlds include Second Life, Active Worlds, Kaneva, Smallworlds, Onverse and OpenSimulator (Virtual Worlds 2010).

Virtual worlds first attracted 'gamers' – people interested in engaging in online activities involving goals and skill levels, then social networking aficionados and now, business, enterprise, designers, science and industry. Space within the virtual environment is typically purchased/dedicated for particular use such as research, business outlets or social venues. Within those areas, the owner can build and own its property. Participants are visible within the environment as avatars that, as representatives of the physical self in digital form, can be shaped and dressed according to choice. Interaction with other participants is by keyboard or voice and can be public or private.

The use of virtual worlds in surgical education is still in its infancy. This is largely due to limitations within current virtual worlds including lack of flexible interaction, poor quality of graphical and 3D representations, non-intuitive navigation and slow response. However, its potential has been demonstrated through online E-learning applications (Toro-Troconis 2010), virtual classrooms (Wiecha et al. 2010) and virtual hospitals/clinics (2ndHealth 2010).

8.5 The Simulation Journey

Surgical education has witnessed a considerable paradigm shift over the last decade. Working time directives, economic and financial constraints, changing practice patterns and patient safety issues have resulted in alternatives to the traditional apprenticeship model. Surgery has experienced an equally significant change with the adoption of new technologies and techniques in routine surgical practice. All of these changes have created a significant challenge for surgical educators, forcing them to rethink how to educate the present-day surgeon, as well as the surgeons of the future. Whilst this challenge is considerable, it represents a unique opportunity for revolutionising surgical education and dramatically improving patient safety.

According to Satava, the revolution has already started and is being spearheaded by simulation science, which he regards as including not only the technology of simulators but also new curricula, objective assessment methods and criterion-based requirements (Satava 2010). Pugh et al. also point out the major impact that the Internet and online technologies have had on surgical education, suggesting that surgical educators should take advantage of the possibilities offered by the Internet in order to adapt to the changing needs and abilities of today's learners, whilst at the same time not forgetting core experiences and skills that must be acquired by more traditional means (Pugh et al. 2009).

Competency-Based Medical Education (CBME) is another major driving force in this revolution. Recently defined by the International CBME collaboration as 'An outcomes-based approach to the design, implementation, assessment, and evaluation of medical education programs, using an organizing framework of competencies' (Frank et al. 2010), competency-based (or proficiency-based) training in surgery has resulted in residents no longer being trained for a specified time, but rather trained for whatever length of time is required to reach or maintain pre-specified benchmark measures (Satava 2010).

Whilst competency-based frameworks are more readily applicable to postgraduate specialty training where performance can be closely linked to the relevant specialty (Iobst et al. 2010), ongoing changes to the undergraduate curricula and the establishment of national accreditation standards have enabled the introduction of competency-based frameworks at this level (Harris et al. 2010). Such frameworks can provide a useful and direct linkage between the postgraduate and undergraduate stages, offering increased opportunities for undergraduate students to make decisions about their own learning by emphasising formative assessment and structured learning activities that lead to explicit, assessed competency outcomes.

Simulation and E-learning are ideally placed to support competency-based training and assessment at undergraduate and postgraduate levels by allowing educators to devise outcomes-based programmes, using a range of different types of simulation and learning technologies that enable trainees to gain the required knowledge and skills, interact with other learners, practise and rehearse repeatedly until the required outcome or competency level is attained. However, they must be viewed as educational resources meant to enhance teaching and learning, and not as substitutes for high-quality teaching and mentoring. This requires a thoughtful educational programme that incorporates suitable simulation and E-learning applications into specific section(s) of the curriculum in order to satisfy the learning needs of a student as he or she progresses through it. Educators need to have a good understanding of the individual and combined affordances of available simulation and E-learning applications, as well as be willing to participate in the design, development and implementation of new simulations and E-learning tools.

We refer to this continuum as the Simulation Journey to reflect the potential for increased use of simulation techniques in E-learning packages, the further interaction and interdependence between simulators, simulation sessions and E-learning, as well as to highlight the need for a unified and coherent approach to the use of simulation and E-learning across the surgical curriculum. Thus, in our view, an undergraduate medical student may commence their simulation journey making use of a range of basic online E-learning tools in combination with simple benchtop models. As they progress through the undergraduate curriculum and into postgraduate training, the fidelity, complexity, interactivity and collaborative opportunities of the online tools, simulators and simulations evolves accordingly, but in a carefully planned, gradual and structured manner.

The concept of a simulation continuum has been discussed by several authors, but mainly in relation to simulator fidelity, and without reference to the potential for integrating simulation and E-learning, progression in computer-based representations, level of complexity, interactivity and collaboration as we are proposing. Maran and Glavin suggest the use of different levels of simulation from low to high fidelity in a continuum of training (Maran and Glavin 2003). Aggarwal et al. point out that the teaching of technical and non-technical skills should be comprehensive and sequential, suggesting that junior trainees could learn basic surgical skills on a low-fidelity VR simulator, progress to learning the specific steps of an operation on a high-fidelity VR-procedural simulator and, ultimately, refine their skills in a simulated operating room (Aggarwal and Darzi 2009). Windsor uses a musical analogy to illustrate the hierarchy of surgical skills that needs to be considered when using simulation in surgical education and training, and highlighting the need to match simulation to surgical skills (Windsor 2009). Scalese et al. recognise the role of simulation for teaching and assessment across the continuum of educational levels and different healthcare professions (Scalese et al. 2007).

More recently, Brydges et al. advocate a progressive learning approach that exposes students to simulators using stepwise increases in simulator characteristics (e.g. fidelity, information content – fidelity plus number of clinical skills integrated into the simulation experience) from simple to complex that are matched to the student's current skill level (Brydges 2010). Based on results from an experimental study, they suggest that the question is not which level of simulator fidelity to use, but rather how the range of different simulator fidelities should be incorporated into a progressive training programme. They go on to recommend that simulation modalities should be integrated into curricula using evidence-based theoretical principles, and that educational research intensity must match the rate at which simulation modalities are introduced.

In addition to the simulator fidelity and information content continuum recognised by the above authors, we relate the Simulation Journey to a progression in computer-based representations used, level of complexity, interactivity and collaboration of simulators and E-learning applications, which are mapped onto the individual changing requirements of a surgeon as they progress through their training.

We now present a case study to illustrate this progression, as well as to demonstrate how an iterative software development process can identify and support the needs of surgical trainees.

8.6 Case Study

The case study is taken from an ongoing project at Imperial College London funded through the London Deanery's STeLI initiative (STELI 2010). It aims at supporting all aspects of learning for open hernia repair operations and currently consists of a 3D tutorial and an online simulation.

8.6.1 3D Tutorial

User centred design prioritises the needs and limitations of users (Dix et al. 2004). In practice, this means studying how users interact with, and learn from, a software system, by means of interviews, observations and other techniques that help building a contextual understanding of how the software is used.

It is important to involve users early on in the design process. Therefore, one month into the project we conducted a pilot interview study with a junior registrar specialising in plastic surgery; a computer scientist specialising in surgical graphics; a fifth-year medical student with an interest in surgery, and a year 2 specialist registrar in general surgery. The purpose of the study was twofold: (1) comparing two different types of 3D anatomical representations offering distinct levels of fidelity and interaction in order to determine which one might be more suitable for use in the 3D tutorial and online simulation; (2) elucidating the value of the 3D anatomical representations for each of the target groups (medical student, junior registrar and specialist registrar).

A software interface was created allowing interaction with eight examples from the high-quality commercial 3DScience 3D anatomical collection (3DScience 2010). Each image can be rotated through 360° and on some examples anatomical layers can be stripped away/built up (Fig. 8.8; Station 2). Respondents were asked to rate each representation out of ten for 'visual quality' and 'level of realism'. Equivalent images from Primal Pictures (Primal 2010) were also rated to provide a comparative benchmark (Fig. 8.8; Station 1).

All respondents agreed that the 3DScience representations were superior to Primal Pictures in terms of realism and quality (average rating of 7.6/10 compared to 6/10 for Primal Pictures). However, it was pointed out that some important structures were missing and may need to be added before the models could be used. Interviewees also agreed that 3D representations are probably most valuable at the start of surgical training to introduce an operation, or act as a 'just-in-time' revision

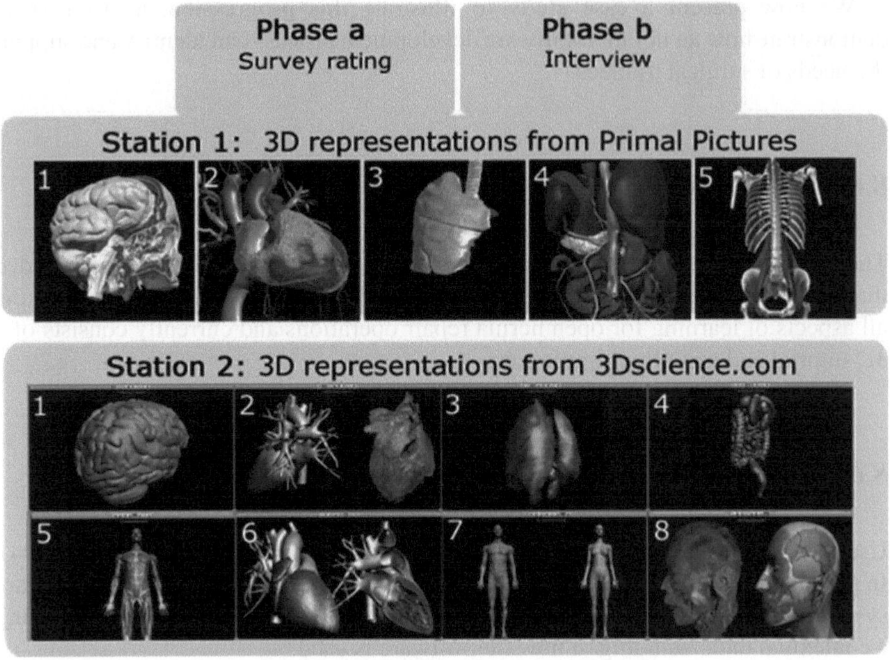

Fig. 8.8 Study comparing 3D representations from 3DScience and Primal Pictures

aid before a surgical case. They should be presented according to the 'surgical mindset':

1. Anatomy should be grouped in the same way that surgeons are taught, such as dividing the abdomen into supracolic and infracolic compartments.
2. Surgically salient anatomy should be presented in the order it is encountered during an operation.
3. Danger points during an operation should be indicated including downstream muscles, which may be affected by nerve injury.
4. Anatomical variation and pathology should be shown where it is surgically relevant. The aesthetic qualities of a 3D representation are appreciated, but the relevance and clarity of the information they contain is more important.

User personas are fictional characters modelled on the behaviour of an archetypal user (Cooper 2004). Personas help software developers to focus their attention on the needs of the user and not get sidetracked with technical and implementation issues.

The primary persona in this project was Anne, a 27-year old Foundation House Officer 2 (FHO2; equivalent to PGY-2). Anne is familiar with the salient anatomy (although she is not aware that she has forgotten some of it). She has observed four hernia operations but not assisted in any. She requires a clear account of the

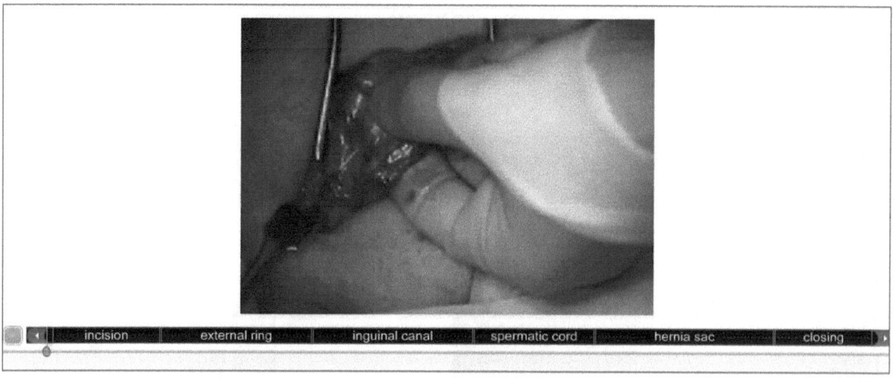

Fig. 8.9 Open hernia repair 3D tutorial prototype version 1

key stages of a hernia operation and an opportunity to revise the surgically salient anatomy. There are two secondary personas: (1) Mark, a 34–year-old second-year specialty registrar (equivalent to PGY-4) who has performed several operations and wants a quick revision aid before going into theatre; (2) Professor Baker, a consultant in a teaching hospital who wants a visual aid to help teach trainees.

Having decided to focus on an inguinal open hernia repair operation following suggestions from the pilot interview participants and discussions with senior surgeons, who confirmed that this operation requires an understanding of conceptually difficult 3D anatomy, the first stage was to assemble illustrations and photographs. These allow a designer to see how illustrators have 'solved' the problem of visually communicating an open hernia operation. Paper prototypes were drawn to experiment with different screen layouts and navigation controls. These were shown to a surgeon who suggested that a video should be used to complement the 3D representations, allowing the trainee to navigate the key stages in the operation (Fig. 8.9). The key stages were taken from a hierarchical task analysis (HTA) that examined 130 operations to determine the principal tasks and sub-tasks performed during a hernia repair (Sarker et al. 2008).

As the application developed, the operation timeline indicating the key stages and allowing the trainee to navigate through the tutorial was refined. A 3D representation that displays relevant anatomy in synchrony with the video was also added (Fig. 8.10). An important part of the design process is to impose constraints upon the system that help a user to 'unlock' relevant information. These constraints come in various forms, from graphical overlays that draw attention to a region of the screen (e.g. the labels in Fig. 8.11), to camera angles that lock a 3D representation into an appropriate viewing angle.

Several additional versions were created, discussed with users and then revised. During this cycle of generation and testing, the software was gradually adapted to meet the requirements of the three user personas described above. For example, midway through the process, it became clear that surgically important blood vessels

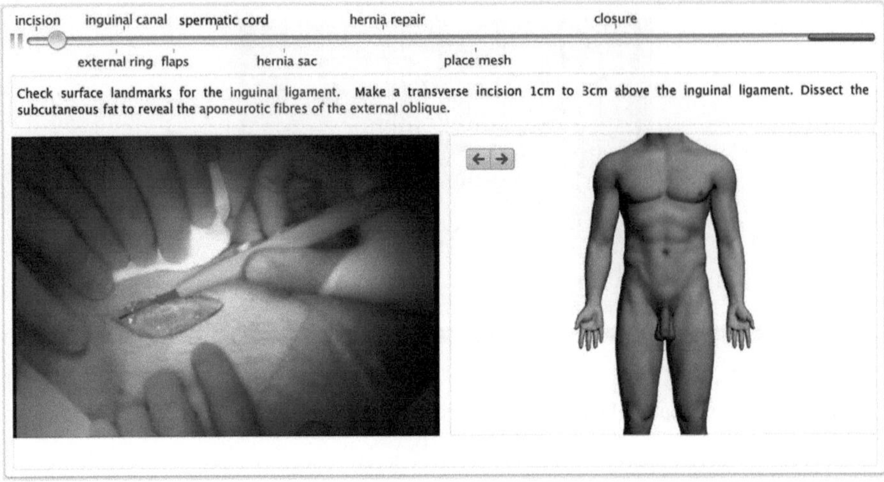

Fig. 8.10 Open hernia repair 3D tutorial prototype version 2

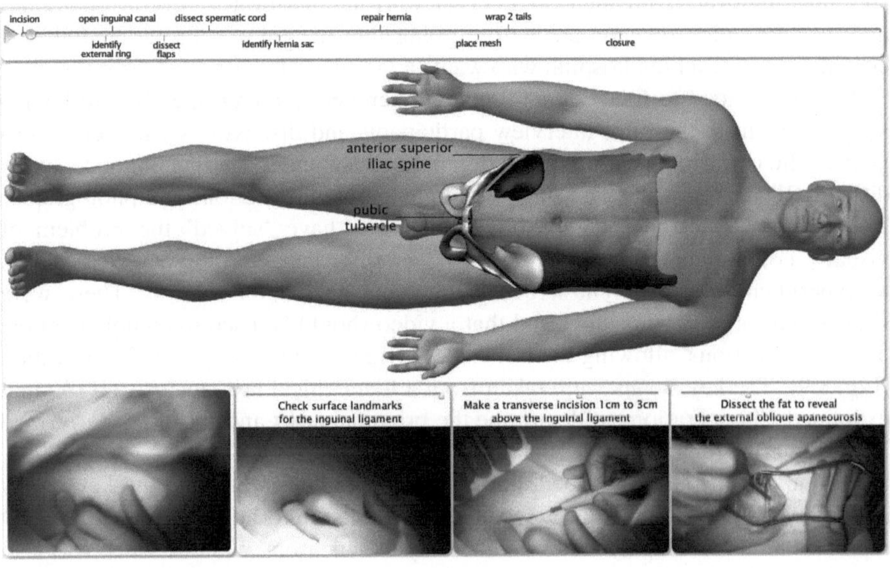

Fig. 8.11 Open hernia repair 3D tutorial final prototype

(inferior epigastrics) were missing from the available 3D representations. These were then built using a 3D modelling application and added to the final version of the tutorial.

Evolutionary software development works on the principle that designers are fallible and they won't get everything right the first time round. By designing for

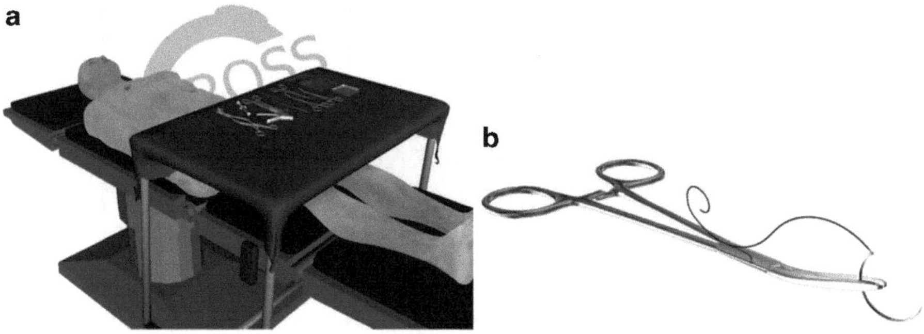

Fig. 8.12 (**a**) Virtual operating theatre; (**b**) Representation of surgical tool

a user persona (Anne), and generating and testing multiple prototypes, the software can be incrementally adapted to the requirements of the surgical trainee.

8.6.2 Online Simulation

Our goal was to develop an online open hernia repair simulation system that can contribute to the confidence, skills and knowledge of trainee surgeons, making them progress faster up the learning curve. The emphasis was on teaching the anatomy and its spatial relations, as well as the tasks involved in the repair procedure.

The system was designed based on the hierarchical task analysis mentioned above (Sarker et al. 2008), as well as in continuous correspondence with expert surgeons and observations made in the operating theatre. Using the HTA as a foundation, we compiled an implementation plan detailing (A) the virtual environment, (B) the user interactions and (C) the requirements of deformable models. The implementation plan was then used to guide the iterative system development according to the overall specifications outlined above. The final version of the implementation plan encompasses the 46 subtasks of the HTA itself, input from the literature review, observations from video recordings of inguinal hernia repair surgery (open and laparoscopic), observations from hernia repair procedures (three laparoscopic, two open) and continuous feedback, discussions and input from expert surgeons.

3D models are ideal for teaching the spatial relations of the inguinal region as they can minimise the level of mental abstraction required by the trainee. A virtual operating theatre that is a close but simpler recreation of a real operating theatre was built to further minimise the level of abstraction. This involved building high-quality 3D models of the necessary tools and equipment in the operating theatre (Fig. 8.12a, b).

The 3DScience models were used as a basis for the anatomical models of skin, muscles, intestine, ligament, bone, blood vessels and nerves. Whilst these models

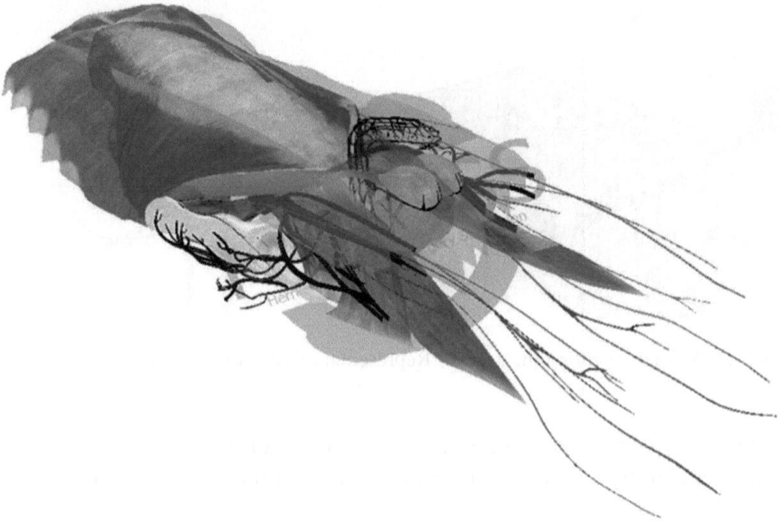

Fig. 8.13 Modified 3D models of relevant anatomy

are of high quality and suitable for general visualisation and rendering purposes, the level of anatomical detail present does not accurately reflect the anatomy of the inguinal region. This required careful modification and extension of the models in close collaboration with expert surgeons to correctly reflect this anatomy (Fig. 8.13).

Our implementation plan contains a wide range of different user interactions, from selection and application of the correct tool, selection from multiple interaction choices (e.g. location of incision), 3D navigation and manipulation, to exploring the anatomy. We carefully designed the individual interactions to focus on the key elements to be taught to the trainees. For instance, when incising the external oblique muscle, we focus on teaching the trainee where to cut, not how to cut. As a result, rather than cutting freely, the user is presented with a series of incision sites, thus allowing the system to easily detect and feedback to the user when they try to perform an erroneous incision. Other tasks such as the mobilisation of the spermatic cord give the user full freedom to drag, twist and explore the spermatic cord. When the execution of the procedure comes to an end, the user is given feedback on her/his performance. This includes highlighting any incorrect action and explaining how to execute it properly. Figure 8.14 shows the open hernia repair online simulation prototype being used to perform an operation.

The design and implementation of the above 3D tutorial and online simulation prototype have occurred simultaneously. This has allowed us to exploit the synergies between them, including the 3D anatomical models, the detailed procedural task analysis, the expert knowledge from surgeons and the user feedback from students. Whilst the 3D tutorial supports a more directed learning experience, providing limited visualisation interactions (i.e. zooming, rotation, selection), and serving as a general reference for the open hernia repair operation, the online simulation allows

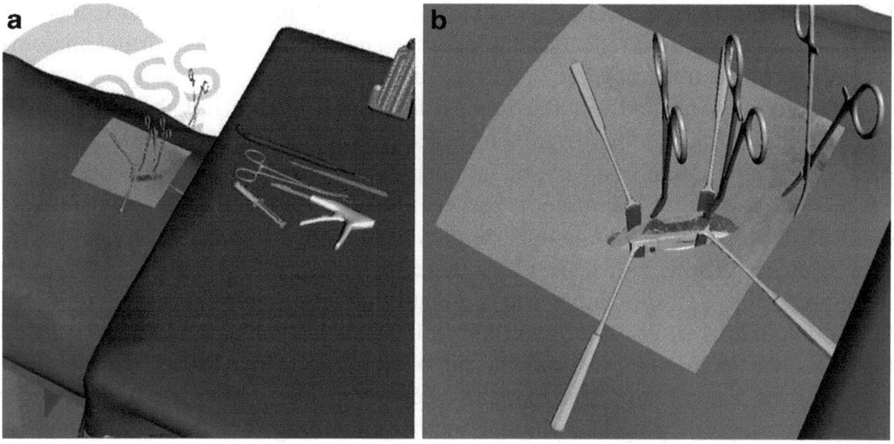

Fig. 8.14 Open hernia repair online simulation prototype: (**a**) peripheral view; (**b**) close-up view showing the dissected anatomy

for the manipulation of the anatomical structures, as well as the performance of the tasks involved in the repair procedure. The next step in this Simulation Journey would be a benchtop hernia repair model allowing the trainee to further rehearse the surgical anatomy and tasks learned in the 3D tutorial and online simulation, before assisting in a real-life procedure.

8.7 Future Developments

There seems little doubt that the role of simulation and learning technologies in surgical education will continue to increase. Trainees will expect to be provided with an evolving collection of online E-learning applications and simulation encounters, and will carry on leading the way in exploiting the collaborative opportunities of Web 2.0. The seamless integration between online E-learning and simulation across the surgical curriculum will progress towards a fully integrated, individualised Simulation Journey, with E-learning applications and simulations developed in tandem to support each other.

Virtual learning environments will evolve towards personalised learning environments (PLEs), able to track each trainee's progress along their simulation journey, providing them with consistent, coherent and timely formative and summative feedback throughout. Trainers will be assisted by the PLE giving them much needed insight into overall trainee performance, and allowing better coordination across educational activities.

Improved medical imaging will lead to better 3D models, resulting in increased use of 3D/4D (3D + time) representations across E-learning and simulation. Models will be patient specific, leading to a library of cases being available for E-learning applications, simulation rehearsal and practice and highly detailed virtual anatomy supporting prosection, dissection and evolutionary anatomy.

Faster computers and graphic processing units (GPUs), together with better software algorithms and hardware interfaces, will enable enhanced and more complex virtual simulations, capable of supporting a greater range of procedures (e.g. SILS – single incision laparoscopic surgery; NOTES – natural orifice transluminal endoscopic surgery), including open surgery operations.

Advanced prosthetics will result in more realistic physical models that will be integrated with VR simulators and simulated patients into a new generation of hybrid simulators offering a much higher level of realism that will also be used to try out new techniques, instruments and operations in silico.

Increased acceptability and patient safety concerns will bring a new, more affordable range of plug-and-play simulators consisting of a core platform with different modules for different procedures offered by competing vendors and no longer restricted to a single specialty.

8.8 Conclusion

These are truly exciting times for surgical education. Carefully designed strategies for the development, evaluation, implementation and integration of simulation and learning technologies into the surgical curriculum promise to revolutionise the fabric of surgical education and fundamentally enhance training and practice, leading to an unprecedented level of quality of care and patient safety. This will require a huge amount of effort and coordination between educators, trainees, practising surgeons and technology developers, but the opportunity must not be missed or it may be many years before it occurs again.

References

2ndHealth (2010) http://secondhealth.wordpress.com/. Accessed 18 Oct 2010.

3DScience (2010) http://www.3dscience.com/. Accessed 18 Oct 2010.

Aggarwal, R., & Darzi, A. (2009). From scalpel to simulator: A surgical journey. *Surgery, 145*(1), 1–4.

Blackboard (2010) www.blackboard.com. Accessed 18 Oct 2010.

Bradley, P. (2006). The history of simulation in medical education and possible future directions. *Medical Education, 40*, 254–262.

Brown, J. S., & Adler, R. P. (2008). Minds on fire: Open education, the long tail, and learning 2.0. *Educause Review, 43*(1), 16–32 (Online).

Brydges, R. (2010). Coordinating progressive levels of simulation fidelity to maximize educational benefit. *Academic Medicine, 85*(5), 806–812.

Chenkin, J., et al. (2008). Procedures can be learned on the web: A randomized study of ultrasound-guided vascular access training. *Academic Emergency Medicine, 15*, 949.

Choi, A. R., Tamblyn, R., & Stringer, M. D. (2008). Electronic resources for sur- gical anatomy. *ANZ Journal of Surgery, 78*, 1082.

Clark, D. (2002). Psychological myths in e-learning. *Medical Teacher, 24*, 598–604.

Cook, D. A., & Dupras, D. M. (2004). A practical guide to developing effective web-based learning. *Journal of General Internal Medicine, 19*(6), 698–707.

Cooper, A. (2004). *The inmates are running the asylum: Why high-tech products drive us crazy and how to restore the sanity*. Indianapolis: Sams.

Corrigan, M., et al. (2008). "SURGENT" – student e-learning for reality: The application of interactive visual images to problem-based learning in undergraduate surgery. *Journal of Surgical Education, 65*, 120.

Criley, J. M., et al. (2008). Innovative web-based multimedia curriculum improves cardiac examination competency of residents. *Journal of Hospital Medicine, 3*, 124 (Online).

Cronbach, L., & Snow, R. (1977). *Aptitudes and instructional methods: A handbook for research on interactions*. New York: Irvington Publishers.

De Rouck, S., Jacobs, A., & Leys, M. (2008). A methodology for shifting the focus of e-health support design onto user needs. *International Journal of Medical Informatics, 77*(9), 589–601.

Deladisma, A., et al. (2008). Medical student satisfaction using a virtual patient system to learn history-taking and communication skills. *Studies in Health Technology and Informatics, 132*, 101–105.

Dix, A., et al. (2004). *Human-computer interaction*. Harlow: Prentice Hall.

Downes, S. (2005). E-learning 2.0. *eLearn Magazine* (Online).

Frank, J. R., et al. (2010). Competency-based medical education: Theory to practice. *Medical Teacher, 32*(8), 638–645.

Garg, A., et al. (1999). Learning anatomy: Do new computer models improve spatial understanding ? *Medical Teacher, 21*(5), 519–522.

Garg, A., Norman, G., & Sperotable, L. (2001). How medical students learn spatial anatomy. *Lancet, 357*, 363–364.

Garg, A., et al. (2002). Is there any real virtue of virtual reality? The minor role of multiple orientations in learning anatomy from computers. *Academic Medicine, 77*(10), S97–S99.

Gaumard (2010). http://www.gaumard.com/. Accessed 18 Oct 2010.

Ghali, F., Cristea, A. I. (2009). Authoring for e-learning 2.0: A case study. In Ninth IEEE International Conference on Advanced Learning Technologies (pp. 170–174), ICALT 2009, Riga, Latvia.

Grant, T., McNeil, M. A., & Luo, X. (2008). Absolute and relative value of patient simulator features as perceived by medical undergraduates. *Simulation in Healthcare, 3*(3), 133–137.

Greenhalgh, T. (2001). Computer assisted learning in undergraduate medical education. *BMJ, 322*, 40–44.

Gutierrez, F., et al. (2007). The effect of degree of immersion upon learning performance in virtual reality simulations for medical education. *Studies in Health Technology and Informatics, 125*, 155–160.

Harris, P., et al. (2010). Competency-based medical education: Implications for undergraduate programs. *Medical Teacher, 32*(8), 646–650.

Heylings, D. (2002). Anatomy 1999–2000: The curriculum, who teaches it and how? *Medical Education, 36*(8), 702–710.

HPS (2010). http://www.meti.com/. Accessed 18 Oct 2010.

i>clicker (2010). http://www.iclicker.com/. Accessed 18 Oct 2010.

Iobst, W. F., et al. (2010). Competency-based medical education in postgraduate medical education. *Medical Teacher, 32*(8), 651–656.

Januszewski, A., & Molenda, M. (2008). *Educational technology: A definition with commentary*. New York/London: Erlbaum/Taylor & Francis.

Jurgaitis, J., et al. (2008). The comparison of 2-dimensional with 3-dimensional hepatic visualization in the clinical hepatic anatomy education. *Medicina Lithuania, 44*(6), 428–438.

Kalet, A. L., et al. (2007). Preliminary evaluation of the Web Initiative for Surgical Education (WISE-MD). *American Journal of Surgery, 194*, 89.

Kemp, M., & Wallace, M. (2000). *Spectacular bodies*. Berkeley: Hayward Gallery Publishing and University of California Press.
Kneebone, R., et al. (2010). Distributed simulation-accessible immersive training. *Medical Teacher, 32*, 65–70.
Krummel, T. M. (1998). Surgical simulation and virtual reality: The coming revolution. *Annals of Surgery, 228*, 635–637.
Lamata, P., et al. (2010). In Soha Maad (Ed.) *Augmented Reality for Minimally Invasive Surgery: Overview and Some Recent Advances*, Augmented Reality. Croatia: InTech (Online).
LapMentor (2010). http://www.simbionix.com/. Accessed 18 Oct 2010.
LapSim (2010). http://www.surgical-science.com/. Accessed 18 Oct 2010.
Levin, A. (2004). *Fewer crashes caused by pilots* (p 2). USA Today (Online), March 2nd.
Levinson, A., et al. (2007). Virtual reality and brain anatomy: A randomised trial of e-learning instructional designs. *Medical Education, 41*(5), 495–501.
Limbs (2010). http://limbsandthings.com/. Accessed 18 Oct 2010.
Luursema, J., et al. (2006). Optimizing conditions for computer-assisted anatomical learning. *Interacting with Computers, 18*(5), 1123–1138.
Luursema. J., Verwey, W., Kommers, P., & Annema, J. (2008) The role of stereopsis in virtual anatomical learning. *Interacting with computers, 20*(4–5), 455–460.
Maran, N. J., & Glavin, R. J. (2003). Low- to high-fidelity simulation – A continuum of medical education? *Medical Education, 37*(Suppl 1), 22–28.
Masters, K., & Ellaway, R. (2008). E-learning in medical education Guide 32 Part 2: Technology, management and design. *Medical Teacher, 30*(5), 474–489.
Meier, A. H., et al. (2005). Implementation of a Web- and simulation-based curriculum to ease the transition from medical school to surgical internship. *American Journal of Surgery, 190*, 137–140.
Minasian-Batmanian, L. C. (2002). Guidelines for developing an online learning strategy for your subject. *Medical Teacher, 24*, 645–647.
MIST (2010). http://www.mentice.com/. Accessed 18 Oct 2010.
Moodle (2010). http://moodle.org/. Accessed 18 Oct 2010.
Preim, B., Ritter, F., & Deussen, O. (1999). A 3D puzzle for learning anatomy. *Lecture Notes in Computer Science, 1679*, 750–757.
Primal (2010). http://www.primalpictures.com/. Accessed 18 Oct 2010.
PROcedure (2010). http://www.simbionix.com/PROcedure.html. Accessed 18 Oct 2010.
Pugh, C., et al. (2009). Surgical education in the internet Era. *The Journal of Surgical Research, 156*, 177–182.
Pulman, A., et al. (2009). Enabling interprofessional education: The role of technology to enhance learning. *Nurse Education Today, 29*, 232–239.
Reality Surgery (2010). https://www.realitysurgery.com/. Accessed 18 Oct 2010.
Romero, C., et al. (2006). Web-based adaptive training simulator system for cardiac life support. *Artificial Intelligence in Medicine, 38*, 67–78.
Ruiz, J. G., Mintzer, M. J., & Leipzig, R. M. (2006). The Impact of e-learning in medical education. *Academic Medicine, 81*(3), 207–212.
Sarker, S., et al. (2008). Constructing a hierarchical task analysis in surgery. *Surgical Endoscopy, 22*(1), 107–111.
Satava, R. (2010). Emerging trends that herald the future of surgical simulation. *The Surgical Clinics of North America, 90*(3), 623–633.
Scalese, R. J., Obeso, V. T., & Issenberg, B. S. (2007). Simulation technology for skills training and competency assessment in medical education. *Journal of General Internal Medicine, 23*(Suppl 1), 46–49.
Shimizu, S., et al. (2007). Telesurgery system with original-quality moving images over high-speed Internet: Expansion within the Asia-Pacific region. *Journal of Laparoendoscopic and Advanced Surgical Techniques, 17*, 673.
Simbionix (2010). http://www.simbionix.com/. Accessed 18 Oct 2010.
SimMan (2010). http://www.laerdal.com/. Accessed 18 Oct 2010

Simulab (2010). http://www.simulab.com/. Accessed 18 Oct 2010.

Sisson, S. D., Hill-Briggs, F., & Levine, D. (2010). How to improve medical education website design. *BMC Medical Education, 10*, 30.

SMART (2010). http://smarttech.com/. Accessed 18 Oct 2010.

STELI (2010). http://www.simulation.londondeanery.ac.uk/. Accessed 18 Oct 2010.

Tavangarian, D., et al. (2004). Is e-learning the solution for Individual learning. *Electronic Journal of E- Learning, 2*(2), 273–280 (Online).

Temkin, B., et al. (2006). An interactive three-dimensional virtual body structures system for anatomical training over the Internet. *Clinical Anatomy, 19*(3), 267–274.

Toltech (2010). http://www.toltech.net/. Accessed 18 Oct 2010.

Toro-Troconis, M. (2010). Design and delivery of game-based learning for virtual patients in second life: Initial findings. In A. Peachey, J. Gillen, D. Livingstone, & S. Robbins (Eds.), *Researching learning in virtual worlds* (pp. 111–138). London: Springer.

Virtual Worlds (2010). http://en.wikipedia.org/wiki/Virtual_world. Accessed 18 Oct 2010.

Voelter, S., & Kraemer, K. (1995). Virtual reality in medicine: A functional classification. In K. Inamura, H. U. Lemke, C. C. Jaffe, & M. W. Vannier (Eds.), *Computer assisted radiology* (pp. 1297–1298). New York: Springer-Verlag Telos.

Ward, J. P. T., et al. (2001). Communication and information technology in medical education. *Lancet, 357*, 792–796.

Wiecha, J., et al. (2010). Learning in a virtual world: Experience with using second life for medical education. *Journal of Medical Internet Research, 12*(1), e1 (Jan 23).

Windsor, J. A. (2009). Role of simulation in surgical education and training. *ANZ Journal of Surgery, 79*, 127–132.

Yip, G., & Rajendran, K. (2008). Snapanatomy, a computer-based interactive tool for independent learning of human anatomy. *Journal of Visual Communication in Medicine, 31*(2), 46–50.

Chapter 9
The Role of Patients in Surgical Education

Debra Nestel and Lesley Bentley

9.1 Introduction

The key ideas in this chapter have historical precedence, since the centrality of patients in education has long been recognised. Osler wrote at the beginning of last century, "For the junior student in medicine and surgery it is a safe rule to have no teaching without a patient for the text, and the best teaching is that taught by the patient himself" (Bliss 1999). We use the term *patient* to describe individuals who are in or have recently completed an episode of treatment. *Simulated patients* (SPs) are individuals trained to portray real patients. The term, *standardised patient* is widely used in Canada and the United States (US) probably reflecting the prevalence of SPs in high-stakes assessments of clinicians where there is a need for repetitions of 'standardised' performance (Wallace 2007). However, we adopt the term 'simulated patient' reflecting the more generic role. Here *trainee* refers to medical students, surgical residents or trainees. *Medical education* includes all under- and post-graduate training while *surgical education* refers to teaching and learning on surgical rotations (undergraduate or residency) or in specialist surgical training. We do not draw a distinction between education and training. Surgical examples are provided where they exist; otherwise we draw on illustrations from other areas of clinical practice. We frequently take a United Kingdom (UK) perspective, as below.

D. Nestel (✉)
Medical Education, Gippsland Medical School, School of Rural Health, Monash University, Melbourne, Australia
e-mail: debra.nestel@monash.edu

L. Bentley
Patient Liaison Group, Royal College of Surgeons, England, UK

H. Fry and R. Kneebone (eds.), *Surgical Education: Theorising an Emerging Domain*, Advances in Medical Education 2, DOI 10.1007/978-94-007-1682-7_9,

9.2 The Role of Patients in Healthcare Services

Since its inception over 60 years ago, the UK National Health Service (NHS) has undergone significant changes. Current policy documents place the patient at centre stage in the NHS (Darzi 2008). Patients may be involved as informant, consultant or partner in drafting strategic healthcare service policy, in service development and at the level of individual care (NHS Modernisation Agency 2005). There is a legal responsibility for NHS Trusts, Primary Care Trusts and Strategic Health Authorities to involve and consult patients and the public in proposals for change. There has also been a shift away from simply seeking the views of patients (as expert advisor) to maintaining their involvement across the life of projects (as partners; NHS Modernisation Agency 2005; Coulter 1999).

Professional medical standards have come under scrutiny with high-profile cases of poorly performing and unethical clinical practice of doctors. The Kennedy Report on high mortality rates in a paediatric surgical unit makes several recommendations for embedding patient and public involvement in the NHS. Healthcare service organisations must make efforts to systematically obtain feedback from patients and professional organisations and must involve the public in their decision-making processes about education and training (Kennedy 2001).

Professional associations and licensing bodies increasingly promote active roles for patients and the public. The specialist Medical Royal Colleges acknowledge the importance of patient involvement in education and professional issues via ‘patient liaison representatives’. These are lay members of Patient Liaison Groups (PLGs) who bring patients’ perspectives to college issues. Lay members of the PLG at the Royal College of Surgeons England (RCSE) are volunteers, most are either patients or carers, are not medically qualified, do not represent any organisation and their views are their own as individuals, independent of the college. Terms of reference outline their scope of practice and a maximum term of office.

Broader societal changes have also influenced the role of patients in education. This includes changes in which healthcare is viewed as a commodity with patients as consumers. The NHS Plan (2000) describes a service that is organised around the needs and concerns of patients and not around the convenience of providers (Department of Health 2000). Patients’ charters have been published since the early 1990s and set out patients’ responsibilities. However, those we examined do not mention involvement in education. In contrast to the early writings on the NHS, patient involvement is no longer assumed but invited with many schemes supporting active patient involvement.

9.3 Changes in Medical and Surgical Training

Influential reports on medical education over the last century reveal a shift in perspective away from passive and relatively powerless patient involvement that reflected strong hierarchical structures in clinical settings (Calman 2007). Educational policy documents have also adopted comparable language about patient (and public) involvement to those in service policy documents. Despite contemporary examples of patient involvement in education, much can still be done to increase contributions and ensure their perspectives are routinely considered.

The landscape in which surgical training occurs is constantly changing (see Chap. 1). Increased clinical throughput, specialisation and the number of seriously ill patients all influence the capacity for training (Kneebone and Nestel 2010). Concerns have been expressed about insufficient exposure to patients for trainees. Restricted working hours are having powerful effects on traditional patterns of learning (Reznick and MacRae 2006; Aggarwal 2006). Long but relatively unstructured apprenticeships are no longer feasible. In response, new surgical curricula have been introduced. New educational methods have permeated all levels of training, such as workplace-based assessments and simulation although the latter is limited by accessibility (see also Chap. 3). The focus of healthcare delivery is shifting away from individual clinicians towards clinical teams, and workforce structure and functions (Williams et al. 2007). This team-based but potentially fragmentary approach to care may profoundly impact patients' experiences. Clinicians may not always be aware of this effect as they grapple with the implications for their own role. More than ever, effective communication with patients, their relatives and colleagues is essential for safe clinical practice. This is an opportunity for genuine engagement of patients in all phases of education from planning to evaluation.

In the UK and Ireland, the Joint Committee on Surgical Training (www.jcst.org) has collaborated with the four Surgical Royal Colleges, the specialist associations and the nine Specialty Advisory Committees to produce the Intercollegiate Surgical Curriculum Programme (www.iscp.ac.uk) for post-graduate surgical education and training. The curriculum defines stages in the development of competent surgical practice to consultant level with each stage underpinned by explicit outcome standards. Common and specialty-specific surgical skills are described together with generic professional skills. The curriculum is mapped to the Good Medical Practice Framework of the General Medical Council of the UK and draws strongly upon the CanMEDS roles (Frank 2005). Skills and behaviours associated with the role of surgeon as 'communicator' are specified in Table 9.1.

9.4 Patients' Experiences of Healthcare Services

Capturing patient perspectives on healthcare experiences can provide a deep understanding of what constitutes quality care. This includes individual interactions with surgeons and the ways these encounters fit within the patients' overall experiences of healthcare. Patients are the only source of information regarding some aspects of service reporting on their experiences through formal and informal channels (Ware et al. 1995).

Table 9.1 Surgeons as communicators: communication with patients and their relatives (https://www.iscp.ac.uk/Syllabus/Overview.aspx?spec-GEN)

Skills
Elicits information regarding the beliefs, concerns and expectations of patients with regard to their presenting conditions
Evaluates factors such as the patient's age, gender, ethnic, cultural, socio-economic and spiritual values and the impact that these may have on the management of that patient and condition
Delivers information to the patient and family humanely and in a way that is understandable
Provides the information the patient needs or wants to make a decision by using systematic approach that is empathetic, non-coercive
Works with patients who present significant communication challenges such as anger or confusion, or an ethno-cultural background different from the doctor's own
Supervises the co-ordination of care for hospital patients with terminal illness
Counsels patients effectively
Recognises a situation where a potential complaint is developing and taking the appropriate steps to defuse the situation where possible
Behaviours
Shows empathy
Adapts style and approach to each individual patient's needs
Avoids using technical medical jargon
Gives opportunities for the patient to ask questions, encourages discussion and promotes the patient's participation in decision making to the level appropriate for the situation
Checks patient's and/or relative's understanding throughout the consultation before moving on
Encourages patients who have knowledge about their condition to use this when they are making decisions about their care
Responds to patient's concerns, anxieties or doubts as they arise
Recognises when the limits or his/her competence has been reached and refers to a more senior practitioner

As quality assurance measures, patient satisfaction surveys provide valuable feedback. Patients rate elements of the healthcare experience (Ware et al. 1995) on variables patients are thought to be most concerned about (e.g. making appointments, waiting times, politeness of staff, comfort of facilities). However, they may also include specific judgements on the encounter with the doctor such as interpersonal and professional skills (e.g. listening, explaining, showing interest, friendliness, respect and reassurance) (NHS Modernisation Agency 2005; Thorne et al. 2002; Richards and Coulter 2007).

Aggregate survey data has educational value identifying strengths and areas for development. Surveys may offer insight into a surgical team's performance prompting remedial action and maintenance of valued practice. This type of data also highlights the notion of a patient 'journey' or 'pathway' with events impinging on each other. The encounter with the surgeon is just one interaction in the patient's overall journey. A US-based survey and telephone study of patient satisfaction with surgeons' communication skills suggested effective communication before and during hospitalisation. However, patients were less satisfied after discharge when new questions arose. The authors proposed teaching strategies to improve surgeon communication for the longer-term support of patients (D'Angelica et al. 1998).

Survey data has limitations such as the structure and content of questions, their level of detail, timing and method of distribution. Patients may also find it hard to comment on treatment during their care for fear of reprisals, lack of confidence, pain or low energy.

Patients' experiences of healthcare providers are also evidenced in verbal or written expressions of gratitude or complaints. Although gratitude is often non-specific, complaints vary in specificity. Timing also varies with verbal feedback most often provided at the point of care while written feedback is commonly delayed. Expressions of gratitude are more likely to be offered to clinicians, with complaints sent to a senior and/or administrative officer. Post-discharge complaints make it more difficult for feedback to be acted on in part because of a highly mobile workforce, especially for trainees. The responsibility for dealing with complaints is often removed from the source resulting in little direct action. The severity of the complaint (and its consequences) may influence the extent to which feedback returns to the individuals. Encouraging trainees to reflect on gratitude and complaints is important. The non-specific nature of gratitude makes it harder for trainees to identify attitudes and behaviours that were appreciated. Learning from complaints may be easier since they are more likely to refer to specific events. Again, reflecting on the event, its circumstances and outcome may promote learning and improve quality.

Patients have been asked to keep diaries revealing a longitudinal experience of care (Kielmann et al. 2009). From diaries, it is apparent that patients experience health care differently to those who deliver it, that is, patients have their own perspectives that can be difficult for health professionals to recognise from their position of expertise. Although potentially valuable, it is probably not feasible for trainees to make direct use of patients' diaries. Observing a patient support group may provide frank and immediate insight to the breadth of patients' responses to healthcare services.

9.5 Patient Involvement in Medical and Surgical Education

Patient involvement in medical and surgical education varies widely. We outline examples in and outside clinical settings while acknowledging there are many others. First, we outline relevant theoretical perspectives. Bleakley and Bligh argue for raising the profile of patients as educators (Bleakley and Bligh 2008). Using similar language to Osler, they suggest that patients are 'texts' that can be read to co-produce knowledge to support the development of clinical reasoning. That is, the trainee–patient relationship is not only a starting point but also potentially a continuous source of learning. A critical role for the clinician is in facilitating and valuing trainee–patient learning. Of course, there is value in the trainee–clinician relationship but it has dominated 'knowledge production' and minimises potential and critical learning from patients. Bleakley and Bligh also identify the paradox that patient-centredness is usually not learned from patients but from clinicians and educators.

Table 9.2 Potential content for trainees' learning *with* and *from* real and/or simulated patients in surgical education

Stage	Content
Pre-operative	Patient's ideas (e.g. about symptoms, illness, disease)
	Patient's concerns (e.g. most worrying, other concerns and the reasons why)
	Patients' expectations (e.g. of the consultation, of the surgery, of the eventual outcome of their problem)
	Patient assessment skills (e.g. history-taking, physical examination)
	Information giving skills (e.g. explaining procedures, interventions and operations; obtaining informed consent; explaining risk; giving bad news)
	Negotiation skills
	Investigative and procedural skills (e.g. patient experience)
Intra-operative	Surgical technique (e.g. patient experience)
Post-operative	Patient's ideas (e.g. about their symptoms, illness, disease)
	Patient's concerns (e.g. most worrying, other concerns and the reasons why)
	Patients' expectations (e.g. of the consultation, of the eventual outcome of their problem)
	Patient assessment skills
	Negotiation skills
	Information giving (e.g. explaining post-operative and discharge care; giving bad news; disclosing error)
Overarching	Professionalism
	Patient safety
	Quality
	Clinical reasoning

Constructivist learning theories describe the ways in which individuals create new knowledge by engaging with others through talk, activity and problem solving. Social environments are critical for learning. Wenger locates or situates learning in 'communities of practice' (Wenger 1998; see also Chap. 2 for more on learning theories). Although patients appear in the 'community', they have largely been marginalised in the 'practice', that is in co-construction of clinical knowledge. Patients as full members of the 'community of practice' may enrich and improve the quality of clinical learning.

A systematic review of real patient involvement in medical education identified 47 research papers (Jha et al. 2009). Most studies focused on the role of patients as teachers, with fewer studies reporting roles in assessment and course development. Most studies were set in undergraduate medical education. Authors argued for patient involvement as a means of bringing patient perspectives into education. Patients mainly contributed to teaching of clinical and communication skills. Few studies implemented robust evaluation strategies making it difficult to draw conclusions about educational impact.

Learning from patients may occur in any stage of their surgical pathway – pre-, intra- or post-operatively (Table 9.2). Involvement in education may occur during the routine delivery of care or form part of a formal teaching session. Trainees may be observed interacting with the patient or may observe or assist others. Audiovisual recordings can facilitate later review of performance. A US study exploring empathic communication of surgical trainees in their first visit for oncology consultations used videotapes for analysis of communication behaviours and identified trainees' inattentiveness to patients' expressed emotions providing a clear target for improved behaviour (Easter and Beach 2004).

Patients may participate as experts in their illness/condition in teaching sessions to share their experiences from the perspective of a patient (Nestel et al. 2008d). Although there are many examples for patients with chronic illness and in undergraduate medical education, we could not locate any in surgical education. Negative and high-impact experiences may motivate some patients to contribute to education (Bideau et al. 2006; Blasco et al. 2005). Sensitively facilitated, sharing of these experiences are likely to be rich learning opportunities for trainees, surgical educators and patients.

Clinical skills assessments are often performed with patients such as the Objective Structured Clinical Examination (see also Chap. 5). However, there is a shift to working with SPs in such assessments to achieve standardisation of assessments (Adamo 2003). The patients may be asked to be themselves or adopt a given history. They may also be asked to make a judgement on trainee performance.

Multi-source feedback (see also Chap. 5) offers another way in which patients can contribute to surgical education. Currently, multi-source feedback provides summary assessment data to individual trainees on many facets of professional practice collected from their colleagues. This could be extended to patients who can make judgements on trainee performance from their own perspective.

There are several excellent patient-focused resources in websites, films and books. Audiovisual accounts of patients' illness and healthcare experiences are recorded and made available online. These are often designed for patients but may have relevance for health professionals. The DiPEX resources are a high-quality database of patients' experiences of illness from diagnosis through recovery (Ziebland and McPherson 2006). Videorecorded accounts of patients' experiences have advantages and disadvantages for patients and trainees when compared with in person discussions. The former offers a resource to be accessed at the trainees' convenience and the patient only needs to revisit the experience once. Disadvantages include no opportunity for patient-trainee interaction to seek clarification or further detail.

9.6 The Advantages and Disadvantages of Patient Involvement for Different Groups

9.6.1 Outcomes for Patients

Active involvement of patients in education has diverse outcomes. Although we can ascribe positive or negative value to outcomes, it is really the patient who makes this judgement. The literature reports positive outcomes such as higher levels of engagement in self-care, feeling valued, improved levels of health related knowledge, specific therapeutic benefits and extra attention (Haq et al. 2006; Blasco et al. 2005; Vail et al. 1996; Lehmann et al. 1997; Cowles et al. 2001; Stacy and Spencer 1999). Negative outcomes include the psychological impact of revisiting stressful experiences, feeling burdened by the 'responsibility', distress associated with a lack of insight into their condition and/or deficits in trainees' communication skills, reinforcement of the 'sick role' and time pressures (Walters et al. 2003; Coleman and Murray 2002). Patients may be compromised in consenting to participate and providing honest feedback to trainees whilst receiving care. Ways to ensure that patients can comfortably decline involvement need to be practised. Timing of contribution is also an important issue. At different phases during treatment, remission or recovery the impact on patients may vary. Although emotionally expressive interactions can be powerful they must not cause harm to the patient. Patients may also feel uncomfortable using their experience to improve the care of others questioning their validity in improving quality for others.

9.6.2 Outcomes for Trainees

Positive outcomes for trainees of learning from real patients include making sense of theory, providing a meaningful and memorable context for knowledge (Bell et al. 2009). Pattern recognition, communication and physical examination skills develop (Gaver et al. 2005; Klein et al. 2000; Smith et al. 2000). Trainees have also reported improved understanding of social and psychological factors in illness, disease and response to treatment and a temporal dimension often absent from readings about clinical medicine (Bell et al. 2009; Thistlethwaite and Cockayne 2004; Stacy and Spencer 1999). Additionally, trainees have reported an appreciation of the complexity of patients' experiences and clinical practice (Bell et al. 2009; Bideau et al. 2006; Smith et al. 2000; Gaver et al. 2005). Negative outcomes include the inability of trainees to locate patients with conditions about which they must learn. Some trainees lack confidence or skills to seek active patient involvement. Learning from real patients has also left some trainees feeling uncomfortable and incompetent (Bell et al. 2009; Barnes et al. 1980).

9.6.3 Outcomes for Clinicians/Educators

Positive outcomes may include greater knowledge, greater personal satisfaction, improved relationships with patients, development of attitudes commensurate with patient-centred care and improved interpersonal skills. In response to specific patient involvement there may be acquisition of new and important information to assist diagnosis and management. Trainees may also value the professionalism of consultants who are willing to teach and learn with and from patients. Negative outcomes for clinicians may include balancing and slowing the delivery of care with education, compromising relationships with patients who may ask for favours for participating in teaching, managing relationships with patients whom trainees may have upset or created difficulties.

9.7 Simulated Patient Involvement in Medical and Surgical Education

SPs involvement in medical education was first were reported in 1963, at the University of Southern California. Barrows trained an SP to simulate the history and examination findings of a patient with multiple sclerosis and paraplegia (Barrows 1968). Using a checklist, the SP assessed the performance of the trainee. SPs now make a substantial contribution to medical education. Initially, SP involvement was ancillary; however, there are several drivers to their expansion and centrality in curricula. These include ethical imperatives for learning in simulation, patient safety initiatives, patient empowerment and increased numbers of medical students with reduced access to patients in clinical settings. Additional drivers include growing acceptance of simulation as an educational method, emerging theoretical underpinning and the maturation of SP programmes.

SPs work as a 'proxy' for real patients coached to portray patients and to provide feedback to trainees. SPs have the potential to raise the profile of patient perspectives, to promote the development of professionalism and effective communication in trainees. Additional benefits of trained SPs include the provision of predetermined scenarios of given levels of challenge that reflect specific goals of training programmes, the opportunity to tailor learning to individual trainee needs, ease of scheduling as required and the provision of standardised scenarios for assessment of trainees in clinical and surgical skills. Unlike real patients, SPs are trained to provide structured feedback to trainees on their performance.

In undergraduate medical education, SPs usually play the role of a patient in supporting the development of a range of interpersonal and professional skills. Guidelines for roles are provided by clinicians and educators or designed with participants at the time of the session. SPs also play 'standardised' roles in high-stakes assessments in which they may be asked to make judgements on trainee performance. *Unannounced* or *incognito SPs* enter clinical practices with the purpose of assessing the actual practice of individual clinicians. Interventions usually take place in primary care and often go undetected by the clinician. Several excellent papers outlining the breadth of work undertaken by SPs have been published (Barrows 1968; Vu et al. 1992; Ker et al. 2005; Petrusa 2002; Adamo 2003; May et al. 2009; Rethans et al. 2007; Wallace 2007).

The scope of SP methodology is rapidly expanding. For example, SPs have worked in diverse and complex educational activities. In Chap. 3, Kneebone describes the concept of patient-focused simulations (PFS), where SPs are linked with simulators (benchtop models such as suture pads) in simulated clinical settings to support the development of procedural skills. Trainees are expected to integrate psychomotor, dexterity, patient-centred and professional skills essential for safe clinical practice as they perform 'procedures'. No longer are trainees expected to learn discrete skills separately and removed from the settings in which they will be practiced. Rather, trainees can rehearse the entire set of skills and receive feedback from expert clinical and patient perspectives. The approach has been applied with undergraduate medical students, junior doctors, surgical trainees and new roles practitioners (Kneebone et al. 2006a; Nestel et al. 2010b; LeBlanc et al. 2009; Moulton et al. 2009).

In the developments described above, SPs work directly with real patients to write and perform authentic roles (Nestel et al. 2008c). Actors (SPs) play the roles of healthcare professionals in team simulations in the operating theatre, the interventional suite and at handover (Black et al. 2006; Nestel et al. 2005, 2008b; Kassab et al. 2010). Handheld computers and other technologies have been introduced for SPs to provide feedback to trainees (Nestel et al. 2008a; Kneebone et al. 2008). SPs lead some aspects of teaching sessions such as briefing and debriefing students, training them in managing emotions and performance anxiety, and orientating them to role-play. SPs are often called to work in scenarios that are sensitive, highly charged and for which high-stakes judgements are made.

In surgical education, SPs support trainees in learning history-taking, physical examination, procedural skills, operative skills, to give information, to explain risk, to obtain informed consent, clinical decision making, ethics and professionalism (Moulton et al. 2009; LeBlanc et al. 2009). SPs also contribute to training in managing 'difficult' interactions such as those involving patients with strong emotions, cultural differences and communication deficits, and in disclosing error and making apologies when things have gone wrong (Chan et al. 2005; Chipman et al. 2007).

SP-based education is becoming increasingly professionalised with professional associations although no professional licensing exists. In order to work in demanding scenarios, SPs require an understanding of education, interpersonal skills theory, patient-centred communication skills and performance. They may be placed in highly emotive scenarios with diverse groups of individuals (SPs, students, tutors, clinicians, researchers). Responding to these complex demands, 'professional' responsibilities for all those involved in SP work have been developed by stakeholders (trainees, tutors, administrators and SPs) in SP-based teaching (Table 9.3). Reciprocal guidelines were also developed for trainees, tutors and administrators, illustrating the partnership and collaborative nature of this work (Nestel et al. 2010a).

9.8 Patient-Focused Simulations (PFS)

PFS in surgical education provide the opportunity for trainees to integrate the skills required for safe clinical practice of procedural (e.g. intravenous cannulation, urinary catheterisation) and operative skills on conscious patients (e.g. lipoma

Table 9.3 Expectations of SPs in professional education

1.	Possess a range of qualities such as self-awareness, sensitivity, empathy, vigilance, respect, enthusiasm, curiosity, warmth and a good memory
2.	Possess facilitation skills
3.	Work in partnership with other SPs and teachers to support trainee learning
4.	Show respect to trainees
5.	Have knowledge of basic educational principles
6.	Have knowledge of principles of patient-centred communication
7.	Model behaviours for effectively managing difficult situations
8.	Use knowledge and experience to support trainee learning
9.	Use acting expertise to portray roles – avoid stereotype or caricature
10.	Actively participate in training and teaching sessions
11.	Invite feedback on performance (e.g. role-play and feedback)
12.	Critique scenarios and SP roles
13.	Follow programme guidelines in giving feedback to trainees
14.	Participate in session/programme evaluations
15.	Keep information about trainees' confidential although incidents or concerns should be reported to the programme director in a timely fashion
16.	Be familiar with the prescribed SP roles

excision and wound closure, carotid endarterectomy). The physical, psychological and social fidelity of real work environments is recreated, enabling trainees to integrate the broad sets of skills (e.g. professional, psychomotor, communication) that are often taught separately but all required in real clinical practice. Having a 'patient' at the centre of the scenario creates a sense of reality that is absent in manikins or simulator kit. PFS can be used flexibly to support learning. Trainees are first encouraged to reflect on their prior relevant experiences and to identify their learning needs. Immediately after the scenario, trainees self-assess and receive feedback from clinical assessors and SPs in approximately equal measure (Kneebone and Nestel 2005; Kneebone et al. 2008; Nestel et al. 2008a). Scenarios are videotaped enabling facilitated feedback or trainee-led reflection. Results from several studies suggest that trainees benefit from these experiences and that PFS offers learning opportunities different from traditional approaches to skills teaching (LeBlanc et al. 2009; Moulton et al. 2009). Although studies have shown that trainees found the scenarios and SP roles realistic, convincing and richly complex for learning (Kneebone et al. 2006b, 2007), real patients were not involved at any stage.

9.9 Authenticity in Simulated Patient Methodology

We have stated that SPs can function as proxies for real patients. Given the emphasis of healthcare service and education policy documents of involving patients as partners, they are notably absent from the realm of SP work. In part, this is for obvious reasons, that is, SPs are working instead of real patients because of their many advantages (e.g. standardisation, repeatable performance, feedback etc). However, we have a responsibility to ensure that SPs' performances are derived from real patient experiences, that the voice of the SP is that of a 'real' patient. Otherwise, SPs may simply serve to recreate clinicians' and educators' perceptions of patients' experiences (Nestel et al. 2008c; Morris 2006).

There is little published literature on the processes adopted for writing SP roles and scenarios. Common practice is that roles are crafted by clinicians and educators often derived from an individual patient's history or an amalgam of several patients' records. There are important reasons for this including the pressure to produce new roles for teaching and assessments, the desire to tailor learning experiences to trainees' individual needs and to align roles with other curriculum activities. But clinician or educator-generated roles may be quite different from the authentic experiences of individuals (Black et al. 2006) that they are interpretations of a patient's history and without direct patient involvement. However, it is challenging for those immersed in teaching and the delivery of healthcare to see through the eyes of someone who is not. The literature reports many examples of clinicians experiences as patients (Klitzman 2007; Jones 2005; O'Brien 2008). Clinicians and patients think differently about many facets of healthcare (Morris 2006; Temple et al. 1998; Lazarus 2007). Because of this gap between clinical and patient perspectives and the implicit assumption that SPs are representing real patients, there is an obligation to explore authenticity in all aspects of SP work.

Here we summarise three SP-based projects in which real patients have been invited to participate. The first project explored the feasibility of immersive simulated-based training for surgical trainees in carotid endarterectomy (Black et al. 2006). During the operation, patients are conscious contributing to progress by maintaining some speech and motor movements in order for the anaesthetist and surgeon to assess cerebral perfusion. In the simulation, a carotid model was aligned with an SP lying on the operating table in a simulated theatre with a full operating team. The trainee was required to perform the operation. Pre-operatively, the trainee obtained an informed consent from the SP (and partner) and made a follow-up visit in the recovery room. Audiovisual recordings were made and used to provide feedback to trainees on all aspects of surgical expertise. In order to base the SP role and scenario in reality, patients who had undergone this operation were interviewed exploring their experiences, concerns and information needs pre-, intra- and post-operatively. Experiences as reported by patients differed from those that the research team had considered, adding a richness and a genuine patient perspective in the crafting of the SP role (Black et al. 2006).

In the second project, patients in the emergency department who had undergone procedural and examination skills (e.g. intravenous cannulation, ECG) were interviewed. SP roles and scenarios were then constructed based on these individual patients' histories and experiences. This information was used to develop SP roles for patient-focused simulations. SPs were asked to rate the realism of these real patient and faculty-generated roles for procedural skills. Although differences in

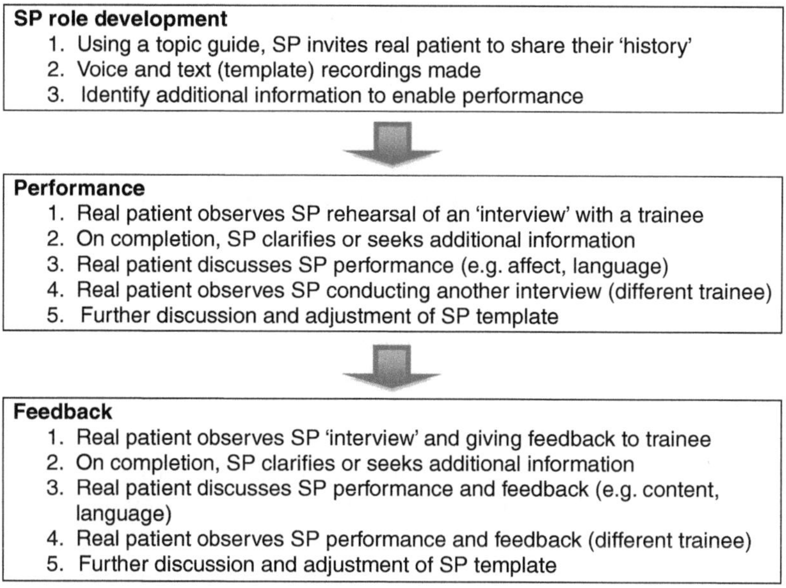

Fig. 9.1 Process for including real patients in SP role development and training

ratings were not statistically significant, analysis of free text comments showed the benefits of providing authentic patient language derived from interviews with real patients (Nestel et al. 2008c).

In the third project, patients with complex histories were recruited to participate in SP training for role performance and feedback. There were three parts to the project (Fig. 9.1). First, crafting the SP role was based on individual patients working with two SPs to obtain the patient's perspective of the "facts" (~60 min). Faculty observed and facilitated where it was thought to be necessary. Although a template was used to record information, the patient's story was first heard in full. Additional information was discussed including the patient's attitudes towards their illness, clinicians and the healthcare service. SPs noted the real patients' use of language, accents and mannerisms. Discussions were also voice-recorded for later reference. Second, the real patient then observed the SPs in consultations with trainees. After the encounters, the real patient coached the SPs on their performance with respect to authentic representation. Several iterations and discussions resulted in what the real patient deemed authentic performance (~60–90 min). Third, SPs were observed by real patients giving feedback to trainees. The SPs were consistently more critical and provided more detailed feedback than the real patients whom they were portraying. SPs also emphasised different points. The SP adopted the language of a professional communications expert (e.g. "There were few open ended questions") compared with the real patient (e.g. "I did not have a chance to really tell you what was happening to me"). The process proved salutary to the SPs involved, reminding them of the realities of the people they represent.

The educational impact of these approaches to involving real patients in SP-based work needs further evaluation, but it was already very clear how easy it was to make inaccurate assumptions about patients' attitudes and experiences.

9.10 Simulated Patient Involvement in High-Stakes Assessments

SPs now regularly participate in high-stakes assessments. SPs have the responsibility of performing consistently according to a prescribed role and of making judgements about trainees. Although checklists are sometimes used, rating scales are reported to have greater reliability and validity. SPs commonly make judgements about interpersonal skills but this may be from a technical perspective (e.g. use of open-ended questions, empathy, transition statements). They are sometimes trained to assess clinical decision making, examination and other professional skills. Despite the statistical reliability and validity, it is important to remember that often these judgements are made from the perspective of the 'professional' SP as proxy for a clinician assessor rather than as proxy for a real patient. We need to be clear about the nature of the assessment the SP is offering. In many instances, it appears that these perspectives become one rather than appreciated and valued for their diversity.

9.11 Concluding Remarks

Real and simulated patients have important contributions to make to medical and surgical education. Many opportunities go untapped. Whether patient surveys on healthcare experience or active involvement of patients in the process of care delivery, patients have much to offer. While healthcare service policy has embraced patient and public involvement, education policy has been slower and less committed.

Following Bleakley and Bligh (2008), we argue for a shift in prominence of the trainee–patient learning dyad, facilitated rather than led by clinicians. Similarly, we argue for real patient–SP dyads facilitated by educators to create authentic SP roles, performance and feedback, which can then be incorporated into patient-focused training programmes. We propose that patients be considered as full (although transient) members of the 'community of practice' promoting learning for clinicians, trainees and patients.

There are benefits and challenges of involving patients at all stages of education. Of course, not all patients will be suited to such work. Ways need to be found to ensure that a breadth of patient perspectives can be represented. The emphasis on educational interventions of patient involvement at the undergraduate level is noteworthy. However, there are very few examples in specialty training, where the dominant learning sphere seems to be the clinician-trainee with the patient ancillary. Of course, we will need to evaluate the educational impact on trainees of real patient and SP methodologies. There is much to be done to explore the breadth of possibilities for both.

References

Adamo, G. (2003). Simulated and standardized patients in OSCEs: Achievements and challenges 1992–2003. *Medical Teacher, 25*, 262–270.

Aggarwal, R. (2006). Technical-skills training in the 21st century. *The New England Journal of Medicine, 355*, 2695.

Barnes, H., Alabanese, M., & Schroder, J. (1980). Informed consent: The use of inpatients as teaching-patients for sophomore medical students. *Journal of Medical Education, 55*, 698–703.

Barrows, H. S. (1968). Simulated patients in medical teaching. *Canadian Medical Association Journal, 98*, 674–676.

Bell, K., Boshiuzen, H., Scherpbier, A., & Dornan, T. (2009). When only the real thing will do: Junior medical students' learning from real patients. *Medical Education, 43*, 1036–1043.

Bideau, M., Guerne, P., Bianchi, M., & Huber, P. (2006). Benefits of a programme taking advantage of patient-instructors to teach and assess musculoskeletal skills in medical students. *Annals of the Rheumatic Diseases, 65*, 1626–1630.

Black, S., Nestel, D., Horrocks, E., Harrison, R., Jones, N., Wetzel, C., & Kneebone, R. (2006). Evaluation of a framework for case development and simulated patient training for complex procedures. *Journal of Simulation in Healthcare, 1*, 66–71.

Blasco, P., Kohen, H., & Shapland, C. (2005). Parents as teachers: Design and establishment of a training programme for residents. *Medical Education, 33*, 695–701.

Bleakley, A., & Bligh, J. (2008). Students learning from patients: Let's get real in medical education. *Advances in Health Sciences Education, 13*, 89–107.

Bliss, M. (1999). *William osler: A life in medicine*. New York: Oxford University Press.

Calman, K. (2007). *Medical education, past, present and future*. Edinburgh: Churchill Livingstone Elsevier.

Chan, D. K., Gallagher, T. H., Reznick, R., & Levinson, W. (2005). How surgeons disclose medical errors to patients: A study using standardized patients. *Surgery, 138*, 851–858.

Chipman, J. G., Beilman, G. J., Schmitz, C. C., & Seatter, S. C. (2007). Development and pilot testing of an OSCE for difficult conversations in surgical intensive care. *Journal of Surgical Education, 64*, 79–87.

Coleman, K., & Murray, E. (2002). Patients' views and feelings on the community-based teaching of undergraduate medical students: A qualitative study. *Family Practice, 19*, 183–188.

Coulter, A. (1999). Paternalism or partnership?: Patients have grown up and there's no going back. *BMJ, 319*, 719–720.

Cowles, R. A., Moyer, C. A., Sonnad, S. S., Simeone, D. M., Knol, J. A., Eckhauser, F. E., Mulholland, M. W., & Colletti, L. M. (2001). Doctor-patient communication in surgery: Attitudes and expectations of general surgery patients about the involvement and education of surgical residents. *Journal of the American College of Surgeons, 193*, 73–80.

D'Angelica, M., Hirsch, K., Ross, H., Passik, S., & Brennan, M. F. (1998). Surgeon-patient communication in the treatment of pancreatic cancer. *Archives of Surgery, 133*, 962–966.

Darzi, A. (2008). *High quality care for all*. London: TSO

Department of Health. (2000). *The NHS plan – Summary*. London: Department of Health.

Easter, D. W., & Beach, W. (2004). Competent patient care is dependent upon attending to empathic opportunities presented during interview sessions. *Current Surgery, 61*, 313–318.

Frank, J. (2005). *The CanMEDS 2005 physician competency framework. Better standards. Better physicians. Better care*. Ottawa: The Royal College of Physicians and Surgeons of Canada.
Gaver, A., Borkan, J., & Weingarten, M. (2005). Illness in context and families as teachers: A year-long project for medical students. *Academic Medicine, 80*, 448–451.
Haq, I., Fuller, J., & Dacre, J. (2006). The use of patient partners with back pain to teach undergraduate medical students. *Rheumatology, 45*, 430–434.
Intercollegiate Surgical Curriculum Project (2010). https://www.iscp.ac.uk/. Last accessed 1 Jan 2010.
Jha, V., Quinton, N., Bekker, H., & Roberts, T. (2009). Strategies and interventions for the invovlement of real patients in medical education: A systematic review. *Medical Education, 43*, 10–20.
Jones, P. (2005). *Doctors as patients*. Oxford: Radcliffe.
Kassab, E., King, D., Hull, L., Arora, S., Sevdalis, N., Kneebone, R., & Nestel, D. (2010). Actor training for surgical simulations. *Medical Teacher, 32*(3), 256–258.
Kennedy, I. (2001). The Inquiry into the management of care of childrenreceiving complex heart surgery at the Bristol Royal Infirmary. London: Crown Publishing.
Ker, J. S., Dowie, A., Dowell, J., Dewar, G., Dent, J., Ramsay, J., Benvie, S., Bracher, L., & Jackson, C. (2005). Twelve tips for developing and maintaining a simulated patient bank. *Medical Teacher, 27*, 4–9.
Kielmann, T., Huby, G., Powell, A., Sheikh, A., Price, D., Williams, S., & Pinnock, H. (2009). From support to boundary: A qualitative study of the border between self-care and professional care. *Patient Education and Counselling, 79*(1), 55–61.
Klein, S., Tracy, D., Kitchener, H., & Walker, L. (2000). The effects of the participation of patients with cancer in teaching communication skills to medical undergraduates: A randomised study with follow-up after two years. *European Journal of Cancer, 36*, 273–281.
Klitzman, R. (2007). *When doctors become patients*. New York: Oxford University Press.
Kneebone, R., & Nestel, D. (2005). Learning clinical skills - the place of simulation and feedback. *The Clinical Teacher, 2*, 86–90.
Kneebone, R., & Nestel, D. (2010). Learning and teaching clinical procedures. In S. E. Dornan (Ed.), *Medical education: Theory and practice* (pp. 172–192). London: Elsevier.
Kneebone, R., Nestel, D., Wetzel, C., Black, S., Jacklin, R., Aggarwal, R., Yadollahi, F., Wolfe, J., Vincent, C., & Darzi, A. (2006a). The human face of simulation: Patient-focused simulation training. *Academic Medicine, 81*, 919–924.
Kneebone, R. L., Nestel, D., Chrzanowska, J., Barnet, A. E., & Darzi, A. (2006b). Innovative training for new surgical roles–the place of evaluation. *Medical Education, 40*, 987–994.
Kneebone, R. L., Nestel, D., Vincent, C., & Darzi, A. (2007). Complexity, risk and simulation in learning procedural skills. *Medical Education, 41*, 808–814.
Kneebone, R., Bello, F., Nestel, D., Mooney, N., Codling, A., Yadollahi, F., Tierney, T., Wilcockson, D., & Darzi, A. (2008). Learner-centred feedback using remote assessment of clinical procedures. *Medical Teacher, 30*, 795–801.
Lazarus, P. A. (2007). Patients' experiences and perceptions of medical student candidates sitting a finals examination. *Medical Teacher, 29*, 478–483.
Leblanc, V. R., Tabak, D., Kneebone, R., Nestel, D., Macrae, H., & Moulton, C. A. (2009). Psychometric properties of an integrated assessment of technical and communication skills. *American Journal of Surgery, 197*, 96–101.
Lehmann, L., Brancati, F., Chen, M., Roter, D., & Dobbs, A. (1997). The effect of bedside case presentations on patients' perceptions of their medical care. *The New England Journal of Medicine, 336*, 1150–1155.
May, W., Park, J., & Lee, J. (2009). A ten-year review of the literature on the use of standardized patients in teaching and learning: 1996–2005. *Medical Teacher, 31*, 487–492.
Morris, P. (2006). The patient's voice in doctor's learning. In J. Thistlethwaite & P. Morris (Eds.), *The patient doctor consultation in primary care: Theory and practice*. London: Royal College of General Practitioners.

Moulton, C.-A., Tabak, D., Kneebone, R., Nestel, D., Macrae, H., & Leblanc, V. R. (2009). Teaching communication skills using the integrated procedural performance instrument (IPPI): A randomized controlled trial. *American Journal of Surgery, 197*, 113–118.

Nestel, D., Kneebone, R., & Barnet, A. (2005). Teaching communication skills for handover: Perioperative specialist practitioners. *Medical Education, 39*, 1157.

Nestel, D., Bello, F., Kneebone, K. A. R., & Darzi, A. (2008a). Remote assessment and learner-centred feedback using the Imperial College Feedback and Assessment System (ICFAS). *The Clinical Teacher, 5*, 88–92.

Nestel, D., Black, S., Kneebone, R., Wetzel, C., Thomas, P., Wolfe, S., & Darzi, A. (2008b). Simulated anaesthetists in high fidelity simulations for surgical training: Feasibility of a training programme for actors. *Medical Teacher, 30*, 407–413.

Nestel, D., Cecchini, M., Calandrini, M., Chang, L., Dutta, R., Tierney, T., Brown, R., & Kneebone, R. (2008c). Real patient involvement in role development evaluating patient focused resources for clinical procedural skills. *Medical Teacher, 30*, 795–801.

Nestel, D., Tierney, T., Muir, E., & Kubacki, A. (2008d). Learning to talk with patients: Feasibility of a volunteer simulated patient programme for first year medical students. *International Journal of Clinical Skills, 2*, 121–128.

Nestel, D., Clark, S., Ashwell, V., Tabak, D., Muir, E., & Higham, J. (2010a). Defining responsibilites of simulated patients in medical education. *Simulation in Healthcare, 5*(3), 161–168.

Nestel, D., Kneebone, R., Barnet, A., Tierney, T., & Darzi, A. (2010b). Evaluation of a clinical communication program for peri-operative and surgical care practitioners. *Quality and Safety in Healthcare, 19*(5), e1. April 21, 1–7.

NHS Modernisation Agency. (2005). *Improvement leaders guides: Involving patients and carers*. London: Department of Health Publications.

O'Brien, C. (2008). *Never say die*. Sydney: HarperCollinsPublishing.

Petrusa, E. (2002). Clinical performance assessments. In G. Norman, C. van der Vleuten, & D. Newble (Eds.), *International handbook of research in medical education* (pp. 673–710). Dordrecht: Kluwer Academic.

Rethans, J., Gorter, S., Bokken, L., & Morrison, L. (2007). Unannounced standardised patients in real practice: A systematic literature review. *Medical Education, 41*, 537–549.

Reznick, R., & Macrae, H. (2006). Teaching Surgical Skills – Changes in the Wind. *The New England Journal of Medicine, 355*, 2664–2669.

Richards, N., & Coulter, A. (2007). *Is the NHS becoming more patient-centred? Trends from the national surveys of NHS patients in England 2002–07*. Oxford: Picker Institute Europe.

Smith, M., Henry-Edwards, S., Shanahan, E., & Ahern, M. (2000). Evaluation of patient partners in the teaching of the musculoskeletal examination. *The Journal of Rheumatology, 27*, 1533–1537.

Stacy, R., & Spencer, J. (1999). Patients as teachers: A qualitative study of patients' views on their role in a community-based undergraduate project. *Medical Education, 33*, 688–694.

Temple, W., Toews, J., Fidler, H., Lockyer, J. M., Taenzer, P., & Parboosingh, E. J. (1998). Concordance in communication between surgeon and patient. *Canadian Journal of Surgery, 41*, 439–445.

Thistlethwaite, J., & Cockayne, E. (2004). Early student-patient interactions: The views of patients regarding their experiences. *Medical Teacher, 26*, 420–422.

Thorne, L., Ellamushi, H., Mtandari, S., Mcevoy, A. W., Powell, M., & Kitchen, N. D. (2002). Auditing patient experience and satisfaction with neurosurgical care: Results of a questionnaire survey.[see comment]. *British Journal of Neurosurgery, 16*, 243–255.

Vail, R., Mahon-Salazar, C., Morrison, A., & Kalet, A. (1996). Patients as teachers: An integrated approach to teaching medical students about the ambulatory care of HIV-infected patients. *Patient Education and Counselling, 27*, 95–101.

Vu, N., Barrows, H., Marcy, M., Verhulst, S., Colliver, J., & Travis, T. (1992). Six years of comprehensive, clinical performance-based assessment using standardized patients at the Southern Illinois University School of Medicine. *Academic Medicine, 67*, 43–50.

Wallace, P. (2007). *Coaching standardized patients for use in assessment of clinical competence*. New York: Springer Publishing Company.

Walters, K., Buszewicz, M., Russell, J., & Humphrey, C. (2003). Teaching as therapy: Cross-sectional and qualitative evaluation of patients' experiences of undergraduate psychiatry teaching in the community. *BMJ, 326*, 740–745.

Ware, J., Davies, A., & Connor, E. (1995). Patients assessments of quality. In M. Lipkin, S. M. Putnam, & A. Lazare (Eds.), *The medical interview: Clinical care, education, and research*. New York: Springer.

Wenger, E. (1998). *Communities of practice: Learning, meaning and identity*. Cambridge: Cambridge University Press.

Williams, R. G., Silverman, R., Schwind, C., Fortune, J. B., Sutyak, J., Horvath, K. D., Van Eaton, E. G., Azzie, G., Potts, J. R., 3rd, Boehler, M., & Dunnington, G. L. (2007). Surgeon information transfer and communication: Factors affecting quality and efficiency of inpatient care.[see comment]. *Annals of Surgery, 245*, 159–169.

Ziebland, S., & McPherson, A. (2006). Making sense of qualitative data analysis: An introduction with illustrations from DIPEx (personal experiences of health and illness). *Medical Education, 40*, 405–414.

Chapter 10
Self-monitoring in Surgical Practice: Slowing Down When You Should

Carol-anne Moulton and Ronald M. Epstein

10.1 Background

Every profession relies on the ability of its members to self-regulate their performance in order to achieve excellence and to retain the trust of the public. This ability to self-regulate is the key to autonomy and takes place at two levels – the systems level and the individual level (Epstein et al. 2008; Regehr and Eva 2006) On the systems level, there are numerous authorities that set standards to ensure that individuals within that profession are competent, in what could be conceptualized as a top-down process. National or state governing bodies dictate acceptable standards required of each member of that profession. This will usually include entrance examinations to ensure a minimum level of competence and ongoing involvement in continuing education programs that will ensure the professional remains up to date. Individuals might answer to a local administrative chief, although this more immediate level of control might only arise in some centres if questions of incompetency arise. Authorities also are responsible for setting limitations on practice as necessary and providing support for re-education or retraining when needed. On the individual level, each professional monitors or regulates his or her own performance; it is up to the individual to decide what new training he or she requires, to seek out that training and to incorporate new information into his or her practice. It is also up to the individual to appreciate and acknowledge when he or she is at the limits of his or her competence and to seek help from external sources when necessary.

C.-a. Moulton (✉)
Wilson Centre, University of Toronto, Toronto, ON, Canada
e-mail: Carol-anne.Moulton@uhn.on.ca

R.M. Epstein
Rochester Center, University of Rochester Medical Center, Rochester, NY, USA

H. Fry and R. Kneebone (eds.), *Surgical Education: Theorising an Emerging Domain*, Advances in Medical Education 2, DOI 10.1007/978-94-007-1682-7_10,

The surgical profession is a classical example of a self-regulating professional body. Standards are set at national, state and hospital levels; surgeons are required to pass fellowship exams to practice surgery and are required to satisfy local administrators of their level of competence in operating within their scope of practice. At an individual level, surgeons monitor their own performance on a moment-by-moment basis – they make decisions about whether they are skilled enough to do a particular procedure, whether they are out of their depth, whether they will call for help. Surgeons often operate alone or in the presence of less-experienced staff who may not have the skills or confidence to challenge what they are doing. Incisions are closed and their handiwork is no longer accessible – for admiration or criticism – to the outside world. Owing to the nature of surgery, the surgeon is not uncommonly met with situations he or she has not confronted before, both in and out of the operating room, or is offered new technology he or she has not tried before. Challenging and novel situations present themselves in the moment-by-moment activities of their daily lives. The ability of the surgeon to recognize and accept the limits of their own competence is paramount to patient safety as well as to the public's trust in the surgical profession. For these reasons, the surgical profession relies upon, arguably more than any other profession, effective individual self-regulation.

This chapter focuses on and explores the concept of individual self-regulation of the surgeon. How does the surgeon self-regulate his or her performance? When does a surgeon decide to call for help? What are the factors that influence surgeons in their moment-by-moment activities? This chapter explores various literatures that inform the way surgeons think during these more critical aspects of practice. A language will be offered that will encourage surgeons to be, or surgeon educators to develop surgeons who are, more critically self-reflective and metacognitively mindful in the moment-by-moment activities of their daily practices.

10.2 How Surgeons Think

When considering how surgeons self-regulate their own performance, it is paramount that we understand how surgeons think in practice. Various literatures have explored the ways professionals or 'experts' think in the course of their daily activities, and this section explores the key concepts and theories within these literatures and consider them in the context of a surgical practice (see also Chap. 7 for another consideration of expertise.)

10.2.1 Capacity Model of Attention

There are various models to explain why humans cannot attend to an infinite number of stimuli in their environment at any one time. One model, the Capacity Model, describes the human mind as having a limited capacity for attention (Kahneman 1973). There is a threshold beyond which we cannot attend to further stimuli. We have the capacity to multitask, paying attention to several stimuli at one time, provided we do not exceed the threshold. For a stimulus to receive attention once we are at our threshold, attention has to be taken away from another stimulus. Likewise, if a stimulus that is already receiving attention requires more attention, then attention has to be taken from either the spare capacity or from existing stimuli. This withdrawal of attention can be demonstrated in the operating room when a surgeon engaged in an extraneous conversation is suddenly confronted by something unusual or dramatic in the surgical field demanding of his attention. He or she will, out of necessity, withdraw from the conversation and focus on the surgical task (Moulton et al. 2010b). Along similar lines, music that was not bothering him 2 s before the event may suddenly become a distraction; he or she loses the ability to dual-task.

10.2.2 Automaticity and Expertise

Importantly, the development of automaticity diminishes the amount of attention that is required for any particular task. As we become 'expert' at doing a task or solving a problem, we no longer need the same amount of attention to complete the task or solve the problem. We 'automate' the activities or thought processes. An example to illustrate this concept in the surgical arena is to consider the relatively simple task of suturing an abdominal wound. The surgeon who has been doing this for many years can close the wound and be engaged in many other activities at the same time – listening to music, talking about last night's favourite television show or teaching (or all of the above!). The junior surgical trainee, on the other hand, is completely focused on the task of closing the wound and is not able to pay attention to other stimuli. If you ask him or her to talk about the patient who was admitted the night before, he or she will find it difficult to engage in the dual tasking activities of suturing and talking simultaneously. Interference produced through the mechanism of dual tasking as a function of expertise has been studied within the surgical context (Hsu et al. 2008). In this study, participants at the novice and expert level were challenged by a cognitive task while performing a basic laparoscopic skill. Participants in the expert group were not affected by the addition of the cognitive task, whereas participants in the novice group demonstrated a significant deterioration of performance in their cognitive skill results. This study suggested that experienced surgeons had achieved automaticity to a level that cognitive distraction did not affect performance, while less-experienced surgeons had not achieved the same degree of automaticity.

This concept of automaticity has formed the basis for many theories of expertise. Dreyfus and Dreyfus (1986), for example, suggest a five-stage model for expertise – novice, beginner, competent, proficient and expert. A novice, they argue, is predominantly rule-based and relies upon lists and rules to solve the problems of the field. As the novice acquires more experience he or she works his or her way through the various stages to become an expert, functioning largely in an automatic – or intuitive – manner. He or she simply knows the right answer or knows what to do in any particular scenario confronting his or her in the realm of his or her expertise – the general surgeon quickly makes the diagnosis of appendicitis in the emergency room, or the vascular surgeon 'intuitively' puts a finger over a hole in a major vessel to stop the bleeding. In this sense, the development and utilization of automatic resources are adaptive, enabling the expert to get through their daily activities as quickly and efficiently as possible. Several automatic resources – cognitive scripts and schemas, pattern recognition, heuristics and biases – have been described in the cognitive psychology literature (Kahneman 1973; Kahneman et al. 1982) and explored in the medical education literature (Epstein 1999; Norman 2005).

Gigerenzer (2007) in his book 'Gut Feelings: The Intelligence of the Unconscious' reminds us that simple cognitive heuristics are essential for accurate and quick choices and suggests they be celebrated for their role in our successes. Similarly, this concept of automaticity is central to Reyna and Lloyd's (2006) 'Fuzzy Trace' Theory where her work in the medical field has demonstrated that expert clinicians use less information than we might expect when making decisions and judgements relying instead on their 'gut feelings' or as she describes the 'gist' of the situation (Reyna and Lloyd 2006, 2009). Recent work suggests that emotions and sensory experiences are packaged with our learning experiences and knowledge and form part of our memory; when the memory is retrieved, the emotions and sensory experience is automatically retrieved as well potentially influencing behaviour and decision-making (Damasio 1999; Schmidt et al. 1990). While automaticity is, as Gigerenzer suggests, an important part of expertise, the expert is unable to stay in this mode all the time, transitioning when appropriate to a more effortful or analytic model (Eva 2004; Moulton et al. 2007). Practitioners describe, as does Polanyi (1998), a level of 'subsidiary awareness' even when in this automatic processing mode that permits the practitioner to recognize when situations are aberrant and require more attention and focus.

10.2.3 Effortful Modes of Cognition

Effortful modes of cognition have been studied using various terms: decision-making, problem solving, critical thinking and clinical reasoning. When faced with uncertainty or novel situations, we use more effortful, more deliberate, analytical cognitive processes. A surgeon, for example, is confronted by a liver abscess and acute cholecystitis when opening for an elective pancreaticoduodenectomy (Whipple) procedure to treat pancreatic cancer. The biliary stent that was positioned a few weeks prior to relieve jaundice has obstructed the cystic duct causing sepsis. Should he or she go ahead with the Whipple operation at this setting or just deal with the gall bladder problem? A surgeon experiences a stapler misfire during a routine low anterior resection of the colon. How is he or she going to manage the situation? Will he or she attempt to fire another stapler or will he or she perform a hand sewn anastomosis? This slower mode of thinking is distinct from the non-analytic and rapid processes of the automatic mode described above using different neural pathways to get to the answer or to complete the task. Both modes – the automatic and the effortful – are incorporated into what is often referred to as the 'dual-processing model' in the cognitive psychology and broader judgement literatures (De Neys 2006). Rather than thinking of either the automatic or effortful mode as being superior over the other, it is obvious in practice that each mode has an important role in clinical practice. Just as a surgeon could err by remaining in automatic mode when they should not, attributing severe back pain, for example, to musculoskeletal pathology rather than considering an aortic dissection, the surgeon could also err by being too analytical, being forced to consider all the options of a dermatological condition rather than relying on his or her 'gut feelings' (Chan Kulatunga-Moruzi et al. 2001; Gigerenzer 2007). Thus, the ideal is applying the right cognitive modality to the task at hand, being automatic or effortful as appropriate.

10.3 Transitioning from the Automatic to the Effortful in Practice: 'Slowing Down When You Should'

While experts spend most of their time in automatic mode, just doing what they know how to do, what are the factors that allow an appropriate transition into the effortful mode? When a surgeon is performing a 'routine' gall bladder dissection what determines whether he or she transitions appropriately to the more effortful if the actual situation is not 'routine'. The ability to make this transition appropriately in clinical practice has been suggested to be the hallmark of expertise (Moulton et al. 2007) and has been studied recently by Moulton in a surgical context. Surgeons across various specialties were asked to describe their experiences with the transitions in their own surgical practice. When surgeons were operating in their routine or 'automatic' mode what were the circumstances that caused this transition into a more 'effortful' mode of functioning? What does this transition into the more effortful 'feel' like, what does it 'look like' and what are the factors that influence this transition? All surgeons recognized the phenomenon and were able to provide examples of it in practice; 'the change to that sort of state usually goes along with where I stop talking to the resident and focus very intently on what's going on and I may, again, ask for quiet in the room or to reduce distractions, that sort of thing' (Moulton et al. 2010a, b). Participant surgeons described two main initiators of this transition in their operative surgical practice (see Fig. 10.1).

The first referred to the 'proactively planned' initiators – essentially the transitions that were anticipated or planned prior to surgery. Surgeons described

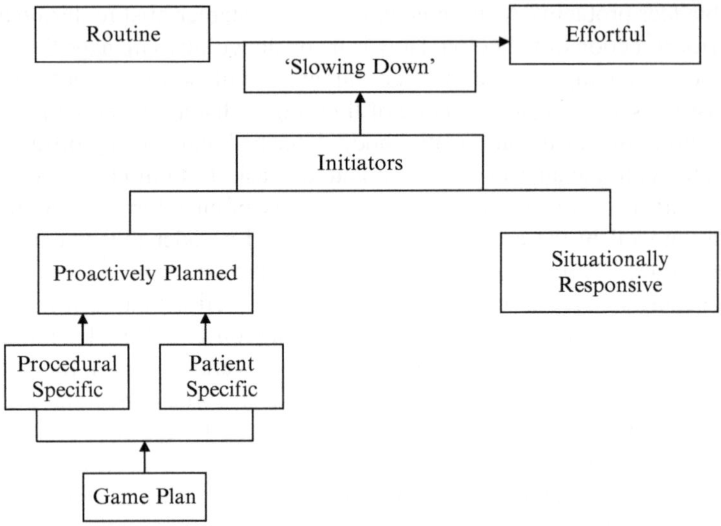

Fig. 10.1 Conceptual framework including the initiators of the 'Slowing Down' phenomenon (With permission from Springer, *Journal of GI Surgery*)

'slowing down' moments that occurred intra-operatively that had been planned pre-operatively. A colorectal surgeon when studying the abdominal CT scan prior to surgery might predict a potentially troublesome dissection around the pancreas and alert his or her hepato-biliary colleague pre-operatively to be prepared to remove part of the pancreas if required. When approaching this part of the dissection, he or she might become particularly focused, 'slowing down' appropriately as planned. To anticipate the 'slowing down' moments, surgeons in this study talk about using mental rehearsal and visual imagery in what many termed the 'game plan' (Moulton et al. 2010b). 'Slowing down' moments were anticipated based on details that were either specific to the procedure (e.g. the superior thyroid pedicle ligation in a thyroidectomy) or the patient (e.g. an anatomical variant). The attention literature refers to this process of 'proactive planning' as 'priming' or 'pre-cueing'. Humans are more likely to pay attention to a stimulus if they have been 'primed' to expect the stimulus (Folk et al. 1992; Kahneman 1973). If you know what you are looking for, you are more likely to notice it when it appears – like a blip on a visual monitor (Folk et al. 1992), or a sound in your headphones (Kahneman 1973). In this paradigm, the attentional set – what you are looking out for – determines what you see and perceive in a top-down process (Treisman 2006). Neurocognitive researchers suggest there is no 'immaculate perception' (Matthews 1989), that descending neural pathways can alter what our primary sensory organs are telling us, setting up a 'perceptual tension' between what 'is' and what we think the world 'should be' (Hawkins and Blakeslee 2004). The higher cortical areas are more concerned with interpretation and regulation of information with the potential therefore to alter, modify, and inhibit incoming signals to the sensory cortices. It is likely that practitioners learn to pay attention to perceptions from the sensory organs through these top-down processes in what is referred to as 'priming' (or planning). In addition, though, they learn to inhibit sensory input that is considered irrelevant – for better (by avoiding cognitive overload) or for worse (by ignoring data that do not comport with their self-image or expectations). Although these processes are largely unconscious, they can be brought to attention through development of greater subsidiary (Siegel 2007) awareness.

Several new paradigms have found that, quite often, unexpected objects fail to capture attention – a phenomenon known as 'inattentional blindness' (Simons 2000; Theeuwes et al. 1998; Yantis and Hillstrom 1994). If we rely on bottom-up processes, that is, the cue or stimulus to 'grab' our attention, literature suggests we often fail to take notice. Simons and Chabris (1999) demonstrates this in a video where two superimposed teams, one wearing white shirts and the other wearing black shirts, pass a basketball to other members of the team. Halfway through the video, a person in a gorilla costume walks right through the centre of the field, taking 5 s to walk from one side of the screen to the other. When people are asked to view the video and count how many times either the white team or black team passed the basketball, over half will fail to notice the gorilla. When it is brought to their attention, many find it difficult to believe they had watched the same video.

When unanticipated situations arise in the operative room – the tumour is more adherent than expected, the artery to be used for a bypass procedure is calcified, the anatomy is abnormal – the surgeon must transition into a more effortful mode and deal with the issue. In the language provided by the 'slowing down' study (Moulton et al. 2010b), the surgeon must be 'situationally responsive', attending to the dynamic situation and slowing down when he or she should. This requires an awareness (situation awareness) of the surgical environment. The attention literature discusses other factors that aid in our ability to transition or notice a stimulus or cue when it is not expected. One factor is the saliency of the cue. We are more likely to notice a cue that is loud, fast-moving or bright. They are hard-wired as part of our make-up and fit under the category of 'involuntary attention'. As surgeons, seeing a gush of blood will 'grab' our attention whether we are looking for it or not. Sometimes the cue that needs attention, however, is not as obvious as a 'gush of blood' but is a vague cue coming from within – what Reyna and Lloyd (2009) refer to as a 'gist' feeling, the feeling that 'something is not quite right' but is unable to be characterized more precisely at that moment in time. Another factor in whether we 'notice' a cue is the novelty of the cue'. Novel cues – seeing something we have never seen before – are likely to get our attention. As non-experts, there are many situations we have not seen before. Over time we develop pattern recognition, an automatic resource that enables us to quickly and appropriately understand many clinical situations. When we are then exposed to something 'novel' – a rare tumour, unusual anatomy – we take notice. Learning how to manipulate this, through making familiar situations novel, making 'facts' seem conditional, and persons seem unique forms one of the central tenets of mindful practice (Langer 1990). Our capacity for awareness and control over our cognitive processes will determine our ability to 'slow down' appropriately.

10.4 How Surgeons Monitor How They Think – Self-monitoring

So far we have discussed the cognitive aspects of how surgeons think – using automatic or effortful modes with appropriate transitioning between the two when required. We have briefly discussed the importance of maintaining awareness of, and having control over these cognitive processes. But how does this awareness develop? How do surgeons assess or monitor their thinking? What information or cues do they use to assess whether they are making the right decisions or are on the right track? How do they know when they have reached the limits of their ability and need to call for help?

10.4.1 Self-assessment and Self-monitoring

The ability to assess the environment and maintain an accurate picture of the situation at all times, that is, situation awareness – both in automatic and effortful modes of thinking – is key to expert performance. Self-assessment can be regarded as *summative* (an assessment of how one performed on the task, e.g. I did well today), *predictive* (an assessment of how one will do on a task, e.g. I will perform well tomorrow), or *concurrent* (an assessment of how well one is doing right now, e.g. I am performing well right now on this task) (Epstein et al. 2008; Eva 2004). The act of monitoring one's performance in-the-moment relies on the activities of *concurrent* self-assessment. Self-monitoring can be defined as 'an ability to attend, moment to moment, to our own actions; curiosity to examine the effects of those actions; and willingness to use those observations to improve behaviour and patterns of thinking in the future' (Epstein et al. 2008). Self-monitoring is a metacognitive process that involves 'thinking about thinking' (Flavell 1979) and includes monitoring of one's emotions as well as one's performance. An understanding of one's emotions might lead to an understanding of one's behaviour. A surgeon feeling guilty about a complication, for example, might be avoiding direct contact and communication with that patient. Monitoring one's situation is also important for maintaining situation awareness. Investing energy and attention towards monitoring what is unfolding in a surgical field is important to avoid 'drifting' or loss of situation awareness – both potentially leading to error (Moulton et al. 2010c). Therefore, self-monitoring involves monitoring of not only one's thoughts, emotions and feelings but also one's situation, actions and environment. Although this may sound relatively easy to do, there are several factors that might limit or prevent us from adequately engaging in these self-monitoring activities.

First, if one considers the various models of attention, there seems to be a limit to the amount of attention or pathways for paying attention at any given time (Kahneman 1973). To engage in these monitoring activities then requires some available capacity that in stressful or uncertain situations might not seem readily available. Second, monitoring mental processes and activities assumes that we have access to them and have some control over them. By definition, automatic functioning takes place without effort through processes that are thought to be beyond our control (Eva and Norman 2005; Nisbett and Wilson 1977). Cognitive heuristics are tendencies in human judgement that enable fast and efficient functioning typical of expert performance (Kahneman et al. 1982). Without access to these processes, it is difficult to monitor or manipulate them. In this sense, quick automatic judgements that are normally adaptive become maladaptive, potentially leading to erroneous presumptions or conclusions. Third, our ability to accurately assess our performance at any given moment relies on high-quality external and internal data. As surgeons, once trained, we rarely receive high quality 'external' in-the-moment feedback about our performance. If we do, there are many psychological and neurocognitive mechanisms in place to counteract negative feedback we receive (Festinger 1957).

Borrell-Carrió and Epstein (2004) call for self-awareness on the part of physicians to prevent errors in clinical practice, focusing the spotlight on individual factors, such as emotional factors and distractions as the causes of error. They propose a 'rational-emotive' model that may help develop physician's insight and self-awareness. An important aspect of this training is the development of a tolerance to ambiguity and uncertainty and a cultivation of certain 'habits' that enable this to occur, such as the 'habit of self-questioning' or the 'habit of reframing'. This mindful approach appears not to be focused on any particular aspect of practice, such as diagnostics, and does not appear to be related only to the 'automatic' functioning of an expert. Rather, it stresses the importance of an alternative way of practicing, one that emphasizes an approach characterized by 'habits of the mind' – such as self-questioning – that can be applied to all aspects of practice, and includes overriding automatic behaviours (Borrell-Carrió et al. 2004; Epstein 1999; Epstein et al. 2008).

10.4.2 Mindful Practice

Mindfulness has its roots in the philosophical-religious tradition (Kabat-Zinn 1994; Langer 1990) yet the underlying philosophy is essentially pragmatic, based on the 'interdependence of action, cognition, memory and emotion' (Epstein 1999). Rather than being viewed as an exercise in meditation, which many people perceive as a practice that 'empties the mind', mindful practice is 'conscious and intentional attentiveness to the present situation – the raw sensations, thoughts, and emotions as well as the interpretations, judgments, and heuristics that one applies to a particular situation' (Epstein et al. 2008).

Epstein argues that habits can be developed, which will improve our ability to be mindful during our clinical activities. These habits include the following: (1) attentive observation, (2) critical curiosity, (3) beginner's mind and (4) presence. *Attentive observation* includes vigilance and openness to the unexpected, both in details pertaining to the external world, for example, the surgical field, the patient or the CT, and within ourselves, for example, our perception and responses to cues in our environment and to our emotions. In surgery, how are the time pressures affecting the progress of the case, or, how is the desire to preserve ego getting in the way of calling for help? *Critical curiosity*, or 'seeing the world as it is and not as we would like it to be' is another habit of mindful practice. Here, doubt and uncertainty has to be tolerated and welcomed into practice. Rather than withdrawing from emotionally or cognitively difficult situations (e.g. an angry patient and a surgical mishap) or blaming the situation on others, the surgeon can approach the situation with openness: 'How did this come to be? Are there factors that I haven't considered?' The adoption of a *beginner's mind* – to see a situation freshly – with a willingness to set aside assumptions that have previously been made – is a healthy state that allows for 'contradictory ideas to be held simultaneously' (Epstein et al. 2008) and for new ideas to emerge. For a surgeon, this might mean that a rule might invite an exception that the diagnosis needs revisiting or the tumour that he or she thought was resectable is not. More importantly, is that observations are considered conditional – that the certainty of fact is replaced with a subjunctive 'might-be', recognizing that all conflicts and dilemmas do not need to be reconciled immediately. The habit of *presence* means avoiding preoccupation and distraction and being 'in-the-moment'. Cognitive resources are invested back into the situation. When this is achieved, clinicians may be more likely to appropriately 'respond' to the slowing down moments focusing and remaining purposeful in a productive manner – rather than miss the cue altogether or inappropriately 'react' with unproductive anxiety (Asher and Epstein 2005). Engaging in the state of mindful practice assists us in our efforts to seek, integrate, and respond to both 'external' and 'internal' data about our own performance (Epstein et al. 2008). This state of mindful practice is linked to the ability to adequately engage in the process of *self-monitoring* in practice.

If this state of mindful practice is essential for self-regulating professionals, it is important to ask, 'Can mindful practice be taught?' Recently, Krasner et al. (2009) completed a study in which primary care physicians were trained to be more mindful in everyday practice, using brief meditative, interpersonal and teamwork exercises that focused on awareness of one's internal landscape as well as awareness of interpersonal interactions in health care. Participants in the intensive 50-h course over a year subsequently reported lower burnout, greater emotional stability and well-being, and better ability to be present with patients, express empathy and attend to their concerns (Krasner et al. 2009). These changes were mediated by increases in mindfulness, as measured using a self-report survey. While clearly in a different context than surgical practice, these results suggest that mindfulness can be learned even by experienced practitioners, and that subjective difference in physicians' practices (which often correlate with observational measures) can result. Similar programs are being offered for surgical residents. Training and practice might increase one's ability to tune into the emotions, thoughts, bodily sensations and images when they emerge and provide an opportunity to assess and modulate how they might be impacting actions and behaviours.

In recent years, researchers using functional magnetic resonance imaging have demonstrated focal increases in cortical thickness (Lazar et al. 2005) and changes in neural pathways that accompany mindfulness training (Farb et al. 2007); these changes correlate to areas of the brain that regulate sensory input, executive function and emotions. Researchers propose that mindful awareness can be developed that will disentangle set pathways of automatic responses, engaging some activities and disengaging others so that information flow is altered. This has been proposed to offer benefits of personal well-being (Siegel 2007) and professional practice (Epstein et al. 2008).

10.4.3 The Mindful Surgeon

Interestingly, the 'surgical culture' seems to foster habits that might undermine the habits of 'mindful practice'. Cassell (1991) noted that 'the surgical ethos stresses decisiveness, control, confidence, and certitude' (Cassell, p. 57). Given that uncertainty is part of surgical practice she described an unavoidable tension surgeons experience between certainty and uncertainty. She postulates this tension is stronger and more stressful in surgery than other specialties because of the simultaneous need to manifest 'overwhelming self-confidence' to be effective in the operating room (Cassell, p. 57). Engaging in habits of mindful practice may assist surgeons in their efforts to remain clear despite this tension.

The journey of one surgeon towards mindful practice can be appreciated with the following excerpt from the Ph.D. thesis of one of the authors (Moulton 2010). A participant surgeon who during the course of the study had taken an interest in both the phenomena of 'slowing down when you should' as well as 'the concepts of mindful practice' wrote the following:

> *As a senior surgeon caring for complex cancer patients for over 15 years, I have often thought about my reaction to unexpected crises before, during and after surgery. We are taught to be confident and decisive, with an apparent lack of regard for our behaviour or feelings in times of stress or crisis during surgery. Though I have been aware of heightened moments of tension that occur in the operating room and elsewhere, I have not had words to describe or discuss my reactions to such events . . . The simple act of giving words to this phenomenon – 'slowing down' – seems to have altered my subjective reaction while I am in this transition. I feel a sense of comfort knowing that this phenomenon – and all of its associated subjective emotions and reactions individual to the surgeon – is not only a common component of surgical practice but also an essential one. Previously, without awareness of what I was experiencing, my efforts during these moments of crises were consumed with the anxiety I was feeling and intermixed with feelings of inadequacy, uncertainty, reputation and ego. Perhaps it is best explained by saying that I no longer feel anxious about being anxious and I can now focus my efforts appropriately on the immediate task at hand. The awareness of this phenomenon has evolved into a challenge in every case to not only 'slow down' but to 'slow down when I should' – appropriately marshalling the cognitive resources in a timely manner. I now 'look for the traps' and have found myself being more mindful 'in the moment' to avoid injury and error.*

It is possible that introducing a recognizable phenomenon that serves to flag potential critical aspects of practice encourages a more explicit approach to self-reflection, self-monitoring and therefore self-regulation in practice. It has been suggested that 'the language people use both makes possible and constrains the thoughts they can have. More than just a vehicle for ideas, language shapes ideas – and the practices that follow from them'. (Burke 1969; Lingard and Haber 1999). In this sense, our description of the mental processes that accompany attention, deliberation, automatic processing and mindfulness has the potential to make explicit an activity that was, at best, implicit in the surgeon's practice, and help surgeons be more intentional about these important aspects of surgical practice.

Recent views of expertise propose a juxtaposition of two different types of experts: Bereiter and Scardamalia (1993) distinguish between the 'true expert' and the 'experienced non-expert', Hatano and Inagaki (1986) compare the 'adaptive expert' with the 'routine expert' and Epstein (1999) describes the 'mindful practitioner' and the 'mindless practitioner'. The important consideration in all of these models of expertise is not how automatic, routine or intuitive the expert has become but rather how they allocate and reinvest their freed up attention to be more aware and in control of their cognitive processes no matter what attentional mode is being used – the automatic or effortful. Do they need to recruit additional cognitive resources right now? What is influencing their thoughts and actions? Are they *purposefully* paying attention to their environment or surgical field, looking out for cues that may alter their plan? Are they examining their assumptions, applying a 'beginner's mind' to the situation when necessary? This maximally efficient recruitment and reinvestment of limited attention and cognitive resources offers a challenge to the expert to approach their practice in a 'mindful' way.

With increasing evidence from outside literatures and an increased awareness and interest in self-assessment, self-reflection, self-monitoring and self-regulation, it may be the right time to consider realigning our efforts in surgical education towards a different model of expertise – one that focuses not on the fast and efficient expert, but rather on the mindful and adaptive expert. The experts in this model require certain 'habits of the mind' – a tolerance of uncertainty, a critical curiosity, a beginner's mind, a purposeful attentiveness and an ability to critically reflect on one's thought processes and actions.

References

Asher, B., & Epstein, R. (2005). *Managing the stress of surgical complications*. Boca Raton: Taylor & Francis/CRC Press.

Bereiter, C., & Scardamalia, M. (1993). *The need to understand expertise*. Chicago and La Salle: Open Court.

Borrell-Carrio, F., & Epstein, R. M. (2004). Preventing errors in clinical practice: A call for self-awareness. *Annals of Family Medicine, 2*, 310–316.

Borrell-Carrió, F., Suchman, A. L., & Epstein, R. M. (2004). The biopsychosocial model 25 years later: Principles, practice, and scientific inquiry. *Annals of Family Medicine, 2*, 576–582.

Burke, K. (1969). *A rhetoric of motives*. Berkeley: University of California Press.

Cassell, J. (1991). *Expected miracles: surgeons at work*. Philadelphia: Temple University Press.

Damasio, A. R. (1999). *The feeling of what happens: body and emotion in the making of consciousness*. New York: Harcourt Brace.

De Neys, W. (2006). Dual processing in reasoning: Two systems but one reasoner. *Psychological Science, 17*, 428–433.

Dreyfus, H. L., & Dreyfus, S. E. (1986). *Mind over machine*. New York: The Free Press.

Epstein, R. M. (1999). Mindful practice. *JAMA, 282*, 833–839.

Epstein, R. M., Siegel, D. J., & Silberman, J. (2008). Self-monitoring in clinical practice: A challenge for medical educators. *The Journal of Continuing Education in the Health Professions, 28*, 5–13.

Eva, K. (2004). What every teacher needs to know about clinical reasoning. *Medical Education, 39*, 98–106.

Eva, K. W., & Norman, G. (2005). Heuristics and biases - a biased perspective on clinical reasoning. *Medical Education, 39*, 870–872.

Farb, N. A., Segal, Z. V., Mayberg, H., Bean, J., McKeon, D., Fatima, Z., & Anderson, A. K. (2007). Attending to the present: Mindfulness meditation reveals distinct neural modes of self-reference. *Social Cognitive and Affective Neuroscience, 2*, 313–322.

Festinger, L. (1957). *A theory of cognitive dissonance*. Evanston: Row, Peterson and Company.

Flavell, J. (1979). Metacognition and cognitive monitoring: A new area of cognitive-developmental inquiry. *The American Psychologist, 34*, 906–911.

Folk, C. L., Johnston, J. C., & Remington, R. (1992). Involuntary covert orienting is contingent on attentional control settings. *Journal of Experimental Psychology. Human Perception and Performance, 18*, 1030–1044.

Gigerenzer, G. (2007). *Gut feelings: the intelligence of the unconscious*. New York: Penguin Group.

Hatano, G., & Inagaki, K. (1986). *Two courses of expertise*. New York: W.H. Freeman.

Hawkins, J., & Blakeslee, S. (2004). *On intelligence*. New York: Times Books.

Hsu, K. E., Man, F. Y., Gizicki, R. A., Feldman, L. S., & Fried, G. M. (2008). Experienced surgeons can do more than one thing at a time: Effect of distraction on performance of a simple laparoscopic and cognitive task by experienced and novice surgeons. *Surgical Endoscopy, 22*, 196–201.

Kabat-Zinn, J. (1994). *Wherever you go, there you are: Mindfulness meditation in everyday life*. New York: Hyperion.

Kahneman, D. (1973). *Attention and effort*. Englewood Cliffs: Prentice-Hall.

Kahneman, D., Slovic, P., & Tversky, A. (1982). *Judgment under uncertainty: heuristics and biases*. Cambridge: Cambridge University Press.

Krasner, M. S., Epstein, R. M., Beckman, H., Suchman, A. L., Chapman, B., Mooney, C. J., & Quill, T. E. (2009). Association of an educational program in mindful communication with burnout, empathy, and attitudes among primary care physicians. *JAMA, 302*, 1284–1293.

Kulatunga-Moruzi, C., Brooks, L. R., & Norman, G. (2001). Coordination of analytic and similarity-based processing strategies and expertise in dermatological diagnosis. *Teaching and Learning in Medicine, 13*, 110–116.

Langer, E. J. (1990). *Mindfulness*. Reading, Mass. Addison-Wesley Publishing Company Inc.

Lazar, S., Kerr, C., Wasserman, R., Gray, J., Greve, D., Treadway, M., McGarvey, M., Quinn, B. T., Dusek, J. A., Benson, H., Rauch, S. L., Moore, C. I., & Fischl, B. (2005). Meditation experience is associated with increased cortical thickness. *Neuroreport, 16*, 1893–1897.

Lingard, L., & Haber, R. J. (1999). Teaching and learning communication in medicine: A rhetorical approach. *Academic Medicine, 74*, 507–510.

Matthews, M. R. (1989). *The scientific background to modern philosophy: Selected readings*. Indianapolis: Hackett Publishing Company Inc.

Moulton, C. A. (2010). *Exploring the role of "slowing down when you should" in operative surgical judgment*. Toronto: Institute of Medical Science, University of Toronto.

Moulton, C. A., Regehr, G., Mylopoulos, M., & MacRae, H. M. (2007). Slowing down when you should: A new model of expert judgment. *Academic Medicine, 82*, S109–S116.

Moulton, C. A., Regehr, G., Lingard, L., Merritt, C., & Macrae, H. (2010a). Operating from the other side of the table: Control dynamics and the surgeon educator. *Journal of the American College of Surgeons, 210*, 79–86.

Moulton, C. A., Regehr, G., Lingard, L., Merritt, C., & Macrae, H. (2010b). 'Slowing down when you should': Initiators of the transition from the routine to the effortful. *Journal of Gastrointestinal Surgery, 14*, 1019–1026.

Moulton, C. A., Regehr, G., Lingard, L., Merritt, C., & Macrae, H. (2010c). Staying out of trouble in the operating room: Remaining attentive in automaticity. *Academic Medicine, 85*, 1571–1577.

Nisbett, R. E., & Wilson, T. D. (1977). Telling more than we can know: Verbal reports on mental processes. *Psychological Review, 84*, 231–259.

Norman, G. (2005). Research in clinical reasoning: Past history and current trends. *Medical Education, 39*, 418–427.

Polanyi, M. (1998). *Personal knowledge: towards a post-critical philosophy*. London: Routledge and Kegan Paul Ltd.

Regehr, G., & Eva, K. (2006). Self-assessment, self-direction, and the self-regulating professional. *Clinical Orthopaedics and Related Research, 449*, 34–38.

Reyna, V. F., & Lloyd, F. J. (2006). Physician decision making and cardiac risk: Effects of knowledge, risk perception, risk tolerance, and fuzzy processing. *Journal of Experimental Psychology. Applied, 12*, 179–195.

Reyna, V. F., & Lloyd, F. J. (2009). Clinical gist and medical education. *Journal of the American Medical Association, 302*, 1332–1333.

Schmidt, H. G., Norman, G. R., & Boshuizen, H. P. (1990). A cognitive perspective on medical expertise: Theory and implication. *Academic Medicine, 65*, 611–621.

Siegel, D. J. (2007). *The mindful brain*. New York: WW Norton.

Simons, D. J. (2000). Attentional capture and inattentional blindness. *Trends in Cognitive Sciences, 4*, 147–155.

Simons, D. J., & Chabris, C. F. (1999). Gorillas in our midst: Sustained inattentional blindness for dynamic events. *Perception, 28*, 1059–1074.

Theeuwes, J., Kramer, A. F., Hahn, S., & Irwin, D. E. (1998). Our eyes do not always go where we want them to go: Capture of the eyes by new objects. *Psychological Science, 9*, 379–385.

Treisman, A. (2006). How the deployment of attention determines what we see. *Visual Cognition, 14*, 411–443.

Yantis, S., & Hillstrom, A. P. (1994). Stimulus-driven attentional capture: Evidence from equiluminant visual objects. *Journal of Experimental Psychology. Human Perception and Performance, 20*, 95–107.

Chapter 11
Learning and Identity Construction in the Professional World of the Surgeon

Alan Bleakley

'With a blend of arrogance and innocence the surgeon makes his incision . . .'

– Richard Selzer (1996: 37).

11.1 Limitations to Studies of Surgeons and Surgical Education

The working life and identity construction of the surgeon has been the subject of three major anthropological studies in North America (Millman 1976; Cassell 1991; Katz 2000), and a further study solely of women entering what is still an overwhelmingly male culture (Cassell 2000). This small, but rich, literature is already an archival curiosity. Surgical education – at least in the UK – is undergoing such a radical transformation that the studies of surgical work and learning – by Marcia Millman in the mid-1970s, Pearl Katz in the late 1970s and Joan Cassell in the early 1980s and again in the early 1990s – are no longer helpful indicators of what a surgical education of the future may look like, other than as reminders of a chronically conservative legacy, where the surgeon was typed – or more often stereotyped – as heroic, macho, aloof, hubristic, impulsive, authoritarian, misogynistic and aggressive, while surgical students were seen to emulate these traits as a central part of their education of character, absorbing them through role modelling as the main form of identity construction.

In *Cultivating a thinking surgeon*, the UK-based surgeon Linda de Cossart and the educationalist Della Fish (de Cossart and Fish 2005: xvi) do not refer to this anthropological literature, although identity is signalled as a major theme, and their text 'is about the surgeon being and becoming a growing professional'. According to de Cossart and Fish, whose book does represent a new wave of thinking about surgical education, there are five critical educational issues in becoming a surgeon for the twenty-first century, which must be considered against the background of a radically reduced training time: first, a previously hit-and-miss apprenticeship

A. Bleakley (✉)
Medical Education, Peninsula Medical School, Plymouth, Devon, UK
e-mail: alan.bleakley@pms.ac.uk

H. Fry and R. Kneebone (eds.), *Surgical Education: Theorising an Emerging Domain*, Advances in Medical Education 2, DOI 10.1007/978-94-007-1682-7_11,

learning-by-doing must be radically restructured to provide educational frameworks for learning on the job; second, these frameworks must be guided by contemporary learning theory, particularly reflective practice; third, what was previously a tacit process – the acquisition of clinical reasoning in surgery – must now be made more explicit through deliberative practice; fourth, learning must be supported by competent teaching, where surgical teachers must deepen their educational expertise to become surgical educators; and fifth, the teaching and learning process must be structured around issues of professionalism, where an agreed set of values is upheld.

Professionalism is a double-edged sword – surgeons in training must be socialized into the wider community beyond the Royal College structure (that focuses on examination and passage through training grades), to include engagement with quality assurance, appraisal, wider trust governance and management and policy issues. Where surgical *trainers* in the past have been restricted to largely opportunistic support of trainees in learning on the job, there will now be an expectation for a shift in identity construction through subscribing to a set of educational values as a surgical *educator*.

At this point, a fault line appears in de Cossart and Fish's model of surgical education, where surgeons who wish to become surgical educators, beyond jobbing surgical teachers or demonstrators, have to shift from the tough-minded culture of surgery to enter what is seen as the alien, tender-minded community of practice of 'education' and adopt its professional values. This is problematic, where the professional identity and values of the education culture are described as if they were transparent and homogenous. In fact, there is as much difference, or heterogeneity, within the educational community as there is between the specialties of medicine, and between medicine and surgery.

For example, de Cossart and Fish (2003: 40) say 'it is broadly agreed by educators that to act educationally is to open minds, liberate thinking, encourage critique, explore the foundations of good practice and develop creativity'. Actually, there is much debate within the educational culture about such claims for emancipation. In the role of the emancipator, educationalists who think that they should be 'open minded' and have 'liberal thinking' may be engaging in a kind of imperialism – the colonizing of a supposedly educationally (and even intellectually) naïve surgical culture, as if to liberate them from their ignorance. Educationalists need not dictate the agenda in this manner, but can work closely with surgeons to develop a responsive and progressive surgical-education culture that benefits patients. In order to resist potential colonizing by any single, inevitably biased set of ideas exported from the mixed culture of education (Bleakley et al. 2008), it is important that a surgical-education culture of the future develops an identity from within its own cultural resources.

What, then, is left as a means of articulating the identity construction of surgeons and surgical educators, if we see previous anthropological studies as historical curiosities, and current educational thinking focused on the consummate 'professional' as a potential form of neo-colonialism? In the remainder of this chapter, I will mine the rich seam of socio-cultural learning theories (Bleakley 2006a) to argue that we must go beyond both ethnography's legacy of focus upon character traits of the heroic individual and reflective practice-oriented education's insistence upon developing the consummate surgical educator in the image of the grown-up 'educationalist'.

11.2 The Dispersal of the Surgical Gaze Marks a New Era for Surgical Education

Michel Foucault's (1976) *The Birth of the Clinic*, first published in 1963, describes the genesis of modern medicine – co-incidentally with the European Enlightenment in the late eighteenth and early nineteenth century – as the development of a particular kind of 'gaze' upon the patient's body. Previously, medicine and surgery had fitted patients into preset systems of classification (such as the four humours), and treated them based on what can now be seen as a spurious system of diagnosis through the odour and colour of urine, the consistency of stools, and so forth, related to an abstract set of categories.

The new clinical gaze was based on close, empirical observation of the individual patient, including intimate examination combined with auscultation, palpation and percussion. This was matched to a growing epidemiological knowledge of the frequency and distribution of illness. Where patients were traditionally visited at home, learning was restricted, but when medical and surgical education was established at the bedside in the hospital setting, as a teaching clinic, this legitimated intimate physical examination in a way that had not been possible in family home settings.

The medical gaze was educated through looking literally into the depths of bodies through cadaveric dissection and pathological anatomy, translating this deep looking, metaphorically, across the surface examination of patients. The doctor's diagnostic gaze was a transposition of anatomical and pathological knowledge into the unseen depths of the patient's body, guided by the text of surface symptoms. The invention of the stethoscope by Laënnec, in 1816, increased the power of the clinical gaze as it provided a necessary 'moral distancing' from the patient. The clinician's gaze into the body was then further augmented by Roentgen's discovery of the X-ray in 1895, and in time, more sophisticated radiological imaging. However, these augmentations have gradually come to *replace*, rather than *amplify*, the clinician's gaze (Bleakley and Bligh 2009). Indeed, the singular 'gaze' in new procedures is already fractured in contexts such as laparoscopic surgery using multiple high-definition screens.

The medical gaze described by Foucault has operated as the dominant discourse of medicine for the past 200 years, but as we progress into the new millennium, it can be argued that a new discourse is emerging in medicine and surgery that is just as radical as the break that Foucault described. This new discourse is educating a different kind of surgical gaze – one that is 'distributed' rather than focused and penetrating. This gaze is creating the conditions for the emergence of a new identity structure for surgeons.

By ‘gaze’, Foucault meant two things – first, a literal looking and seeing. Modern medicine is empirical – based on close noticing and physical examination of symptoms as a basis to diagnosis, prognosis and treatment plan. But Foucault also describes a twin ‘seeing and saying’ that is metaphorical rather than literal. As the surgeon gazes at your posture, asks you about pain levels and mobility and examines your knee outwardly, he is metaphorically, at the same time, gazing into the interior anatomy of the knee, which he knows from anatomical atlases, dissections and surgical operations. He then augments such looking through examining an X-ray. In the new era of non-invasive keyhole surgery, the surgeon can then literally extend his gaze to examine the knee again indirectly, or mediated by the camera, through arthroscopy.

Also, the surgeon in the identity of the ‘interprofessional’ rather than the ‘professional’ – is now more closely implicated in a network of services around a patient, where the surgeon is no longer autonomous. Clinical reasoning is both augmented and dispersed not just by instruments but also by a range of other professionals, such as radiographers, radiologists, physiotherapists, nurses and pharmacists. The personal surgical gaze described by Foucault is mediated, fractured and multiplied to such an extent that Foucault’s era of modern medicine and surgery, that has lasted 200 years, is now eclipsed.

Kenneth Ludmerer (1999) describes a twin crisis in medicine and surgery, concerning a loss of faith by the public, leading to a reformulation of the profession. Doctors and surgeons were judged to be unable to self-regulate adequately enough to inspire public confidence. The profession was also seen to refuse transparency, traditionally closing ranks to cover poor practice. In the UK, the Bristol paediatric heart surgery, and the Alder Hey and Bristol organ retention scandals, followed by the disclosure of Harold Shipman’s mass murder of patients, led collectively to a crisis in legitimacy of self-regulation and the introduction of a monitory democracy (Keane 2009) – a series of quality assurance mechanisms from outside the profession. Where patients were also gradually acquiring greater powers and confidence in challenging medical and surgical practices, so traditional paternalism has been eroded. Finally, the need for change in the way that surgeons share the uncertainties of their practices with patients and colleagues is being addressed.

What does this raft of changes mean for the identity of the surgeon and for surgical education? In short, surgeons must now be democrats rather than autocrats. They must become engaged ‘surgical citizens’, just as they are citizens in everyday, public life. They must shift from traditional vertical, hierarchical structures as they accommodate to horizontal and dialogical collaborative working patterns. They must recognize the importance of non-technical – communication – factors in patient safety. And they must engage with the democratic process whereby a professional community accounts for its activities.

If the surgeon, as citizen, is now a social being, surgical education must switch its attention away from the legacy of *individualistic* learning theories to the application of new *social* learning theories to better shape the surgical apprenticeship. Also, in the area of expertise, the surgeon is no longer just achieving technical proficiency, but also non-technical proficiency, modelling productive communication and appropriate interpersonal behaviour. Indeed, the surgeon's work is not just about producing health or repair, but also about producing the social conditions of communication through which a patient's safety is guaranteed during a period of surgery (Bleakley et al. 2004).

Finally, the surgeon must move beyond reflective practice, or self-direction, to accommodate to the reality of an embodied cognition that is distributed. The surgeon's 'mind' is also 'in' an array of instruments, radiological images and sophisticated technologies including scopes, monitors and robotics, and 'in' the social context in which his work occurs. Cognitive embodiment (Clark 2009) in these distributed resources makes it impossible to talk about a singular surgical gaze in Foucault's terms, and demands that we employ learning theories that comprehend this fractured, multiple and supplemented gaze that is now social.

Traditional reflective practice models describe reflection as inner-directed and not social, privileging introspection over dialogue. This is a safe territory for the conventionally autonomous and monological surgeon, working against the grain of social being that the surgeon must become for safe practice. Rather, the surgeon must become a *reflexive* practitioner – a full participant in a dialogical democracy (Bleakley 1999, 2006b), where he must transparently account for his professional values, surgical practices, communication repertoire and thinking process. The shift from reflective to reflexive practice is then from an internal monologue dwelling on quality of practice to an external dialogue with a variety of others, including patients, colleagues, academics and managers, as a democratic form of quality assurance of practice.

11.3 The Effects of New Work Practices

New working and learning conditions are inevitably reshaping the identity of the surgical education culture, and the identities of surgeons and surgical educators. Structural changes to career pathways have been introduced in the UK through the Modernising Medical Careers (2008) agenda, which will undergo further change as a result of recommendations to overhaul the system from the Tooke Report (2008). Radical reduction in surgical training time, through implementation of the European Working Time Directive, means that the old apprenticeship system has now been transformed.

Surgical educators will now have to ensure that work-based learning is lean and efficient. Rather than an apprenticeship involving a good deal of unproductive watching and waiting, opportunistic learning and demonstrating rather than teaching, surgery will now have to learn from the latest studies and practices in work-based learning concerning acceleration of skills (hot-housing), often through varieties of learning by simulation; optimising conditions of mastery through deliberate or deliberative practice (Colvin 2008); engaging issues of unlearning and overlearning; use of scaffolding and feedback; and collaborative learning.

This demands a new identity construction for the surgical teacher, as supporter and collaborator (see Chaps. 10 and 12). In summary, work modes must shift from traditional vertical, hierarchical structures to horizontal patterns of co-ordination, co-operation and collaboration. Again, this means democratizing surgical work practices. It is quite extraordinary that surgery has for so long been run along autocratic, hierarchical lines, where such a system would never be accepted in our everyday lives. We expect democracy in politics and everyday social discourse, so why not in the operating theatre?

The argument that hierarchies are natural products of technical capability (length of education, complexity of acquired knowledge and skill) is spurious. Evidence demonstrates that patient outcomes are improved where flattened hierarchies are introduced (Borrill and West 2002). Importantly, there is now a good evidence base to show that the majority of surgical errors are not grounded in technical mistakes, but in systems-based collaboration and communication issues (Kohn et al. 1999; Joint Commission 2001; Singh et al. 2007). Surgeons must now be excellent 'non-technical' practitioners (e.g. communicators and team players) to ensure patient safety.

How are work modes changing? There is, first, a wholesale shift from stable surgical teams with continuity, to ad hoc constitution of teams (except in special circumstances such as paediatric cardiac surgery teams, which are now *designed* along the lines of Formula One pit-stop teams, for speed and efficiency (Edmondson et al. 2001)). In parallel, traditional apprenticeship 'family' structures of 'firms' have dissolved, so that junior surgeons must learn to be nomads rather than members of a stable 'house'. As Richard Sennett (quoted in Bauman 2004: 30–31) suggests: 'A flexible workplace is unlikely to be a spot in which one would wish to build a nest'. Rather, we are seeing the rise of 'cloakroom communities' that are 'patched together for the duration of the spectacle and promptly dismantled again once the spectators collect their coats from their hooks in the cloakroom'.

Sennett suggests that 'routine' work, based on stable groups, is crumbling across all sectors and not just health care. Yrjö Engeström (2008) suggests that new professional work settings are even seeing the dissolution of what we have habitually come to call 'team' structures. Rather, we are entering an era of 'collaborative intentionality' and 'negotiated knotworking' – of rapidly pulsating work, where groups of people come together for connected and collaborative tasks, and where there is no stable 'centre', or the centre does not hold. Thus, there is no development of identity as a team member in the sense of passage (and staggered socialization) through the typical stages of group development ('norming', 'storming', 'performing' and 'mourning'). Perhaps 'mourning' is now the default position.

Knotworked sets of professionals (ad hoc 'teams') must tune to the 'pulse' of the work and move straight to 'performing', as threads of activity are tied, re-tied and untied, again with no particular centre that holds. This new, dynamic work pattern – that takes technical proficiency as a given in its organic formation of work groups, but has no such faith in non-technical proficiency, such as skill in communication – suggests that while work itself may have an object or be goal-oriented (benefit to, care of, and safety for the patient; sensitivity to colleagues), identity may not be goal oriented but means oriented. In other words, you work with what you have, not with a planned team where identities are fixed by hierarchy and role.

In these shifting work modes, surgery mirrors the wider culture. Andy Hargreaves (2003: 25) describes a shift in society from 'sustained family conversations and relationships' to 'episodic strings of tiny interactions', and this has also occurred, as noted above, in surgery's transformation of the 'family' or 'firm' structures to more open, complex and fluid arrangements.

Where the centre no longer holds, anarchy does not necessarily break loose. Rather, practices and identities are reinvented dynamically. Such changes mirror what has been termed as wider 'risk society' and 'runaway world' (Giddens 1991) – cultures in which mastery and control seem impossible, and adaptation, flexibility and tolerance of uncertainty are paramount. For example, the new wave of iatrogenic diseases – hospital-acquired infections – seems to be 'runaway' monsters, almost impossible to control, as do new viral infections that evade cures. This does not stop us from attempting to master or nail these runaway objects, but we must recognize that stabilization is sometimes impossible, and adaptive strategies are necessary. Surgery is a culture of both high need for control, and high risk and uncertainty. Do we have learning theories that surgical educators can draw on that recognize and work with such paradoxes, rather than attempt to iron them out with formulaic strategies? In the following three sections, I will briefly consider the contributions of the 'big three' social learning theories.

11.4 Communities of Practice

A major shift in thinking about the identity construction of professionals was introduced by Etienne Wenger's (1998) communities of practice model, originally developed with the anthropologist Jean Lave (1990) to explore apprenticeships. Instead of focusing on learning as sedimentation of knowledge and skills in an individual, Wenger's model describes learning as meaningful participation in a community of practice (such as surgery). Learning is then a work-based activity and 'situated' in a particular context (e.g. the operating theatre or the simulation suite). A novice may experience legitimate participation in a community of practice, such as a surgical trainee on the first rung of a career ladder, but this will be peripheral. As expertise develops, so engagement becomes central, legitimacy is increased and an identity is stabilized.

This model can be seen as a restatement of anthropological rites of passage and socialization models of the sort reported at the beginning of this chapter, where engagement with a community invites initiation into the shared repertoire or history of that community, and consequent identity construction through membership. Cultural histories include stories, rituals, humour, styles of working, effectiveness with key and local artefacts and initiation into 'local knowledge' (the way we do things around here).

The 'communities of practice' model differs from such traditional ethnographic models where it moves beyond description to prescription. The model prescribes the ideal community as receptive, where communication is horizontal, or non-hierarchical, and engagement is mutual or reciprocated by experts (experts do not humiliate or harass). This is a gentle process 'that confers a sense of belonging', but 'more significantly, an increasing sense of identity as a master practitioner' (Lave and Wenger 1990: 111). The tone of the communities of practice model, even in prescribing ideal, horizontal forms of engagement, is undoubtedly tender-minded. It prescribes reciprocal partnerships between novice and expert, and not judgemental initiations. For this reason alone, the model is readily open to scepticism from the characteristically tough-minded surgical community, although the notions of learning by engagement or participation are second nature to such a community, steeped in traditional apprenticeship approaches.

Where the communities of practice model focuses on progressive stabilization of identity, however, it does not have explanatory power to address the new complex, dynamic, unstable work contexts described above as 'liquid' and 'runaway'. Further, the model does not adequately describe how, for example, a surgeon's learning and expertise are constructed, as they are mediated through the use of artefacts such as new surgical technologies. Actor-network theory and activity theory can be seen to be particularly responsive to these issues.

11.5 Actor-Network Theory

Communities of practice models of learning capture how persons – 'actors' – learn collaboratively, but learning also involves persons interacting with material objects. In actor-network theory, these objects are called 'actants' and are afforded a much more active role in shaping learning than in other learning theories (Latour 2007). Where learning theories do describe interactions with the material world, such as learning a skill with an instrument or technology, they tend to focus on human mastery rather than the *interaction* between person and artefact as described by actor-network theory. Such objects, or artefacts, are central to the surgeon's work, as they literally augment and extend identity. Artefacts include traditional instruments such as scalpels, retractors and clamps, and the new technologies of keyhole surgery and robotics.

Actor-network theory specifically analyses people in complex networks, where several actors and artefacts (actants) are in dialogue and mutually engaged. This is not a form of animism. Any surgeon will tell you how the instrument, such as a scalpel, 'speaks back' to the hand and guides the strength of grip or pressure in the cut. As scalpels became more sophisticated through the use of different metals, so the hands of surgeons responded (Sennett 2008).

According to actor-network theory, how we experience the world is as a set of rapidly pulsing and changing associations, over which we attempt to gain mastery. This offers a working definition of surgery. A sense of identity does not emerge out of the mastery but out of the quality of association that is made between person and mediating material artefact as 'types of connections' – ties, bonds, aggregates, forces and assemblages (Latour 2007: 5). A surgeon does not 'learn' through mastery of tasks informed by knowledge, but makes the right kind of connections between the material and the human world, or puts things together in a way that creates both meaning and function. In this sense, through bringing form and function into dialogue, the surgeon is as much a sculptor as a scientist.

This aesthetic identity is clear for aesthetic surgeons, but is disregarded as an important element of identity in other areas of surgery. In short, a surgical education should place emphasis upon how the material world 'speaks back' as surgeons work with it in investigating, suctioning, cutting, clamping, suturing, stapling, and so forth, shaping awareness and senses.

A surgical identity in this view of learning is then not focused on character traits or personality types, but on qualities such as adaptability and sensitivity to the dynamic material world (including another's body). This does not 'objectify' the patient, but does precisely the opposite. A liver becomes 'actant', 'speaking back' to the surgeon, who responds sensitively through close noticing. Work and learning are focused on the quality of attachment to, and perception of, this liver in this particular moment of the operation (Verghese 2009). Latour (2007: 217) suggest that, unlike other learning theories that focus on individual cognition and behaviour, or even upon human social contexts, 'attachments are first, actors are second'.

11.6 Cultural–Historical Activity Theory

Where communities of practice models and actor-network theory tend to analyse any given learning context as stable or static, cultural–historical activity theory focuses on the dynamic aspect of learning activities. This emphasizes the inherent instability of systems (networks) within which people learn, and what may be on the horizon (the unknown) rather than what has been achieved (the known). Activity theory also describes a collective capacity to carry out work, rather than an individual agency and identity at work. Groups of people create transformations and innovations in concert with artefacts, established rules (protocols) and work roles, as this affords identity and meaning. Identity is then an emergent property of the activity system, not a given condition, such as a character trait, and is inherently unstable and in process.

Cultural–historical activity theory (Engeström 1987) – developed from Vygotsky's formulation that 'mind' can never be dissociated from its social and material contexts – then attempts to address learning as a *transformative* process. An activity system (such as an operating theatre team) is temporarily stabilized through sharing a common object (patient care and safety), and through the exercise of protocols or rules. However, division of labour already means that members of the activity system have different sub-goals and agendas, so that how they achieve the shared object of the activity, and how they translate rules and protocols, may produce conflict. For example, the surgeon may be task-oriented ('I will finish the operation'), where the scrub nurse may be time-oriented ('you should never have started this operation, knowing it is close to the end of a shift'). Activity systems – such as an operating theatre team and its artefacts – are then inherently unstable and in states of transformation.

Identities are (trans)formed through the dynamic of the activity system, but are also inherently unstable, and may resist the flow of direction of the activity system, creating further perturbation. Identity formation is not, as the communities of practice models suggests, necessarily about gradual stabilization within a community through increasingly meaningful (peripheral to central) participation, but may result from perturbation, resistance and conflict, and reflects this as a multiple and fractured set of identities. Such an identity complex is not an aberration, where we come to learn how to manage identities as potentially multiple, fractured and labile. In the new, complex and liquid work settings of surgery, what Engeström and colleagues (Kerosuo and Engeström 2003) call 'boundary crossing' – the ability to move across and between activity systems (e.g. anaesthetic room, theatre, recovery and ward) – is hard for those used to the notion of acquiring a stable identity (personal agency, personality, self) within a community of practice, reflecting the classic uniprofessional 'silo' mentality.

In acquiring a 'boundary-crossing' mentality – advertised by flexibility and tolerance – the origins of identity are grounded not in 'selfsame' (identification with my professional group), but in 'difference' (I only know myself in the mirror of the 'other'). Characteristically, selfsame identities exclude the other (intolerance), where identities grounded in difference respect that difference and value the other (tolerance). A powerful example of tolerance of difference is the ability for an operating theatre practitioner to recognize the patient as a guest in the household of surgery, even when anaesthetized, and to offer that patient unconditional hospitality (Bleakley 2006b).

Bounded communities of practice, the basic unit of analysis of which is the 'team', are problematic according to Engeström (2008). Teams present a 'puzzle'. Where exactly 'is' the team? What practitioners experience on the ground is, in Wenger's term, 'participation', and in activity theory, 'intent' to collaborate (although this usually sticks at a lower level of co-ordination or co-operation). At the level of what Wenger calls 'participation' and Engeström calls 'activity', abstract knowledge ('reification' in Wenger's term) or theory is secondary to work experience. A 'team' is actually an abstraction or reification – the noun does not describe what 'teams' might do. Rather, what is experienced in work and learning are complex dynamic *activities*, such as 'teeming'. A new vocabulary for team activity is called for, and Engeström (2008) describes a range of these activities, such as 'swarming', 'knotworking', 'meshworking', 'networking' and 'wildfire activities' (firefighting – a common occurrence in the operating theatre).

This new vocabulary for participation and activity attempts, metaphorically, to grasp what actually happens on the ground in work contexts, in dynamic terms. This may appear to be reactive to situations rather than proactive, but this would be a misunderstanding. Proactivity is inherent to an activity system, as is instability. Proactivity attempts to maintain activity and complexity in the face of instability, in what Searle (1990) calls 'we-intentions', and Engeström (2005) calls 'collaborative intentionality'. Such potential is achieved, again, through open dialogue, the hallmark of a democratic power structure.

According to Ciborra (2000), powerful and successful work collectives do not, paradoxically, seek so much control over their collaborative work as understanding and meaning (returning us to the heart of Wenger's argument about an effective community of practice that generates meaning out of learning and learning out of meaning). Rather, collectives, in Ciborra's view, need not resort to top-down control (the knee-jerk reaction of autocracies), but generate good work practices from 'drift, care, hospitality and cultivation' (in Engeström 2008: 202). Sceptics of such ideas will ask: 'Where is the leadership?' Leadership is distributed according to the changing foci of work activities within an overall collaboration. The 'knot' in knotworking has no single centre or leader, but still holds appropriately to ensure collaboration and the realization of a common object or intention.

11.7 Textualization in Surgical Work

A body of empirical research in work settings shows that medical and healthcare work is changing, leading to 'problematizing identity' (Iedema and Scheeres 2003: 316) and offering what Jackson (2000) calls a new textualization of work, which is both a form of learning in itself and a way of describing learning. Due to the implementation of new work settings such as multi-disciplinary clinical-care pathways, surgeons, allied health professionals and healthcare workers are talking to each other in new ways (first text), talking to patients in new ways (second text), educating in new ways (third text) and talking about this work to academic researchers in new ways (fourth text). As a result of this, surgeons are talking to themselves in new (reflexive) ways about these emergent work conditions, accounting for quality of practice and outcome (see Chap. 12).

The product of new ways of doing things (practices) and describing them to others and to oneself (reflection on practices) promotes a shift in identity. Sometimes, this shift offers not a fine-tuning of practices and the values that inform them, but a reinvention. In this case, reflection shifts to 'reflexivity' – a critical re-examination of what we do, why we do it one way and not another, and importantly 'who am I?' as I engage in these new forms of work.

In the process of negotiating new ways of relating that require new activities (e.g. leading a brief or debrief in theatres) surgeons now have to renegotiate their identities. Surgeons have to recount (speaking and writing) to a wider variety of other people (including patients) why they are doing what they are doing, in ways that were previously unfamiliar. This is not a product of political correctness, bureaucratic management or new forms of surveillance, but a new way of talking about, recounting and accounting for work. Examples include clinically situated work, such as pre-list briefing, and also extra-clinical work, such as incident and accident reporting, appraisal, and, importantly, a spectrum of surgical-education activities. This extends the learning agenda beyond surgical technique to forms of quality assurance of such technique.

In the new, unstable and fluid work settings such as implementing the World Health Authority mandated safety checklist (WHO 2008) prior to surgery, surgeons must speak from positions for which they have uncertain authority, little practice, or do not yet 'know the texts', especially in the non-technical realms of practice that have now been shown to be central to maintaining patient safety (e.g. systems, communication and situational awareness).

Uncertainty is created where identity is de-stabilized by new, fluid work settings, such as work-about-work, or new modes of work-within-work that transcend 'communities of practice' boundaries (e.g. a briefing including members of the ward and recovery teams). Here, subjectivities are not given, expressed and exercised, but are formed through the negotiations that go on within these new textualities of 'speaking about' oneself in relation to a complex of 'others', the details of whose work are actually unknown. Once, it was acceptable for the surgeon to assume what the nurse or physiotherapist did, and not to be accountable to them. Now, doctors must sit down as interprofessionals to learn with, from and about 'others', as they are also accountable to others and to self. These are new forms of democracies, requiring the exercise of authentic democratic participation, producing the new identity of the surgeon as 'surgical citizen'. The 'surgical citizen' is a member of a collaborative, democratic structure of interprofessional work activity centred on the patient – aiming for the best technical result, effective overall care and follow-up, and supportive communication.

As Iedema and Scheeres (2003: 334) suggest, such new work settings are 'volatile, political, and confronting'. This challenges the assumed certainties of a surgeon's role and places traditional identity at risk. The common textual practices in surgery of 'telling' and informing' (monologue) that Atkinson (1995) described as 'the liturgy of the clinic' are being replaced by conversing, negotiating, collaborating, and supporting – again, participative dialogue or engagement, rather than authoritative monologue or telling.

11.8 Construction of Identity Through Public Textual Practices

Perhaps eclipsing, rather than supplementing, the ethnographic studies described at the beginning of this chapter, there is a rich seam of autobiographical and auto-ethnographic accounts by surgeons themselves of what they do and how their culture may be characterized. Richard Selzer (1996), writing since the early 1970s, has led the way in this social-realist genre that has recently been refined by Atul Gawande (2002, 2007), and the fictional work of writers such as Abraham Verghese (1998, 2009). These accounts do not specifically focus on the *education* of surgeons other, again, than by reference to traditional apprenticeship immersion in work. However, they should be on the reading list of any surgical education programme for the insights they promote into a new mode of identity construction – that of *textual construction of identity through public engagement.*

The new generation of physicians and surgeons writing on medicine and surgery (e.g., Abraham Verghese 1998, 2009; Vincent Lam 2006; Kevin Patterson 2007; Nick Edwards 2007; Gabriel Weston 2009) is doing something quite different from the previous generation of writers like Selzer. Selzer lauds surgery, where a writer, like Atul Gawande, admits to its limitations, uncertainties, hubris and pitfalls (while productively suggesting remediation). Gawande – surgeon, educator, researcher and also staff writer on medicine for *The New Yorker* – offers the public education service that the historian of medical education, Kenneth Ludmerer (1999) had demanded as a primary responsibility of the twenty-first century medicine.

As mentioned earlier, Ludmerer, in a North American context, suggested that medicine, as a previously self-regulating profession, had to win back the faith of the public, lost through its inability to disclose, or admit to, error and its closing of ranks in cases of poor practice, and find a productive way to discuss uncertainty with patients. Gawande – in sharp contrast to this legacy – openly shares such issues with his reading audience. In doing so, he sets out a new agenda for surgical educators, intimately linked with the construction of identity as 'surgical educator' focused first on learning with, from and about patients.

Surgeons do not have to be literary writers to engage in textual practices that construct identities. As described in the previous section, they will find themselves increasingly writing and speaking about their work (again, as 'textual practices') to a broadening audience, many of whom they previously may not have had to have contact with, in accounting for what they do, why they do it and how they judge the quality of their practice. Some of these texts will be pre-prepared by hospitals and trusts and posted on the internet, as public information concerning surgical outcomes. The audience now includes patients and families (increasingly demanding more quality of contact and openness in consultations); a wider range of medical and healthcare colleagues in multidisciplinary team meetings, audits, 360° appraisals, briefings and debriefings, and incident and accident reporting; management; policy makers; academics researching their work; and educationalists supporting their work.

The previously isolated world of the operating theatre is now the subject of almost prurient public interest – however distorted its representation – through 'medi-soaps', television medical soap operas such as *E.R.* and *Grey's Anatomy* in the USA and *Holby City* and *Casualty* in the UK. Whatever clinicians think of these representations, and however much they may mislead as well as educate, such programmes are increasingly being used as 'infotainment' or 'edutainment' to provide the public with opportunities to glimpse into worlds to which they previously would not have had easy access, or would have entered already anaesthetized.

In brief, surgeons are now required to account for their work in ways that were once unthinkable. This goes beyond the professional practices of 'accountability' (governance of work rates, meeting targets, ethical governance) that are now often summarized in appraisals and will form the basis for revalidation. Such activities include accountability to colleagues through practices of equality and equity, and to patient safety through collaborative practices such as briefing and debriefing, governance practices such as close call (near miss) incident reporting, and compulsory accident reporting.

These new practices radically expand and democratize the previously insular, restricted practices of closed mortality and morbidity departmental meetings. They offer, collectively, a form of 'monitory' democracy (Keane 2009). This is the newly emerging 'democracy of democracies' – including monitoring and quality assurance – a super-ordinate governance arrangement that no longer allows previously self-regulating bodies of professionals, such as surgeons, to engage in restrictive or closed practices. A new era of surgical education – as 'reflexivity' – is emerging, and this has powerful implications for the identity construction of the surgeon and the surgical educator.

References

Atkinson, P. (1995). *Medical talk and medical work: The liturgy of the clinic*. London: Sage.

Bauman, Z. (2004). *Identity*. Cambridge: Polity.

Bleakley, A. (1999). From reflective practice to holistic reflexivity. *Studies in Higher Education, 24*(3), 315–330.

Bleakley, A. (2006a). Broadening conceptions of learning in medical education: The message from teamworking. *Medical Education, 40*(2), 150–157.

Bleakley, A. (2006b). A common body of care: The ethics and politics of teamwork in the operating theater are inseparable. *The Journal of Medicine and Philosophy, 31*(3), 305–322.

Bleakley, A., & Bligh, J. (2009). Who can resist Foucault? *The Journal of Medicine and Philosophy, 34*(4), 368–383.

Bleakley, A., Hobbs, A., Boyden, J., & Hobbs, L. (2004). Safety in operating theatres: Improving teamwork through team resource management. *Journal of Workplace Learning, 16*(1/2), 83–91.

Bleakley, A., Brice, J., & Bligh, J. (2008). Thinking the post-colonial in medical education. *Medical Education, 42*(3), 266–270.

Borrill, C., & West, M. (2002). *Team working and effectiveness in health care: Findings from the health care team effectiveness project*. Birmingham: Aston Centre for Health Service Organisation Research.

Cassell, J. (1991). *Expected miracles: Surgeons at work*. Philadelphia: Temple University Press.

Cassell, J. (2000). *The woman in the surgeon's body*. New Haven: Harvard University Press.

Ciborra, C. (2000). A critical review of the literature on the management of corporate information infrastructure. In C. Ciborra (Ed.), *From control to drift: The dynamics of corporate information infrastructure* (pp. 15–40). Oxford: Oxford University Press.

Clark, A. (2009). *Supersizing the mind: Embodiment, action, and cognitive extension*. Oxford: Oxford University Press.

Colvin, G. (2008). *Why talent is overrated: What really separates world class performers from everybody else*. London: Nicholas Brealey.

De Cossart, L., & Fish, D. (2005). *Cultivating a thinking surgeon: New perspectives on clinical teaching, learning, and assessment*. Shrewsbury: TFM.

Edmondson, A. C., Bohmer, R., & Pisano, G. P. (2001). Speeding up team learning. *Harvard Business Review, 79*(9), 25–32.

Edwards, N. (2007). *In stitches: The highs and lows of life as an A & E doctor*. London: Friday Books.

Engeström, Y. (1987). *Learning by expanding: An activity-theoretical approach to developmental research*. Helsinki: Orienta-Konsultit.

Engeström, Y. (2005). Knotworking to create collaborative intentionality capital in fluid organizational fields. In M. M. Beyerlein, S. T. Beyerlein, & F. A. Kennedy (Eds.), *Collaborative capital: Creating intangible value* (pp. 307–336). Amsterdam: Elsevier.

Engeström, Y. (2008). *From teams to knots: Activity-theoretical studies of collaboration and learning at work*. Cambridge: Cambridge University Press.

Foucault, M. (1976). *The birth of the clinic*. London: Tavistock Publications.

Gawande, A. (2002). *Complications: A surgeon's notes on an imperfect science*. London: Profile Books.

Gawande, A. (2007). *Better: A surgeon's notes on performance*. London: Profile Books.

Giddens, A. (1991). *Modernity and self-identity*. Cambridge: Polity.

Hargreaves, A. (2003). *Teaching in the knowledge society: Education in the age of insecurity*. Milton Keynes: Open University Press.

Iedema, R., & Scheeres, H. (2003). From doing work to talking work: Renegotiating knowing, doing, and identity. *Applied Linguistics, 24*(3), 316–337.

Jackson, N. (2000). Writing-up people at work: Investigation of workplace literacy. *Literacy and Numeracy Studies, 10*(1/2), 5–22.

Joint Commission on Accreditation of Healthcare Organizations (2001). A follow-up review of wrong site surgery. *Sentinel Event Alert, 24*, 1–3.

Katz, P. (2000). *The scalpel's edge: The culture of surgeons*. New York: Prentice Hall.

Keane, J. (2009). *The life and death of democracy*. London: Simon & Schuster.

Kerosuo, H., & Engeström, Y. (2003). Boundary crossing and learning in creation of new work practices. *Journal of Workplace Learning, 15*(7/8), 345–351.

Kohn, L., Corrigan, J., & Donaldson, M. (Eds.). (1999). *To err is human: Building a safer health system*. Washington, DC: National Academy Press.

Lam, V. (2006). *Bloodletting & miraculous cures*. Toronto: Doubleday Canada.

Latour, B. (2007). *Reassembling the social: An introduction to actor-network-theory* (2nd ed.). Oxford: Oxford University Press.

Lave, J., & Wenger, E. (1990). *Situated learning: Legitimate peripheral participation*. Cambridge: Cambridge University Press.

Ludmerer, K. M. (1999). *Time to heal: American medical education from the turn of the century to the era of managed care*. Oxford: Oxford University Press.

Millman, M. (1976). *The unkindest cut: Life in the backrooms of medicine*. New York: William Morrow.

Modernizing Medical Careers (2008). www.mmc.nhs.uk/. Accessed 3 Jan 2011.

Patterson, K. (2007). *Consumption*. Toronto: Vintage.

Searle, J. R. (1990). Collective intentions and actions. In P. R. Cohen, J. Morgan, & M. E. Pollack (Eds.), *Intentions in communication* (pp. 401–415). Cambridge: MIT Press.

Selzer, R. (1996). *Mortal lessons: Notes on the art of surgery* (2nd ed.). San Diego: Harcourt, Harvest.

Sennett, R. (2008). *The craftsman*. Harmondsworth: Allen Lane.

Singh, H., Thomas, E. J., Petersen, L. A., & Studdart, D. M. (2007). Medical errors involving trainees: a study of closed malpractice claims from 5 insurers. *Archives of Internal Medicine, 167*(19), 2030–2036.

Tooke, J. (2008). *Aspiring to excellence: Findings and final recommendations of the independent inquiry into modernising medical careers*. London: Aldridge Press.

Verghese, A. (1998). *The tennis partner*. New York: HarperCollins.

Verghese, A. (2009). *Cutting for stone*. London: Chatto & Windus.

Wenger, E. (1998). *Communities of practice: Learning, meaning and identity*. Cambridge: Cambridge University Press.

Weston, G. (2009). *Direct red: A surgeon's story*. London: Jonathan Cape.

World Health Authority (2008). www.who.int/patientsafety/safesurgery/ss_checklist/en/index.html. Accessed 3 Jan 2011.

Chapter 12
Beyond "Communication Skills": Research in Team Communication and Implications for Surgical Education

Lorelei Lingard

12.1 Introduction

Team communication has been embraced as central to a competent surgical performance. It has been linked to safe practice, sound leadership, and expert judgement, in a broad array of professional domains (Sexton and Helmreich 2000). Further, increasing evidence has firmly established a link between how teams communicate and their patients' outcomes. In one report, patients had increased odds of complications or death when their surgical teams exhibited three communication behaviors less frequently: information sharing during intraoperative phases, briefing during handoff phases, and information sharing during handoff phases (Mazzocco et al. 2009). A recent succession of efforts to reengineer communication routines in the operating room has demonstrated that improvements in team communication result in better patient care (Haynes et al. 2009; Lingard et al. in submission, Awad et al. 2005; Rivers et al. 2003; Altpeter et al. 2007; Backster et al. 2007).

Research from a host of disciplines and perspectives, ranging from organizational psychology, human factors engineering, and adult education, underpins the recent wave of exploration around surgical team communication. This chapter offers a close study of one dimension of this work, stemming from the discipline of rhetoric. It examines our emerging understanding of how communication "works" in surgery, using a rhetorical perspective to map its influence on surgical work, team relations, and the complex-coordinated actions that constitute a successful surgical procedure. Our emphasis will be on how the knowledge emerging from team communication research can inform surgical education, from our concept of the "expert surgeon," our training objectives, our curricular approaches, and our assessment frameworks.

L. Lingard (✉)
Department of Medicine, University of Western Ontario, London, ON, Canada
e-mail: Lorelei.Lingard@Schulich.uwo.ca

H. Fry and R. Kneebone (eds.), *Surgical Education: Theorising an Emerging Domain*, Advances in Medical Education 2, DOI 10.1007/978-94-007-1682-7_12,

12.2 A Rhetorical Approach to Communication

Rhetoric belongs to the social theories of learning (see Chap. 2 for a short introduction to these) due to its attention to how language shapes relationships, identity, and action (Burke 1969). A rhetorical approach to medical communication expands our attention "from what *goes into* the communication to what *goes on in* the communication" (Lingard and Haber 1999: 509). While the content of any communication is certainly important, it is shaped by three other essential components: the context or occasion – the physical and temporal situation of the communication event; the audience – the persons being addressed and their relationship to both speaker and information; and the purpose – the social action being attempted or accomplished by the communication. Underpinning this basic four-part model is the rhetorical concept of "identification," which Burke posits as a central force within all social acts of communication (Burke 1966). Any attempt at communicative connection or persuasion involves a positioning of the speaker/writer in relation to the audience. Such positioning is conceptualized in rhetorical terms as "identification," the cultivation of similarities for the purposes of persuading the listener to some desired attitude or action. This concept provides a basis for exploring communication acts among divergent social groups as found in interprofessional healthcare teams, and for understanding the socialization process as one of trying out, discarding, and negotiating rhetorical positions.

Another relevant rhetorical notion is the theory of genre, which takes the concept of language as social action and applies it to standardized or routine discourse practices in a discourse community. Rhetorical genre theory treats standard discourse forms, such as the case presentation, as dynamic, socially constructed and disputed, and historically evolving. To a rhetorician, genres function as "sites of social and ideological actions" (Schryer 1993). Applied to medical education, rhetorical genre theory extends our attention beyond the mere form of a genre, such as the order of elements in a case presentation, to consider the social values and goals that are both reproduced by that form, and reflected in it. Taking this theoretical perspective, language is a key window onto socialization in surgical education, because attitudes and values are acquired through language, often as part of the "hidden or tacit curriculum" and strongly influenced by role modeling. Therefore, one way to shape the socialization process is to explicitly draw attention to communication practices, to excavate them for educational discussion. Rhetoric is useful to educators because it attends to the role of language in establishing professional identities by orienting speakers and articulating values. It provides a vocabulary for operationalizing the differences between (and the social implications of) "effective" and "ineffective" communication. And it draws attention to the social relations embodied in all language acts, relations underpinning the collaboration and conflict that play out daily in healthcare communication (Lingard 2007).

12.3 Key Findings in Surgical Team Communication Research

Each of the following sections reviews a key area of the study of team communication from a rhetorical perspective. In turn, these sections consider the powerful interpretive facet of communication, the patterns of communication failure in the OR setting, the complexities of silence in the communication spectrum, the notion of collective competence in matters of team performance, and the question of how to reengineer habitual communication routines for improved practice. Each section proceeds with a summary of core findings and a discussion of their relationship with other literatures, followed by a consideration of their implications for teaching and assessing communication practices in the context of surgical training.

12.3.1 Language is Not Self-evident: Interpretation is (Almost) Everything

This phenomenon is broadly apparent across all social situations, and surgical teams reproduce it. Naturalistic investigations of team communication have revealed it to be a complicated social phenomenon regularly punctuated with tension-filled events that are provoked by recurrent catalysts (Lingard et al. 2002a, b, 2004a; Espin and Lingard 2001). For example, observations of operating room (OR) teams in diverse institutional contexts suggest that regular patterns of OR team tension arise, provoked by recurrent catalysts such as issues of time, professional relationships, teaching, and resource use. Tension is neither inherently good nor bad: it can help the individual to productively focus on a problem or it can undermine group collaboration. Of particular importance, however, are tense communicative events that have a "ripple effect," extending a negative influence across time (i.e., resurfacing to disturb the subsequent case), space (i.e., spreading tension to the next OR theatre), and participants (i.e., extending to include individuals not involved in the originating event). Our research has suggested that such tension can accumulate during the case or the day, building toward open conflict and contributing to poor collaborative relations among team members.

Interviewed team members vary in their perceptions of team roles and motivations underlying communication events, while they agree that communicative tension negatively affects administrative, educational, and clinical outcomes (Lingard et al. 2002b). Not only do team members interpret such moments of tension and related communicative events differently but also professional perspective strongly influences these interpretations. In one study, nurses, surgeons, and anesthetists, who rated video scenarios of communicative tension in the operating room, frequently differed by profession in their perceptions of the various professions' level of responsibility for creating and resolving the tension (Lingard et al. 2005). Often team members rated their own profession as having relatively less responsibility for creating the tension compared to the ratings by and for the other professional groups. Furthermore, the pattern of data seen in the ratings of responsibility for creating tension was mirrored in the pattern of data seen in the ratings of responsibility for resolving tension. This suggests an "if you broke it, you fix it" approach to tension resolution among team members, which highlights the problem of differing perceptions regarding who is the cause of the tension.

Situations of communicative tension can pose particular challenges to novices. One study found that trainee surgeons were particularly affected by tension in team communication and responded with behaviors that intensified rather than resolved conflict. When they found themselves involved in a tense situation, trainees evinced two dominant communication strategies: they either mimicked their preceptor's communication approach or withdrew from the communicative sphere. Unfortunately, neither proved a particularly effective tactic. Because the success of a preceptor's communicative style is linked to history, status, and personal relationships, a trainee's adoption of that style in the absence of such history, status, and personal relationships is problematic. Similarly, the tactic of withdrawal from the communicative sphere, while it may reduce overt conflict in the short term, may not protect trainees from "hangover" tension the next time the trainee engages in the communicative exchange in the room (Lingard et al. 2002b).

Divergent perceptions of team communication have also been reported in surveys of safety culture. Communication behaviors, such as cross-checking and questioning in the face of potentially unsafe decisions, are a key dimension of a safe team culture. Surveys of OR team members suggest that team members perceive these aspects of team culture differently, with surgeons rating the likelihood of such communication behaviors more highly than surgical trainees, nurses, or anesthetists. For instance, one survey study found that consultant surgeons had more positive views on the quality of surgical leadership and communication in theatre than trainees and theatre nurses (Flin et al. 2006), while another found that the percent of operating room caregivers rating collaboration and communication as high quality was different by caregiver role and whether they were rating a peer (surgeon–surgeon) or another type of caregiver (nurse–surgeon) (Makary et al. 2006).

That team members differ in their perceptions and interpretations of communication is a finding with powerful educational implications. First, it challenges us to rethink the "content and delivery-focus" of current communication skills training. While accuracy of content and clarity of delivery are important, they do not ensure an effective communication exchange. Equal emphasis must be placed on assessing the context and considering how the needs and orientations of the audience will influence interpretation of the intended message. Furthermore, interprofessional educational efforts should be focused on addressing the influence of profession on disparity of perspectives. Existing communication training initiatives, such as the SBAR tool (Leonard et al. 2004), reflect the reality that certain healthcare environments privilege particular modes of communication; more attention could also be paid to the varied ways that different professional groups communicate. Training in this area might provide novices with the ability to predict other team member's communicative expectations, thus equipping them to diffuse or avoid tense communicative situations rather than exacerbating them. Such abilities would contribute to novices' development of situational awareness and their understanding of how to adapt their communicative responses to the social, emotional and organizational cues in their environment. For example, one interprofessional workshop used videos of team tension to provoke reflective debate among surgical and anesthesia trainees and staff nurses regarding their differing interpretations of communicative conflict, and the implications for both their interpersonal relations and their collaborative work (Lingard et al. 2005).

12.3.2 Communication Problems Aren't Just a Matter of Individual 'Skill': they emerge from rhetorical situations

Recently there has been increasing emphasis on improving team communication for improved patient safety. Root cause analysis often reveals communication problems as a factor in sentinel events: according to the Joint Commission on Accreditation of Healthcare Organizations, communication is a root cause in over 70% of all reported events, and that rises to 85% in specific event categories, such as wrong site surgery (Joint Commission 2004). Improvement, however, requires a precise understanding of the nature of the problem.

Traditionally, the medical education community has focused on communication skills development, based in an individualist emphasis on the communicative actions of individuals. For example, trainees are taught heuristics for delivering bad news to patients in order to facilitate effective performance of this communicative event (Rosenbaum et al. 2004; Colletti et al. 2001) (see also Chap. 9). By contrast, the literature on team performance has tended to take a more situated view of communication, characterizing communication failure in particular as embedded within an intricate web of individual, group, and organizational factors. In an ongoing project to characterize for measurement the nontechnical skills of surgeons (Flin et al. 2006; Yule et al. 2008), communication "skill" is conceptualized as interfacing with situation awareness, decision-making, task management, leadership, and teamwork skills to produce effective surgical performances. Efforts to understand how communication acts within – and is acted upon by – a situational context are based on the premise that cognitive abilities (communication "skills") are but one feature of the situation; others include authority gradients, diffusion of responsibility, and transitions of care (Dayton and Henriksen 2007).

Our effort to explore the situated nature of communication breakdown in the surgical domain has yielded a rhetorical model of communication failure (Table 12.1).

In one observational study, we found that communication failures happened in approximately 30% of communicative exchanges, suggesting both the pervasive nature of communication breakdown in the operating room and the ability of the model to capture these events for closer analysis. Of the four failure types, the most common in the operating environment has been "occasion." Communicative

Table 12.1 Communication failure types

Failure type	Definition
Occasion failure	Problems in the communicative situation, such as timing of delivery
Content failures	Insufficiency/inaccuracy in the information being communicated
Audience failures	Not all relevant team members present for the communication
Purpose failures	Communication events in which the purpose is unclear or not achieved

events in this category usually involve suboptimal timing of an exchange such that information is requested or provided too late to be maximally useful. The "content" category encompasses two types of communication exchange: those in which relevant information is absent and those in which inaccurate information is exchanged. "Audience" failures involve the absence of a key team member during the communication event, most commonly the absence of a surgical representative in discussions regarding the preparation for surgery. And the "purpose" category includes exchanges in which participants fail to achieve their communicative objectives due to lack of resolution of an issue raised.

In summary, we found communication failures to be based in strikingly simple factors: communication is too late to be effective, content is not consistently complete and accurate, key individuals are excluded, and issues are left unresolved until the point of urgency. Furthermore, one third of communication failures resulted in visible effects on system processes, which included inefficiency, team tension, resource waste, workaround, delay, patient inconvenience, and procedural error (Lingard et al. 2004b).

Over the course of a series of research studies, this rhetorical model of communication failures has retained its explanatory power, with the single refinement of one added failure type: style failures, in which the nature of the delivery is problematic. Style failures capture those instances in which the communicative occasion, content, audience, and purpose are unproblematic, but the communication is fraught in terms of the impact of its delivery; for example, an instrument request articulated in a tone that implies the listener is an idiot.

What the model drives home is the lesson that, when communication fails, it is not just a matter of an individual communicating poorly. Communication events are social interactions rather than performances of individual skill, and therefore their effectiveness can only be judged with reference to the social situation. A surgical trainee may have the right information and deliver it to the anesthetist for the right reason at the right time – but if they do not understand enough about the situation to know that the circulating nurse's absence from the discussion is a fatal communication flaw, their communication will fail. Similarly, the delivery of the right information to the right individuals at the wrong time in the team's workflow may also produce a communication failure, with a potential outcome of tension or resource waste.

A rhetorical conceptualization of communication failure has implications for both *what* we teach about communication and *how* we teach and learn about communication. First, our traditional curricular focus on the content of communication, exemplified by an emphasis on teaching the *structure* of communication genres and how to populate that structure with *content*, is necessary but insufficient. While trainees need to learn how to organize an oral presentation of the next surgical case for preoperative information exchange, command of the structure of a case presentation and knowledge of this particular patient's details will not guarantee success if the trainee cannot also gauge what details are relevant, for whom, and at what point in the preoperative planning.

Determining "relevance" and appropriateness requires an understanding not only of communicative *structure* and *content* but also of communicative *context*. Studies of trainees in ward settings suggest that determining relevance is a most difficult and elusive communicative "skill," yet absolutely necessary for success (Lingard and Haber 1999). What would a communication curriculum that teaches trainees to adapt structure and content to context look like? First, it would embrace situated learning: the notion that learning happens in and emerges from participation in authentic situations (Lave and Wenger 1991) (see also Chaps. 2 and 11). Based on this premise, it would maximize opportunities for practice and feedback on not only correctness of structure and content but also fluency in adapting "rules" of structure and content to context. Whether novices can translate their communicative understanding to new and emerging contexts is a central educational question. Studies of workplace communication across a variety of settings have found that expert communicators know more than the rules of a genre; they know when and how to "play jazz" with those rules, adapting them to emerging exigencies (Dias and Pare 2000; Schryer et al. 2005). This aspect of communicative development can be supported by explicit attention to what safety scientists have called "situational awareness": a team member's ability to track what's going on in their complex environment and to modify their own behaviors, plans, and cognitive attention accordingly (Leonard et al. 2004).

Opportunities for practice will be helped significantly by recent advances in high-fidelity simulation for OR team training, such as scenario-based training for interprofessional teams using a mobile mock OR (Paige et al. 2009) or simulated scenarios that combine laparoscopic technical skills and team communication training for residents (Gettman et al. 2009) (see also Chaps. 3 and 8 for further consideration of simulation). Faculty development to promote appropriate feedback will also be required, to enable faculty to draw explicit attention to how trainees are adapting communicative content and structure to the context of the communication event. Currently, faculty may not possess a language for talking about issues such as "relevance" with trainees; indeed, research suggests that, while faculty feedback is littered with comments, such as "Just tell me what's relevant," very rarely is the notion of "relevance" operationalized with reference to the rhetorical situation or context of the exchange (Lingard and Haber 1999). The importance of developing faculty's ability to give constructive feedback regarding trainees' communication abilities cannot be overstated, as the assessment of communication often serves as a more global assessment of general trainee ability. As Kennedy et al. (2008) found, clinical faculty reported using communication "fluency" as a reflection of general knowledge and competence, such that communication "red flags" in trainee communication were a common basis for higher faculty supervision and alertness.

12.3.3 *Meaning Emerges not only from Spoken Discourse, but also from Silence*

So far, we have been focused on communication as, generally, what is said and understood by participants in a particular situation. But spoken discourse – the communicative presence – is only part of the communicative spectrum. Silence also communicates meaning. Silence abounds in the operating room: in fact, some might equate a silent OR with a highly functional team. Therefore, a careful accounting of team communication must grapple with the meanings of silence, including both its functional and problematic dimensions. A rhetorical take on silence asks: What does silence *do*? How does it act on the communicative situation and participants?

In a recent Chap. 17 exploring the difficulties of silence for evaluating communication (Lingard et al. 2009), we considered the following example of silence, taken from observational field notes in a research study categorizing communication failures in the operating room:

> The circulating nurse and scrub nurse are doing their count near the end of the case. The surgical resident requests "4-0 Vicryl please" from the scrub nurse. The nurse's back is to him, and she doesn't immediately respond. The resident requests again with a slightly louder voice: "Can I get a 4-0 Vicryl please?" The scrub nurse still does not respond. The surgical resident raises his eyebrow at the junior resident across the table from him. A few moments later, the count is completed. The scrub nurse repeats "4-0 Vicryl", handing the suture. The resident takes it, appears irritated, sighing loudly and shaking his head.

The nurse's silence could mean many things, with different implications for the categorization of this exchange as a communication failure or not. One interpretation is that the silence has no purpose, because it is not a "response" to the request. This is plausible if the request has not been heard due to the nurse's attention to the counting protocol. Alternatively, the nurse may have heard the request, and the nonresponse reflects her prioritizing of the counting activity and subordinating the suture request in her own task management. Also possible is that the request has been heard, and the prioritizing of nursing tasks has happened, but the nurse's silence carries an additional purpose of indirectly delaying the incision closure until the count is complete. She may purposefully avoid explicit articulation of this purpose: her silence may, in effect, be a conflict-avoidance mechanism.

Each interpretation of the silence casts a different light on the communication exchange, the communicative expertise of the team members, and the nature of any communication failure that might be perceived.

With silence, as with spoken discourse, context is the key. To illustrate, consider how a slight shift in the social context of this event could radically change how it unfolds. Imagine that the suture request in this instance comes from a staff surgeon rather than a trainee and that the counting scrub nurse is a less assertive staff member. Then we might see the counting protocol set aside to allow immediate response to the suture request, and the communicative exchange would appear to go smoothly. In this case, however, the responsiveness might itself be the failure – reminding us that absence of communication, silence, is not necessarily always problematic. Sometimes, communication progresses smoothly toward a dangerous outcome.

What this example well illustrates is the premise that silence is not the absence of communication. While some silences reflect linguistic conventions, such as turn taking in conversational speech, other silences contain propositional content, that is, they are "communicative acts" (Glenn 2004; Saville-Troike 1985, 2003). Silence may also be a socially constructed response, as suggested by studies of the communicative constraints on subordinated groups such as nurses (Manias and Street 2001; Riley and Manias 2005; Gillespie et al. 2007; Bradbury-Jones et al. 2007). Across ethnographic studies of culture that explore institutional patterns of silence, silences emerge as meaningful in the sense that people often use silence to communicate in ways that are revealing of social structures and power relations (Linde 2009). The relationship of silence to power is complex and, as Foucault points out, highly ambiguous, as a silence may signify an exertion of power, a resistance to power, or an acceptance of power (Brown 2005; Gardezi et al. 2009). Thus, understanding what silence does – what attitudes it advertises, what purposes it enacts, what relations it reflects – requires subtle interpretive skills. For instance, silence can promote safety when team members "count to ten" and think before acting, or it can undermine safety when team members fail to cross-check and respond to one another's questions. Silence can mean shared tacit knowledge in a team accustomed to one another's expectations and workflow, or it can mask uncertainty and divergent assumptions about how to proceed. Attributing meaning to silence requires close attention to rhetorical context, both for the "objective" observer of team communication and for the trainee who, through participatory trial and error, is trying to negotiate their way to communicative fluency as a team member. Furthermore, such attributions may be extremely fraught in teams with fluctuating membership due to shift working and irregular staff assignment. When team members, trainees or staff, have limited relationships with one another, attempts to decode silence can easily go awry.

While we've only begun to map the role of silence in team communication, it is evident that its sophisticated use and interpretation should be part of the expert surgeon's communicative repertoire. Recent research on clinical judgment suggests that, when experts encounter a difficult or unexpected aspect of a surgical procedure, they commonly call for silence as part of regaining situational control and rerouting cognitive resources to the emergent situation. Similarly, other team members attend carefully to sudden shifts from speech to silence, as these can herald moments of challenge, renewed focus, and explicit problem solving for the surgical team (Moulton et al. 2010). As Moulton suggests, explicit educational attention to these moments is critical if trainees are to perceive their presence, understand their import, and acquire the skills to manage them in their own surgical practice. The implication for surgical education is twofold: first that we acknowledge silence and its interpretation as a core part of communicative competence, and second that we develop an operational language for pointing out silences to trainees and interpreting their meanings in context.

In the course of our observational research, we have found that the communication failures model offers a window onto – and a language for talking about – particular patterns of silence in the operating room (Lingard et al. 2009). The audience category draws attention to silence due to the absence of a team member, while the timing category highlights the absence of proactive communication earlier in the case. The content category makes visible the failure to communicate relevant information, such as when team members do not update one another on the status of outstanding issues. And in the purpose category, silence recurrently manifests itself as apparent nonresponsiveness following questions or requests. Given the preliminary nature of our study of silence, we do not envision this model as an exhaustive catalog of communicative silence; however, it is one tool for excavating silence from the mass of "taken-for-granted" material that surgical faculty currently have no shared language for attending to in their teaching exchanges.

12.3.4 Changing Team Communication Habits is an Intrinsically Relational Activity

Recently there has been a wave of interest in reengineering team communication for improved patient safety. Teams of surgeons, nurses, and anaesthesiologists working in the operating theatre have been some of the first to adopt such structured communication strategies in local, national, and international patient safety initiatives. For example, preoperative "pauses" or "time outs" – explicit verification of the patient's name, site, and side of surgery just before incision – have been mandated many countries, for example, in the United States since 2004 (JCAHO 2004). The World Health Organization's current Safe Surgery Saves Lives campaign promotes a more extensive three-part checklist (before induction of anaesthesia, before incision, and before the patient leaves the operating theatre), establishing interprofessional surgical communication as an international patient safety priority (WHO 2008).

Empirical research has focused on the impact of these interventions. Team checklists (or "briefings") and time-outs, with and without team training, have been associated with improved communication, direct changes to patient care plans, perception of safe collaborative practice, more consistent use of prophylactic antibiotics, and improved morbidity and mortality (Altpeter et al. 2007; Awad et al. 2005; Haynes et al. 2009; Lingard et al. 2008; Rosenberg et al. 2008). Surgical team checklists have recently enjoyed celebratory and high-profile media coverage, which often highlights the powerful simplicity of the practice. The team "briefing" is so intuitively sensible that it is increasingly assumed to be standard, not innovative.

Team briefings may be simple in principle, but inculcating them in routine practice is not. Educators, researchers, and practitioners commonly report resistance to interventions, variable uptake, and the challenges of sustaining even well-received strategies. Despite the promotional hype, team checklists are used inconsistently (France et al. 2008; Marshall and Manus 2007). The WHO acknowledges that uptake of its new checklist will be gradual and that some individuals will consider it "an imposition or even a waste of time" (WHO 2008: 20). Outcomes, then, are only part of the story. We still know little about how, when, and why interventions work (Haynes et al. 2009); we know even less about how, when, and why interventions fail to work. Attention is beginning to shift from demonstrating the value of these interventions to contending with the challenges of changing collaborative behaviors (Allard et al. 2007). While it is commonly agreed that such improvement efforts must be "bottom up" rather than "top down" (Leonard et al. 2004), just what factors shape "bottom-up" adoption of new communication routines is not well articulated in the literature to date. From an education perspective, it is critical to understand this, since in academic settings, "bottom-up" improvement of communication is likely to start with the trainee ranks.

Educators have long been interested in what prompts learners to grow and change, to learn and apply that learning to their everyday practice. Similarly, we have been intrigued by the question of what forces conspire to motivate or constrain the uptake of a new communication routine in the team setting. Given the situated nature of almost all surgical training in communication, which happens through the authentic experience of being a participating member of a surgical team, this question of how communication patterns evolve and change is a critical one for surgical education, from the postgraduate to the continuing education levels.

Our analysis of the process of uptake suggests that a new communication routine like team briefings is not straightforwardly accepted or rejected; rather, it is negotiated, adapted, and articulated anew in each situation (Whyte et al. 2009). The ease of implementing team briefings into teams' existing processes varied widely. In some cases, the briefings were truly a simple practice that fit easily into the team's work. In other cases, the briefing demonstrated an uncomfortable fit with existing processes, drawing our attention to the relationship between communication routines and other ritualized processes in the theatre (Katz 1999).

Overall, a key finding of our analysis of *why* briefings succeeded or failed is that the relational, rather than the instrumental, aspects of the team briefings are likely to drive the uptake of the briefings. Overall, briefings succeeded or failed based on whether the team members had a shared sense of the purpose and utility of the activity, whether their work patterns provided moments of synchronous activity, and whether the briefing activity "fit" with their sense of their professional commitments and scope of practice. With such a range of relational factors shaping the briefing update, it was insufficient to rely on "patient safety" as the single or even dominant argument to motivate participation. The task of effecting change in the social arena of team communication requires a range of resources and strategies for shifting commitments, attitudes, motives, and situations. We understand this as a fundamentally *rhetorical* process: participants require *convincing reasons* to participate, which may derive from strong arguments, or exigencies of situation, or trusted colleagues, and certainly from personal, professional, and cultural values (Whyte et al. 2009).

From an educational standpoint, this directs our attention to the social nature of learning and change: both are negotiated processes that take place not only inside an individual learner's cognition but also in the social arena of practice. Because surgical trainees will play a critical role in "bottom-up" change processes occurring in academic hospital settings, both educators and institutional change leaders need to think strategically about both how to shape surgical trainees' roles in such initiatives and how to use such initiatives to best educational advantage for surgical training.

In our own experience, we found that the responsibility to initiate and lead briefing conversations often fell to surgical residents and fellows, leading to several educational issues – both positive and problematic – requiring our attention. The positive implications were threefold. First, the briefing checklist tool provided a structure that trainees could use to organize their knowledge about the upcoming case. Second, the briefing activity provided a standardized opportunity for trainees to practice strategic, proactive planning conversations with other team members. Third, the briefing provided a recurrent and objective "event" that faculty could refer to when completing in-training evaluations of trainees' "collaborator" and "communicator" competencies, supporting assessment of such nontechnical aspects of expertise. The problematic issues that arose included the fact that, when trainees attempted to gather the team for a briefing, they periodically encountered resistance, tension, and even direct conflict from other team members. This could put a strain on their collegial relations, a strain that they may not be well-equipped to resolve. Further, some trainees were observed leading briefings for patient cases that they were minimally acquainted with, leading to useless (at best) or misleading (at worst) communication about the case and frustrating other team members. This problem might be avoided if trainees are told to expect to lead a briefing on a case – in such a situation, the briefing could provide both a motivation for trainees to learn about the patient and case and a means of testing whether this learning has occurred. Faculty have expressed an expectation that trainees should do such "homework" (Moulton et al. 2010): the briefing routine could formalize this expectation.

In summary, initiatives to reengineer surgical team performance abound. Many focus on standardized communication routines as a mechanism to improve teamwork and patient safety. Where trainees are members of teams engaged in such improvement initiatives, educators should strategize to maximize the educational opportunities afforded by the initiative and minimize the potential risks for both novice socialization and patient safety.

12.4 Conclusions

Research on surgical team communication from a rhetorical perspective emphasizes the situated nature of communication and the way that communication acts on the situation in which it emerges. From this emphasis we are alerted to the way that multiple individuals in a situation can differently interpret communication, and the impact of those differences on the situation as it continues to unfold. We are forced to move beyond the notion that communication problems reside in incompetent individuals to elaborate how the context, audience, and social purposes of communication contribute to communication failures. We are attendant on the spectrum of communication on a social situation, inclusive of forms of speech and forms of silence. And we are reminded that efforts to improve team communication unfold in a system of social relations, such that uptake is less instrumental than relational, less a linear process over the course of a change initiative than a cyclical negotiation from day to day and moment to moment. As educators, these insights ought to draw our eyes past questions of trainees' "communication skill," past curriculum that focuses on templates for content and organization, and past evaluations that are constructed around a notion of a stable set of skills which, once achieved, will serve the trainee across multiple surgical situations.

References

Allard, J., Bleakley, A., Hobbs, A., & Vinnell, T. (2007). "Who's on the team today?" The status of briefing amongst operating theatre practitioners in one UK hospital. *Journal of Interprofessional Care, 21*(2), 189–206.

Altpeter, T., Luckhardt, K., Lewis, J. N., Harken, A. H., & Polk, H. C. (2007). Expanded surgical time out: a key to real-time data collection and quality improvement. *Journal of the American College of Surgeons, 204*(4), 527–532.

Awad, S. S., Fagan, S. P., Bellows, C., Albo, D., Green-Rashad, B., De La Garza, M., et al. (2005). Bridging the communication gap in the operating room with medical team training. *American Journal of Surgery, 190*(5), 770–774.

Backster, A., Teo, A., Swift, M., Polk, H., & Harken, A. (2007). Transforming the surgical "time-out" into a comprehensive "preparatory pause". *Journal of Cardiac Surgery, 22*(5), 410–416.

Bradbury-Jones, C., Sambrook, S., & Irvine, F. (2007). Power and empowerment in nursing: a fourth theoretical approach. *Journal of Advanced Nursing, 62*(2), 258–266.

Brown, W. (2005). Freedom's silences. In *Edgework: critical essays on knowledge and politics* (pp. 83–98). Princeton: Princeton University Press.

Burke, K. (1966). *Language as symbolic action: essays on life, literature and method*. Berkeley: University of California Press.

Burke, K. (1969). *A rhetoric of motives*. Berkeley: University of California Press. (Original work published 1950).

Colletti, L., Gruppen, L., Barclay, M., & Stern, D. (2001). Teaching students to break bad news. *American Journal of Surgery, 182*(1), 20–23.

Dayton, E., & Henriksen, K. (2007). Communication failure: basic components, contributing factors, and the call for structure. *Joint Commission Journal on Quality and Patient Safety, 33*(1), 34–47.

Dias, P., & Pare, A. (Eds.) (2000). *Transitions: writing in academic and workplace settings.* Cresskill: Hampton Press.

Espin, S., & Lingard, L. (2001). Time as a catalyst for tension in nurse-surgeon communication. *AORN Journal, 74*(5), 672–682.

Flin, R., Yule, S., McKenzie, L., Paterson-Brown, S., & Maran, N. (2006). Attitudes to teamwork and safety in the operating theatre. *Surgeon Journal of the Royal Colleges of Surgeons of Edinburgh & Ireland, 4*(3), 145–151.

France, D. J., Leming-Lee, S., Jackson, T., Feistritzer, N. R., & Higgins, M. S. (2008). An observational analysis of surgical team compliance with perioperative safety practices after crew resource management training. *American Journal of Surgery, 195*(4), 546–553.

Gardezi, F., Lingard, L., Espin, S., Whyte, S., Orser, B., & Baker, G. R. (2009). Silence, power and communication in the operating room. *Journal of Advanced Nursing, 65*(7), 1390–1399.

Gettman, M. T., Pereira, C. W., Lipsky, K., Wilson, T., Arnold, J. J., Leibovich, B. C., et al. (2009). Use of high fidelity operating room simulation to assess and teach communication, teamwork and laparoscopic skills: initial experience. *The Journal of Urology, 181*(3), 1289–1296.

Gillespie, B. M., Wallis, M., & Chaboyer, W. (2007). Operating theater culture: implications for nurse retention. *Western Journal of Nursing Research, 30*(2), 259–277.

Glenn, C. (2004). *Unspoken: a rhetoric of silence*. Carbondale: Southern Illinois University Press.

Haynes, A. B., Weiser, T. G., Berry, W. R., Libsitz, S. R., Breizat, A.-H. S., Dellinger, E. P., et al. (2009). A surgical safety checklist to reduce morbidity and mortality in a global population. *The New England Journal of Medicine, 360*(5), 491–499.

Joint Commission on Accreditation of Healthcare Organizations (JCAHO). (2004). Universal protocol for preventing wrong site, wrong procedure, wrong person surgery. www.jointcommission.org/PatientSafety/UniversalProtocol/. Accessed 26 Sept 2008.

Katz, P. (1999). *Scalpel's edge: the culture of surgeons*. Boston: Allyn and Bacon.

Kennedy, T. J. T., Regehr, G., Baker, G. R., & Lingard, L. (2008). Point-of-care assessment of medical trainee competence for independent clinical work. *Academic Medicine, 83*(10), S89–S92.

Lave, J., & Wenger, E. (1991). *Situated learning: legitimate peripheral participation*. Cambridge: Cambridge University Press.

Leonard, M., Graham, S., & Bonacum, D. (2004). The human factor: the critical importance of effective teamwork and communication in providing safe care. *Quality & Safety in Health Care, 13*(Suppl 1), i85–i90.

Linde, C. (2009). Noisy silences. Stories not told. In C. Linde (Ed.), *Working the past: narrative and institutional memory*. New York: Oxford University Press.

Lingard, L. (2007). The rhetorical 'turn' in medical education: what have we learned and where are we going? *Advances in Health Sciences Education, 12*(2), 121–133.

Lingard, L., & Haber, R. J. (1999). Teaching and learning communication in medicine: a rhetorical approach. *Academic Medicine, 74*(5), 507–510.

Lingard, L., Reznick, R., DeVito, I., & Espin, S. (2002). Forming professional identities on the healthcare team: discursive constructions of the 'other' in the operating room. *Medical Education, 36*(8), 728–734.

Lingard, L., Reznick, R., Espin, S., DeVito, I., & Regehr, G. (2002). Team communication in the operating room: talk patterns, sites of tension, and implications for novices. *Academic Medicine, 77*(3), 232–237.

Lingard, L., Garwood, S., & Poenaru, D. (2004). Tensions influencing operating room team function: does institutional context make a difference? *Medical Education, 38*(7), 691–699.

Lingard, L., Espin, S., Whyte, S., Regehr, G., Baker, R., Orser, B., et al. (2004). Communication failures in the operating room: an observational classification of recurrent types and outcomes. *Quality and Safety in Healthcare, 13*(5), 330–334.

Lingard, L., Regehr, G., Espin, S., DeVito, I., Whyte, S., Buller, D., et al. (2005). Perceptions of operating room tension across professions: building generalizable evidence and educational resources. *Academic Medicine, 80*(10 Suppl), S75–S79.

Lingard, L., Regehr, G., Orser, B., Reznick, R., Baker, G. R., Doran, D., et al. (2008). Evaluation of a preoperative checklist and team briefing among surgeons, nurses, and anesthesiologists to reduce failures in communication. *Archives of Surgery, 143*(1), 12–17.

Lingard, L., Whyte, S., Regehr, G., & Gardezi, F. (2009). Counting silence: complexities in the evaluation of team communication. In R. Flin & L. Mitchell (Eds.), *Safer surgery: analysing behaviour in the operating theatre*. Aldershot: Ashgate.

Lingard, L., Regehr, G., Cartmill, C., Orser, B., Espin, S., Bohnen, J., et al. (2011). Evaluation of a preoperative team briefing: a new communication routine results in improved clinical practice. *BMJ Quality and Safety, 20*(6), 475–482.

Makary, M. A., Sexton, J. B., Freischlag, J. A., Holzmueller, C. G., Millman, E. A., Rowen, L., et al. (2006). Operating room teamwork among physicians and nurses: teamwork in the eye of the beholder. *Journal of the American College of Surgeons, 202*(5), 746–752.

Manias, E., & Street, A. (2001). Nurse-doctor interactions during critical care ward rounds. *Journal of Clinical Nursing, 10*(4), 442–450.

Marshall, D. A., & Manus, D. A. (2007). A team training program using human factors to enhance patient safety. *AORN Journal, 86*(6), 994–1011.

Mazzocco, K., Petitti, D. B., Fong, K. T., Bonacum, D., Brookey, J., Graham, S., et al. (2009). Surgical team behaviors and patient outcomes. *American Journal of Surgery, 197*(5), 678–685.

Moulton, C. A., Regehr, G., Lingard, L., & McRae, H. (2010). Operating from the other side of the table: control dynamics and the surgeon educator. *Journal of the American College of Surgeons, 210*, 79–86.

Paige, J. T., Kozmenko, V., Yang, T., Gururaja, R., Hilton, C. W., Cohn, I., et al. (2009). High-fidelity, simulation-based interdisciplinary operating room team training at the point of care. *Surgery, 145*(2), 138–146.

Riley, R., & Manias, E. (2005). Rethinking theatre in modern operating rooms. *Nursing Inquiry, 12*(1), 2–9.

Rivers, R. M., Swain, D., & Nixon, W. R. (2003). Using aviation safety measures to enhance patient outcomes. *AORN Journal, 77*(1), 158–162.

Rosenbaum, M. E., Ferguson, K. J., & Lobas, J. G. (2004). Teaching medical students and residents skills for delivering bad news: a review of strategies. *Academic Medicine, 79*(2), 107–117.

Rosenberg, A. D., Wambold, D., Kraemer, L., Begley-Keyes, M., Zuckerman, S. L., Singh, N., et al. (2008). Ensuring appropriate timing of antimicrobial prophylaxis. *The Journal of Bone and Joint Surgery, 90*(2), 226–232.

Saville-Troike, M. (1985). The place of silence in an integrated theory of communication. In D. Tannen & M. Saville-Troike (Eds.), *Perspectives on silence* (pp. 3–21). Norwood: Ablex Publishing Corporation.

Saville-Troike, M. (2003). *The ethnography of communication: an introduction* (3rd ed.). Malden: Blackwell Publishing.

Schryer, C. F. (1993). Records as genre. *Written Communication, 10*(2), 200–243.

Schryer, C. F., Lingard, L., & Spafford, M. M. (2005). 'Techne' or artful science and the genre of case presentations in healthcare settings. *Communication Monographs, 72*(2), 234–260.

Sexton, J. B., & Helmreich, R. L. (2000). Analyzing cockpit communications: the links between language, performance, error, and workload. *Journal of Human Performance in Extreme Environments, 5*(1), 63–68.

Whyte, S., Lingard, L., Reznick, R., Doran, D., Orser, B., Cartmill, C., et al. (2009). Uptake of a team briefing in the operating theatre: a burkean dramatistic analysis. *Social Science & Medicine, 69*(12), 1757–1766.

World Health Organization. (2008). Implementation manual: surgical safety checklist. www.who.int/patientsafety/safesurgery/ss_checklist/en/index.html. Accessed 25 Sept 2008.

Yule, S., Flin, R., Maran, N., Rowley, D., Youngson, G., & Paterson-Brown, S. (2008). Surgeons' non-technical skills in the operating room: reliability testing of the NOTSS behavior rating system. *World Journal of Surgery, 32*(4), 548–556.

Chapter 13
Surgical Education: Perspectives on Learning, Teaching and Research

Gunther Kress

13.1 Ways of Teaching, Kinds of Learning and Means of Researching

All of us know things that we were never taught: people who 'just picked up' a musical instrument they had never seen before, to play a melody just heard; the person who cooks a dish with only the recollection of look and taste as a guide. In fact, we might agree that most of the things we 'know' and 'know how to do' were learned without being taught. We know that no amount of teaching can guarantee that something to be learned will be learned. Learning needs a willing learner; in many cases it doesn't require a teacher, or at least, not someone formally identified as one.

The sketch put forward here encompasses (1) what is to be taught – the *curriculum*; (2) how learning can be facilitated and what teaching will come to mean; that is, it will deal with the social environment and the social relations of learners and teachers – *pedagogy* and (3) the provision of principles for conducting research in and for this field.

Over the last 25 years or so, there has been a shift in educational attention, marked by a shift in focus from *teaching* to *learning*. Teaching was seen as the passing on of knowledge in a hierarchically ordered social setting; learning was to 'acquire' or 'absorb' knowledge, as accurately as might be done, from those possessing it and designated to pass it on. Knowledge and authority had been linked, tightly, for so long that it seemed entirely reasonable to ask how there could be learning without teaching.

In the early 1980s, I was involved in a debate focused specifically and 'practically' on knowledge and education. It had been provoked by attempts to establish

G. Kress (✉)
Semiotics and Education, Institute of Education, University of London, London, UK
e-mail: g.kress@ioe.ac.uk

H. Fry and R. Kneebone (eds.), *Surgical Education: Theorising an Emerging Domain*, Advances in Medical Education 2, DOI 10.1007/978-94-007-1682-7_13,

a BA degree in Journalism. On the one side, there were ‘academics’ for whom journalism was, quite simply, not a proper subject for academic inquiry. It was a craft, a skill, it was practical; it did not involve distanced, abstracted and de-contextualized knowledge. As a skill-based profession, journalism had no place in an institution of higher learning. ‘Next thing’, it was said ‘we’ll have degrees for undertakers’. The practitioners were equally clear, for different reasons, that journalism could not be taught. They knew that ‘a real journo’ has an ‘instinct’, a ‘gut feeling’, ‘hunches’ and a ‘real nose for news’, developed through experience – ‘chasing fire-engines’. ‘Journalists’, everyone knew, ‘are born, not made’.

On the one hand, authority, power and explicit knowledge were inextricably linked; on the other, in the place of (explicit) knowledge, there were *hunch, intuition* and *natural ability*. As it turns out, journalism *can* be taught. And universities now offer courses in (Creative) Writing. Much of what had been attributed to *hunch* and *intuition* has been made explicit, in significant ways. *Learning* and the *agency* of the learner are now at the centre of attention in education. With hindsight, it is possible to see that those past debates on education, learning and knowing were reflections of larger- level social changes around hierarchy, power and authority, of agency and knowledge: arguments not yet finally settled.

In the debates then, two positions around knowing were at issue: one, overt knowing, ‘knowing *that*’; the other, implicit knowing, ‘knowing *how*’: *explicit knowledge* versus *tacit knowledge*. Germanic languages have distinct words to name each of the two: (in German) *Wissen* for ‘knowing *that*’ and *Koennen* for ‘knowing *how*’. Each of the two has fostered specific conceptions of teaching and learning; and, with these, social valuations. ‘Knowing *that*’ was, by and large, valued more highly than ‘knowing *how*’, with exceptions for certain elite professions and ‘callings’ – surgeons, musicians – and for those judged to be creative – writers, painters.

How societies value each of these positions, where domains of social life and practice, of knowledge, are seen as properly ‘belonging’ to the one or the other, is a question of real importance. How the assignation of this professional domain to *gut feeling* and *hunch* and that other domain to *explicit curriculum* is settled has as much to do with histories of practice, of professions and their present social organization, concerns and values as it has to do with what might be regarded as the ‘real’ substance of the matter. That assignation shapes in each case what we think *knowledge* is, what *learning* is or should be, how *teaching* should or could happen, and it affects which position we choose to adopt. It guides awareness about which variants or admixtures of the two positions we prefer as our models for thinking and acting, and why, in relation to a profession. Having a social and historical sense of practices of teaching and conceptions of knowledge can help establish a clearer understanding in cases where the bases of a profession’s practices and knowledge, its forms of transmitting knowledge and skill, are the focus of present debate and contestation.

Being social and historical, these positions are not fixed, and particularly so now, in a time which is profoundly unsettled and unstable socially. If in the 1980s and 1990s there was an attempt to make the intuitive explicit, there seems now – a ‘now’ of the last decade or so – a tendency in the opposite direction, that is, once again to see learning more in terms of knowledge arising from experience, as 'gained' and 'built-up', by learners in the course of their social/professional lives. Learning now is often seen as an effect of 'being there', the outcome of participating and observing, by working next to and with someone, as 'experiential learning'. Yet at the same time, under the banner of 'effectiveness' and 'efficiency', the drive towards making the intuitive and the tacit explicit continues, as in the profession of surgery. In elite professions, 'experiential learning', 'learning on the job', is now undergoing a move towards explicitness. This is happening for political and social reasons, for instance, for reasons of access and equity; it is happening also under the banner of 'effectiveness' in the use of 'resources' for 'professional training'.

This is a deeply contradictory situation, in which knowledge, learning and the agency of learners, and in particular teaching and the role of teachers need to be rethought, often pretty much from bottom up. It is here that my interest lies, for reasons which have much to do with my background. My first encounter with 'real' work was as an apprentice (furrier) in what was very much an intact version of 'training' and learning in the (German) medieval guild system: an *embodied* version of 'learning by participation, by doing and by reflection': being *told* what had to be done; *shown* how to do it and *why* to do it in this way; *doing* it; and *reflection* on and *evaluation* of what had been done by the other apprentices, in the presence of the master of the apprentice workshop. Much later, at university, I encountered the other pole of teaching and learning: disembodied, explicit, general, (to some extent) de-contextualized knowledge to be 'acquired'. For me it has, I am certain, been significant to come to the experience of de-contextualized learning from the experience of the entirely contextualized and embodied: learning why this seam was done like that; why its tension had to be like this and to *feel* that tension; and to be able to link that *feeling* to a *reason why*.

For me, the earlier approach to learning has shaped my professional life as an academic: the second form of learning became embedded in and integrated into the former. In my academic career another contextual factor has been crucial: namely the shift from a world of stability – stable trades, professions and disciplines interlinked with a world in which they had been shaped – to a world in which that stability has been unsettled and that interlinking disturbed, and in many instances broken. What that meant is that the disciplines which had been established to deal with the former world – literary studies, linguistics in my case – proved to be no longer sufficient to deal satisfactorily with the shapes and the problems of a differently configured and hugely more dynamic world. The demand became that of building theoretical frames, which would deal with that differently configured world and with the questions thrown up by that world. The task in my present job, as I see it, is to find ways of accounting for a communicational landscape which differs profoundly from that of say, 40 years ago, and to apply insights from new frames to an education system so that it can provide the resources-as-tools for young people to be active in all important aspects of their social lives.

With that as a background, I have been involved now for some 3 years in a project focused on surgical education: in meetings, in ongoing research, attending conferences and exhibitions, to see how my perspective might be useful in this setting (Bezemer et al. 2010a, b). It has been hugely productive for me to use one situation to reflect on the other, to recalibrate my thinking and perspective in both directions. It is from that position – anything but expert – that this chapter is written.

One question is how best to think about *surgical education* in the context of present social and political trends. In many ways, *explicitness* serves demands of equitable access as well as efficiency in teaching and learning. That involves explicitness about *curricula* (the (professional) knowledge at issue: what is to be taught) as well as forms of *pedagogy* (ways of teaching, with their implicit and explicit social relations – of teacher–student; expert–novice; cross-professional relations; hierarchies). A big question here is explicitness as generalized abstracted knowledge, taught and 'learned' not in participation, not by 'being there'; how to make 'visible' and 'accessible' the knowledge which it is essential for surgeons to have. Paradoxically, the goal of 'explicitness' might, in effect, make certain kinds of knowledge invisible: that knowledge, for instance, which is difficult to articulate in speech, writing or image. Expert professionals themselves may not be aware of such knowledge, which for them has long since become 'second nature' – hence my reference at the beginning to professions such as journalism with views that 'Journos are born not made'.

And there is the question of research; the means, that is, for producing insight-as-'knowledge' which is essential for a practice – surgical education – to function. What knowledge needs to be produced to serve as a secure foundation on which to build the practice of surgical education? That project needs the means for dealing with problematic issues as they arise and means for producing relevant, essential knowledge. It has to be theoretically and conceptually strong and plausibly applicable in dealing with questions that arise in the continuous development of this field. Even though there will be profound differences in approach, the principal categories of such a theory will need to be relevant for and applicable to all of surgical education, irrespective to some extent, of different conceptions of surgery within that field.

13.2 Making *Learning* Central: A Communicational Frame for a Theory of Learning

If learning has in contemporary theorizing – even if not yet in practice everywhere – become the centre of attention, it does not in any way mean that *teaching* becomes superfluous or irrelevant: quite the contrary. It does require thinking newly and differently about both learning *and* teaching: about the different responsibilities and tasks of learners and teachers, about what each might need to be, do and mean in relation to specific domains of knowledge. One task is to establish 'what is to be taught' – that is, to answer the question what knowledge is considered to be in a specific domain and how it is best shaped and presented for learners. It requires thinking about forms of teaching suited to these conceptions of knowledge and of learning in a (professional) domain. That includes describing what structures of authority obtain in a field – of surgery, say – and how these structures 'play out' in surgical education: how does teaching happen; what differentials of knowledge are there between learners and teachers; and where, in relation to such differentials, the responsibility lies for different aspects of the overall educational process.

It is unlikely that there will be entire agreement around 'what is to be taught' – the question of *curriculum*; nor for that matter around 'how what is to be taught should be taught' – the question of *pedagogy*. There will be much and intense debate on such issues before these can be fashioned into a plausible, effective and applicable framework in the area of surgical education.

Whether for learning or teaching, or for research, the prior and essential issue that needs to be settled is this: How do we see, or what do we see as the field of surgical education? What is in and what is outside the frame of what surgery is (assumed to be)? Is surgery defined in terms of technical competences? Is it seen in terms of the overall organization and effective working of a 'whole team' in the operating theatre? And what it is to be a surgeon?

Clearly, there has to be congruence between what is regarded as essential knowledge about surgery and of being a surgeon, and of what is in the 'frame' of the surgical curriculum: what is to be learned, taught and known about surgical practice (Kuhn 1996). The former – the profession's agreed sense of what it is – shapes the latter. From that follow theories of learning and teaching which are assumed relevant and adequate. That framing will also shape what is seen as essential or appropriate for research and suggest the principles of how it is to be conducted. There are any number of theories of learning; each theory projects, even if implicitly, specific conceptions of learning, of learners, of the matter to be learned, of how that is to be taught and of the environments in which learning happens. What theoretical frame can deal with this integrated undertaking?

The approach put forward in this chapter is characterized by two features. First, teaching and learning are seen as social practices – as is research. Hence, the theory that can account for them has to be a social theory first and foremost, rather than a cognitive-psychological one. Second, teaching and learning are instances of communication, so that a theory of learning and teaching – an *educational theory* – is set within the general frame of a theory of communication, as an instance of that. Meaning is the issue in both learning and teaching: in learning, learners shape meaning for themselves, and in teaching, teachers shape the environment for learning. In interactions, social factors set the conditions for the production of meaning; the social, as it emerges in interaction, is the generative source of meaning.

In all communication, in all domains of the contemporary social world, meanings are made in ensembles consisting of different *modes*: with gestures and speech, objects, writing, images, gaze, posture, actions all contributing to meaning, always with several of these in complex conjunctions (Hodge and Kress 1988; Kress 2010; Kress and van Leeuwen 2001; Kress and Van Leeuwen 2006). Each of these *modes* offers specific *affordances*, that is, potentials for communication. As a simple example, on a chart of garden birds on the wall in my study, *writing* provides the names of birds (in both English and Latin) and defining features

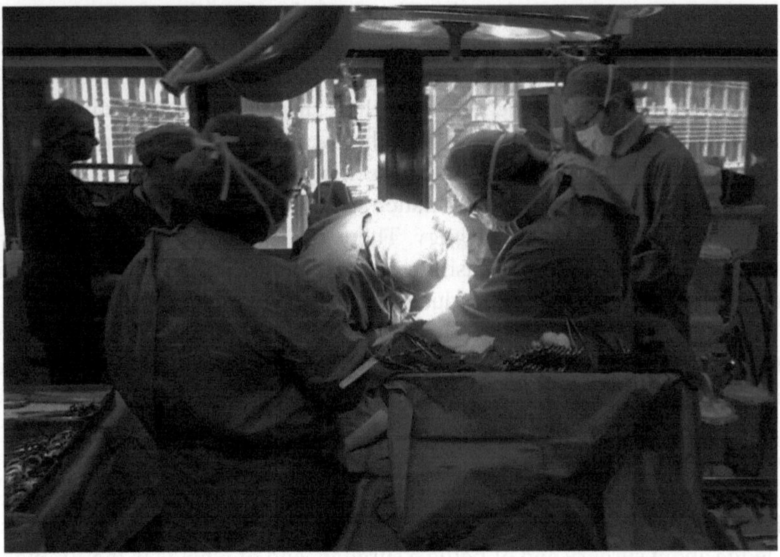

Fig. 13.1 An operation is in its early stage. A scrub nurse is in the foreground. Behind her, to the right, is the lead surgeon; opposite him is the assistant/trainee surgeon. Behind them, separated by a screen, is the anaesthesist; far back on the right and barely visible, stands an operating theatre technician

(breeding period, number of eggs laid, habits, etc.), while *image* provides details which would be difficult or impossible to describe using words: details of colour, markings, shape, the look of the habitat, etc. Without the use of either the one or the other, the information provided by the chart would be severely reduced, differently in the case of each mode. Interactions and the 'texts', which result, draw on a multiplicity of modes, whatever the interaction may be – entirely banal or potent politically, culturally salient, highly valued aesthetically or routinely in surgical practice. Communication is *multimodal*, always.

If *meaning-making* is *learning* (seen from a pedagogic perspective) and is an outcome of communication, then an apt theory of communication is the necessary starting point for developing a theoretical frame for environments and practices of learning (and teaching). To help develop such a theory, I use the example of the operating theatre. While it is a complex site of meaning (-making) and therefore of learning, despite its complexity it is entirely representative of everyday communicational situations, forms and processes.

In developing a sketch of a theory of communication here, I use a multimodal perspective; at the same time, my account here draws on observations made in the ongoing work of a research group (including myself) at St Mary's Hospital in London.

Figure 13.1 shows an operating theatre; an operation is in its early stage. A scrub nurse is in the foreground. Behind her, to the right, is the lead surgeon;

opposite him is the assistant/trainee surgeon. Behind them, separated by a screen, is the anaesthesist; far back on the right and barely visible, stands an operating theatre technician. Four distinct professions are present each with specific traditions, domains of responsibility, ways of talking and of doing, yet with closely interrelated and integrated tasks. This is first and foremost a *clinical* environment and an instance of communication in professional practice. It is also a *pedagogic* site, an environment of learning (and teaching?) for a trainee surgeon.

The site is socially and professionally complex: several distinct and related professions are engaged in a joint task. Communication proceeds through many modes, that is, communication is multimodal: by *speech* at times – with a spoken comment as instruction or request; by *gaze*; by *actions* – the passing of an instrument, or the reaching out for it and by *touch*. Communication is at all times a response to a 'prompt': a *gaze* might be a *prompt* for a *spoken* comment; that might lead to an *action*; *looking* at the screen by both surgeons might produce a spoken comment or a specific action by one, or else a guiding *touch* by one of the other's hand; an outstretched hand is met by an instrument being passed. Communication has happened when the attention of one of the participants has focused on some aspect of the interaction: when she or he has taken some aspect of the interaction to be a message for her or him and has *framed* aspects of that as a *prompt* for her or himself. The *prompt* is *interpreted* by that participant; it, in turn, may lead to further communicational (inter)action. Communication has happened when there has been interpretation (Jewitt 2009).

The notion of *frame* is important for (surgical) education as for communication generally; it provides a means for inclusion and exclusion (Bezemer and Jewitt 2010; Dieckmann et al. 2007; Goffman 1972, 1974). When a painter or film director wants to 'fix' what they wish to represent, they form a rectangle with thumb and fingers of both hands and look at the world through that makeshift frame. What is in the frame now appears separated from what is outside the frame. The elements inside the frame now form a unity in some way. The frame provides unity, relation and coherence for all elements inside the frame. A frame defines the world to be engaged with – it excludes and it includes – and in doing so it shapes and presents the world according to the interest and the principles of those who do the framing. Dramatists and stage designers, painters and filmmakers, architects and urban planners, interior decorators, photographers – amateur and professional – have long exploited the potentials of frames, as indeed have educators. For education, the notion of the frame provides a means for establishing what is to be inside the curriculum and what is to be outside. Frames and means of framing are essential for all meaning-making, in all modes (Bateson 1987; Goffman 1974). A frame defines the world to be engaged with and in doing that it presents the world according to the interests and the principles of those who frame – in the case here, those who establish what is to be considered as surgery and what, therefore, is to be taught.

In the example above, the sequence of *attention* leading to *framing* taken as *prompt* leading to *interpretation* producing *new action* is ceaseless. It involves all the participants, from all the professional groups present, at all times – each from their disciplinary professional perspective, with the distinct responsibility and 'interest' arising from that.

The complex multiple structures of environments of communication demand multiple and layered attention from all participants, that is, the norm rather than the exception. As in all social environments, features of gender, class, generation, 'culture', professional difference and regionality are present and active here, even if their effects are likely to be relatively backgrounded given the over-arching demands of the professional task. One important point is that communication across differences of many kinds is entirely usual and essential – a point that might play into consideration of what should be in the curriculum of surgical education.

If we frame this environment pedagogically, then learning and teaching are in focus. Questions are 'How does learning take place?' 'What is being learned?' 'How does teaching happen?' For the learner, any aspect of the complex dynamic communicational ensemble might at any one time be significant, so that he (in this case) has to be constantly attentive to cues as potential *prompts*: the senior surgeon might give a spoken instruction; the scrub nurse might make a slight movement or an explicit gesture, which the trainee surgeon/learner ought to attend to; the anaesthetist might glance at him to draw his attention to something.

This is by no means a mainstream view of learning: it is not usual to treat 'students' as responsible for framing aspects of the world of the curriculum – whether of the materials a teacher has presented or as here in an instance of a complex and extended period of professional practice. Present methods of assessment stand as guardians against such a view.

In the still dominant models of communication the teacher is the active cause of communication. It is the student's responsibility to ensure that the (meaning of the) message to be 'decoded' is identical with that of the message which was 'encoded'. The power of the teacher was/is not in question. By contrast, in the model outlined above, the responsibility for making meaning *as interpretation* lies with the learner; the authority of the teacher is not diminished but it is differently directed and focused (see Chap. 11).

In the operating theatre model of communication and learning, two concerns are in focus. The first is social interaction: here all aspects of the *environment of learning* are considered. The second is 'what is to be taught': here attention is on the *curriculum* and *resources* available to represent and disseminate the curriculum. A theory of learning needs both. That raises questions such as 'what is the task and the responsibility of the learner and what is the task and the responsibility of the teacher?'.

13.3 Framing: Curriculum and Pedagogy

In principle, it is neither difficult nor implausible to think of learning and teaching in such a frame. The difficulty lies in issues of *power* and in the *complexity* of this framing. If communication – and learning therefore – depends on *interpretation*, then the interest and the power of the *interpreter* as meaning-maker and learner are central. Further, in this model, communication is understood as an always complex interaction embedded in social environments, which are marked by contradiction, contestation and fragmentary social environments. The main point then becomes this: are we prepared to accept, and work with, a theory of learning where the *interpretation* of the learner is taken seriously, as central? Given the fact that this is a clinical environment, it may be thought that the safety of patients may be put at risk by a theory which sees the environment as marked by contradiction, contestation and fragmentation.

A precondition for the design of a coherent, integrated model of surgical education is a clear, explicit articulation of surgical practice with a high degree of consent attached to it. The decision then is whether this is a tenable (as well as a plausible) theory of learning and of learning environments? Is surgical knowledge framed 'narrowly' in terms of technical competence or is it framed in recognition of the complexity of the social conditions in which it is practiced? That decision will permit the framing of *the curriculum – what is to be taught* – and of *pedagogy – how that is to be taught*. On the one hand, there is the recognition and acceptance of the active role of learners; on the other hand, there is the consent of the profession, which lends authority to the teacher who has knowledge of all relevant aspects of surgical practice.

In this approach, the teacher is the designer of an environment of learning, which is most conducive for the students' interpretation-as-learning. The question arises: 'What is an apt environment of learning in any one specific case?' In schools, an environment of learning for sport will differ from one for history or chemistry. Tennis is not best taught from a book; chemistry is not best taught by giving young people tins of chemicals and setting them free to practise. The fundamental question is about the fit between what is to be learned – surgical practice in this case – and the necessary characteristics of environments which are designed for its most efficacious learning.

This is one of *the* big questions for surgical education. Earlier, I had contrasted tacit and explicit knowledge; I had contrasted embodied and general, abstracted knowledge. Embodied knowledge is knowing how to ride a bicycle; changing gears while watching the traffic; playing a drop-shot in squash, with your front foot in the right place, or cooking a meal while listening to the radio: things we know so well that we don't know that we know them. In telling my story of the apprentice workshop, my point was to insist that there is no necessary opposition between embodied knowing on the one hand and explicit knowledge gained from reflection on practice based on embodied knowledge on the other. It may be that surgical practice is one of the cases which is best learned by doing and by reflecting, in environments carefully designed to enable both.

Environments for learning can be designed as *sequences*, where the centrality of the learner's interpretation in practice is followed by overt and explicit reflection, with the help of a teacher/expert. Designed in the frame of a specific theory of *learning-in-simulation*, simulation can offer a route of embodiment and of explicitness. Of course, 'simulation' is a term with a very wide range of uses, even within the frame of surgical education. It is necessary therefore to say that I am referring to forms of simulation, which are based on careful analyses of the kind I have suggested: on what is to be taught – curriculum; on forms of teaching – pedagogy (Kneebone et al. 2010); on the boundaries of what is clinical knowledge and what is knowledge about the social 'setting' of the surgeon's work in relation to co-present participants from other professions and of patients (see Chap. 3). From these, a careful selection is made of those factors which are to be in focus, in this moment of learning. In a specific arrangement, that becomes the environment for learning, enabling maximal focus on learning that which is the teacher–designer's aim to be learned. In the kind of simulation envisaged here, the environment for learning becomes a four-dimensional material realization of 'scripts', in which explicit and embodied knowledge is materialized as *objects*, in *space*, as the *interrelation* of *participants*, 'performed' in *time*. This gets beyond a false (as it turns out) dichotomy of *tacit* and *explicit* knowledge – of *knowing that* and *knowing how*; of *explicit*, *abstract* and *general* versus *embodied* and *specific*; and of a mystification of 'expertise' as natural, 'inborn'.

Simulation offers routes for developing any one of a number of educational approaches; the prerequisite in all cases is clarity about the conception of surgical practice. In simulation, the need for explicitness and precision about what is framed as the curriculum of surgical practice is met not by abstracted categories – transposed, for instance, from *action* in *practice* to *words* or *images* – but by the *materialization* of the *categories*, *participants* and their *relations* in a carefully scripted and staged *practice-as-performance*. The need for precision about knowledge as curriculum is met by the precision of the design in the construction and materialization of the learning environment and in the design of scripts in which curriculum and pedagogy are presented to learners for their engagement through participation in the performing of the script. Curriculum is present as explicit knowledge in spoken and written form as much as in the three-dimensional environment and in the performance of practices, as in the scripting of interpersonal aspects of surgical practices. Precision and explicitness exist not in order to circumvent the interpretative action of learners but rather to shape, guide and focus the process of engagement and interpretation transparently and overtly.

The emphasis on practice in performance brings into focus the importance of *mimesis* as one central means of learning: a focus by the learner on salient actions of others and the learner's inward or outward 'repetition' of those actions (Wulf 1995; Wulf et al. 2010). In other words, in an approach which foregrounds the embodiedness of learning, the embodied means and processes of learning and simultaneous reflection need to be fostered, as in: 'Oh, I see (or feel), that's how that shot is played!'.

Whatever the professional/disciplinary position taken, it will provide a specific 'lens of recognition', at one and the same time making visible particular aspects of surgical practice and making others invisible; each lens producing 'ways of seeing' (to use John Berger's phrase) the subject in a specific fashion. The 'stance' taken will suggest and shape what needs to be in the frame of surgical education. It will have an effect on how learning is seen and where learning is seen to happen.

13.4 Simulation: Designing Environments of Learning

In surgical education, many arguments speak for learning by participation. In simulated settings of the kind envisaged here the learner is placed in a form of the practice designed so as to maximize the possibility of learning a specific aspect of the curriculum (see Chaps. 3 and 8). They are still able to make selections and transformations in framing from that designed environment, to construct prompts which lead to interpretations. As the learner is central, they must be allowed to encounter the environment in its fullest possible form essential for what is to be learned. The teacher's task is now the focus on the specificity of the design of learning environments as the ground which shapes, guides and provides focus for the learner. Because for reasons of patient safety, this cannot happen in an actual operating theatre; simulation can become the tool which, on the one hand, provides the fullest possible environment for learning (providing careful, precise design to guide engagement by the learner), while on the other offering safety. It allows simultaneously embodied and explicit conditions for learning in an environment which is shaped by the teacher as designer and is reshaped by the learner as interpreter.

The teacher–designer's careful, apt framing and preparing of the *ground* for engagement has taken the place of teaching in traditional ways. It enables learning as an instance of communication. Everything that is either conducive or essential to what is to be learned is placed in the frame. Simulation acknowledges and gives 'recognition' to the multiplicity of forms of communication in surgical practice. That recognition can counteract notions that in the operating theatre much meaning is left implicit or depends on the 'intuition' of the participants. In apt simulation, the curricular categories appear in a carefully designed environment that avoids the epistemologically and ontologically distorting reconfiguring of *action* or *object* or *relation* as *word* or *image* or *writing*. In simulation, what is simulated remains as *object* or *gesture*, as *gaze* or *speech*. What is regarded as salient in the site of original performance and action remains salient, in the same mode. The potentials of learning through *mimesis* remain. In apt forms of simulation, learning by participation is made possible, yet with explicitness about what is in the frame, about the knowledge that has been framed, and why.

13.5 Surgical Education as a Field of Inquiry: Research and the Production of Necessary Knowledge

Is surgical education a discipline (see Chap. 1)? Is it a new discipline? The definition of 'discipline' might rest on the presence of *both* a clearly specified domain of inquiry and the establishment and broad acceptance of a set of categories and relations, which provide accounts of salient phenomena in that domain. If the domain of surgical education was taken to be the induction of 'members-to-be' into the established practices of surgery, then the 'domain of inquiry' might be that of describing the knowledge entailed in surgical education together with apt methods for engaging members-to-be with that knowledge, so as to 'make it their own'. Two distinct areas of already existing knowledge are drawn on – general pedagogic knowledge and the knowledge of members of the profession of surgery. In surgical education, the two need to be integrated in a coherent manner: in non-anglophone societies in Europe the domain of 'didactics'. As an example, the didactics of language teaching brings together relevant knowledge about a specific language – its grammar/syntax, lexis, phonology, etc. – with what are regarded as apt means for making that knowledge available effectively to be learned.

In that sense, the development of surgical education constitutes the addition of another instance of didactics, that of surgical education. Its novelty resides not in the novelty of its two main components but in the conjunction and integration of two existing fields. It is not the development of a new discipline, unlike the extension or expansion or the radical remaking of a theory in areas of the Natural or Social Sciences, where a theory might be overthrown in favour of an account which is distinct in fundamental ways – neither a scientific revolution (Kuhn 1996), nor the 'patching up', say by extension, of an existing disciplinary frame.

The emergence of a new 'discipline' usually takes place in conditions where the social, cultural, economic world (including both the Natural and the Social Sciences) has undergone change significant enough to lead to the emergence of newly configured domains, whose features are not addressed by existing disciplines. The emergence of Sociology in the early years of the twentieth century might be such a case; others might be the emergence of Linguistics, also in the previous century, or of Cultural Studies more recently.

The situation of surgical education is, in many respects, similar to developments in other professions in which learning by participation was regarded as the norm, as 'natural'. One essential question is: 'are the felt problems such as to require the production of a new account, a new frame, a new theory?' It may be that the conjunction of factors – the need for different forms of induction into what is at the moment an elite profession; the characteristics of that profession's practices, for instance its large element of 'embodied knowledge'; the considerations of patient safety; and others – may require the development over time of a quite distinct form of education, enough to warrant being treated as a distinct discipline.

Irrespective of that, there are areas in surgical education where research will be required now. Here I can do no more than make suggestions. Two large 'headings' under which this can be thought about are 'apt theories of learning for surgical education' and 'what counts as essential knowledge in this professional field?'

Under the first heading, that of 'apt theories of learning', there is an immediate need for research about requirements for learning in a profession where much knowledge is embodied, and thereby at the moment maybe implicit to a significant extent. Is surgery a field where learning via *mimetic* processes is likely to be more effective or more usual? How do notions of *embodiment* affect perceptions of knowledge in the field? To what extent, and in what areas of surgery, is simulation essential and where is it not? What forms of simulations are required and most efficacious for which aspects of surgical knowledge and surgical practice? How can everything that is conducive or essential to 'what is to be learned' be described, transcribed and established? In terms of *environments of learning* and their *instantiations* what are the best, the most apt representational means?

The second heading implicitly points to the issue of 'framing', in particular, in relation to what might be called 'boundary regions' or 'borderlands' of surgery – on the one hand in relations with those professions which are essential and crucially involved in the performance of surgery, and on the other relations with those who are the subjects and beneficiaries, the patients. What is made visible and invisible by a specific framing of the field of surgery? What is regarded as salient and why? What is in the frame, what is out and why? What problems are produced?

There is a need for an agreed version of what Bernstein (Bernstein 1996) has called a 'language of description', to enable relatively 'secure' communication about surgical education (see Chaps. 11 and 12). What are the limits of such a language of description? If much knowledge is embodied or is conveyed in modes other than speech or writing, can every mode produce a language of description? Associated with this is the issue of 'naming': that is, 'populating' the field with apt and precise terminology, which can provide coherence for the field, precision and general communicability. In that process, theoretical issues will arise which need to be debated, analysed and described. For instance, what actually is *simulation*? What differences of practice and theory inhere in terms such as *assessment*, *evaluation* and *rating*? As compared with *teaching* or *training*, what does a term such as *instruction* offer? Does the term *knowledge* configure the field of surgical education differently to that of (procedural) *skills*? And the big issue of *assessment*, *evaluation* and *rating* certainly requires research: what are apt or requisite forms, metrics and processes?

Lastly, there is the question of research methods: what are apt and necessary methods? And what are apt 'technologies of transcription'? That is, how do we turn the materials to be researched into data and how do we represent that data? Here the idea of simulation as a research tool seems both essential and appropriate. Do the theories that are invoked provide adequate 'languages of description'? Can the forms of simulation referred to here come to constitute an equivalent of 'languages of description?' Other questions circle around: what is made implicit, or (in)visible through technologies of recording and transcription? How does *framing* produce or reduce complexity? What is lost or gained in reducing complexity? How does and should 'research' in this domain deal with complexity?

13.6 Conclusion

Learning beyond the school and other institutional settings has become a widespread concern. In many ways the theories which had been developed were developed largely in relation to 'school' – to children and therefore to the powerless. These have most predominantly been based on psychological theories – the names of Piaget and Vygotsky stand most eminent. Although in part useful, these are largely insufficient. There is a need for focused thinking about the specific issues in professional learning. In part, this chapter is one such attempt. Yet it differs from the more general debate in that surgical education presents a combination of factors which pose a unique challenge to educational thinking and theorizing: it deals with adults in a high-status profession; much of its professional knowledge is embodied and often implicit; it takes place in multiply complex social settings; and it is practised with requirements for patient safety. Contemporary social, political and financial conditions demand the maintenance of certain aspects of professional practices and a radical transformation of others – broadly in the direction of *embodiedness linked with explicitness*; learners who are already expert will need to be seen as central in the educational process; with a high degree of agency therefore given to learners; in carefully and precisely designed environments for learning by participation.

These features make surgical learning a distinct case not just of professional learning but of learning in general. A theory adequate to the demands of surgical learning will have far-reaching implications for all theories of learning, anywhere, at any age, in all social environments. This will be a theory apt to contemporary social conditions, with a high degree of agency given to learners in theories of learning, which make the interpretative work of learners central, in environments marked by the co-presence of teachers as designers of educational environments and processes, who constantly bring *reflection* on work just performed into the centre of practices of learning.

Whether teaching expert learners and learners who are experts; whether teaching high-status learners or the very young, the exploration of this field and its theorization promises a profound transformation of approaches to learning in integration everywhere and anywhere.

Acknowledgments I wish to thank Alexandra Cope, Jeff Bezemer and Roger Kneebone for allowing me to draw on their research and developmental work in surgical education.

References

Bateson, G. (1987). *Steps to an ecology of mind* (Vol. 2). Northwave: Jason Aronson Inc.

Bernstein, B. (1996). *Pedagogy, symbolic control and identity*. London: Taylor & Francis.

Bezemer, J., & Jewitt, C. (2010). Multimodal analysis: Key issues. In L. Litosseliti (Ed.), *Research methods in linguistics* (pp. 180–197). London: Continuum.

Bezemer, J., Cope, A., Kress, G., Kneebone, R. (2010a). 'Do you have another Johan?': Negotiating meaning in the operating theatre. *Applied Linguistics Review* (in press).

Bezemer, J., Murtagh, G., Cope, A., Kress, G., Kneebone, R. (2010b). "Scissors, please": Shared understanding in surgical activity. *Symbolic Interaction* (in press).

Dieckmann, P., Gaba, D., & Rall, M. (2007). Deepening the theoretical foundations of patient simulation as social practice. *Simulation in Healthcare, 2*(3), 183–193.

Goffman, E. (1972). *Encounters: Allen Lane*. London: The Penguin Press.

Goffman, E. (1974). *Frame analysis*. London: Penguin.

Hodge, R., & Kress, G. (1988). *Social semiotics*. Cambridge: Polity Press.

Jewitt, C. (Ed.). (2009). *The Routledge handbook of multimodal analysis*. London: Routledge.

Kneebone, R., Arora, S., King, D., Sevdalis, N., Kassab, E., Aggarwal, R., et al. (2010). Distributed simulation – Accessible immersive training. *Medical Teacher, 32*(1), 65–70.

Kress, G. (2010). *Multimodality: A social semiotic approach to contemporary communication*. London: Routledge.

Kress, G., & van Leeuwen, T. (2001). *Multimodal discourse: The modes and media of contemporary communication*. London: Hodder and Stoughton.

Kress, G., & Van Leeuwen, T. (2006). *Reading Images: The grammar of graphic design* (2nd ed.). London: RoutledgeFalmer.

Kuhn, T. (1996). *The structure of scientific revolutions* (3rd ed.). Chicago/London: University of Chicago Press.

Wulf, C. (Ed.). (1995). *Paragrana* (Vol. 4). Berlin: Akademie Verlag.

Wulf, C., Althans, B., Audehm, K., Bausch, C., Gohlich, M., Sting, S., et al. (2010). *Ritual and identity: The staging and performing of rituals in the lives of young people*. London: Tufnell Press.

Afterword

Roger Kneebone and Heather Fry

We began this book by asserting that surgical education is an emerging field which is establishing its own identity. We pointed out that although the centre of the field may seem obvious, its boundaries are blurred and often indistinct. We framed this blurriness as both a problem and an opportunity. Much of the book has been devoted to exploring where these boundaries might be drawn, bringing greater solidity to the centre by considering the distinctive aspects of surgical practice, and viewing the issues through an educational lens. The distinctiveness of surgical practice, context and culture are sufficient, it seems to us, to constitute a distinct field of learning, training and teaching. Although sharing many points of contact with its older sister medical education, surgical education requires a different and wider horizon.

We acknowledge *craft* as a defining characteristic of what surgeons do. We also point to the danger in allowing the acquisition of technical dexterity (crucially important though that is) to overshadow equally important yet less tangible aspects of what surgeons do. From this perspective, surgery can be seen as socially constructed, an activity where relations between people (and their interactions with material objects and processes) are necessary conditions for success. Unravelling the delicate relationships which constitute this complexity is one of surgical education's major challenges. For this task, education, social and biomedical science must all play a role.

We have sought to show that surgical education is a special case, distinct from medical education. Paradoxically, however, we have also sought to show its interdependency with a much larger range of fields based in the social sciences. As a background to surgical activity we have painted a landscape of continual and far-reaching change powerfully moulded by advancing technology. Even more

R. Kneebone
Surgical Education, Imperial College London, London, UK
e-mail: r.kneebone@imperial.ac.uk

H. Fry
Higher Education Funding Council for England (HEFCE), Bristol BS1b 1QD, UK

H. Fry and R. Kneebone (eds.), *Surgical Education: Theorising an Emerging Domain*, Advances in Medical Education 2, DOI 10.1007/978-94-007-1682-7,

profound, however, may be the fragmentation of traditional patterns and relationships brought about by wider societal and service change and upheaval. If surgical education is to be effective, it must acknowledge and account for these deep-seated forces which are shaping social climate *as well as* clinical and educational practice.

In the introductory chapters of Part I we offered a personal view of how matters stand at present. In Chap. 1 we picked out recent seminal events within the UK health service which are shaping present day practice. In Chap. 2 we introduced the reader to key educational theories and perspectives, aiming to provide the educational non-specialist with navigational co-ordinates to what can otherwise be an unknown and confusing landscape. In Chap. 3 we looked critically at the role of simulation in surgery, framing it not only as a means of gaining procedural dexterity without jeopardizing safety but also as a route to access the complexity and contingency of authentic clinical practice. And in Chap. 4 we juxtaposed methodologies from bioscience, social science and the humanities which a researcher in surgical education may need to recruit when framing and addressing key questions.

In Part II of the book, we have drawn on the views of a range of expert contributors, selected both because of their eminence in their fields and the freshness of their thinking. We made no attempt to be comprehensive, but rather to provide a vivid palette of perspectives.

However, some broad themes cut across these individual chapters and contributions. A central issue is ontological – what it means to *become* a surgeon and how that comes about. Many contributors have highlighted characteristics of the surgical world, such as the need to make rapid decisions in a fast-moving setting where effective team communication is paramount; to detect, accommodate and respond to subtle changes in an environment where much that is conveyed is unspoken; to be mindful and to monitor one's own performance and capacities (slowing down where appropriate and calling for help if necessary); and to manage risk responsibly. A key concept to emerge is 'uncertainty', as a defining characteristic of surgical practice. Seen as a threshold concept, this reappears throughout a surgeon's development, and coming to terms with uncertainty without allowing it to paralyse progress is both a central component of professionalism and a key educational challenge. Learning to do all this (and more) is a tall order, and it is not surprising that the process entails discomfort and resistance as learners progress from one state to another. Nor should it be surprising if the traditional apprenticeship model of training proves inadequate in the face of today's complexities, demands and pressures, and that changes to training have been hard to craft and have had mixed success.

The acknowledgement that surgeons do not function in isolation but are always part of a team lies at the heart of how surgical care is provided. Understanding how people work in teams becomes of central interest. Ideas around communities of practice, team communication, networking, knotworking, empathic interpersonal interaction and a host of others – none of them the exclusive province of surgery but all of them with something to say – can shed light on behaviours that are frequently taken for granted.

Exploring these ontological processes rigorously requires a well-stocked methodological toolbox. Selecting a theoretical framework is essential for making sense of a complexity which could easily become overwhelming. As Anderson points out from his 'outsider's perspective' as an anthropologist, the natural and social sciences differ in many ways, especially in the role played by dominant theories and paradigms (Anderson 2011). He starts by referring to Kuhn's assertion that the natural sciences operate under a single dominant vision of what can be investigated and how, and work that paradigm until it collapses of its own inconsistencies and a new one takes over sole dominance (Kuhn 1996). Anderson goes on to say that 'this is not so in the social sciences, where theory, not universally shared to begin with, is modified and recycled, debated and adjusted, but rarely discarded altogether'. We hope the chapters in this volume have conveyed something of these approaches.

So an awareness of theory is of central importance. Yet deciding which frameworks to choose can be a major challenge. Various lenses have been put forward in this book, and none is right or wrong. Threshold concepts, activity theory, communities of practice, actor-network theory, multimodality, expertise, team communication, assessment theory, e-learning, patient centredness – all these and many others – may help to illuminate particular questions. We are not advocating one above the other, but highlighting the diversity of what is available. It is for each researcher to decide which approach or combination of approaches best meets their needs at a particular moment, and where along the methodological spectrum their work fits most comfortably. It is for curriculum designers, policy makers, assessors and trainers to understand these theories and this research, working through their possible implications for organizing, supporting and assessing learning and training in surgery. What does seem clear, however, is that a setting as rich and complex as surgery requires research methodologies which can do justice to that richness and complexity. Several of the contributors to this book illustrate this point with research from their own experience.

The approach to framing and addressing research questions within surgical education therefore becomes of great importance. No single methodology or paradigm can cover all eventualities, which is why we argue for a broad palette and an awareness of methods used by education as well as by 'hard' science. It is true that many of the complex issues described above resist being confined within an orthodox 'scientific' framework, and capturing the richness of individual experience frequently requires a more descriptive approach. However, we do not subscribe to the notion of a qualitative/quantitative opposition, but believe that judicious selection is needed in order to find the most apt approaches for each question.

We have seen throughout Part II suggestions for and examples of research and theory suggesting ways of changing educational practices. We emphasize that new educational practices and enterprises need critical evaluation and subsequent adjustment (the educational equivalent of the audit cycle); and that evaluation will typically need to draw on mixed method approaches. Efforts to translate research and theory into changed educational practice will not always prove to be feasible or successful. What may work in one set of circumstances may not do so in another, and human resistance or misinterpretation may distort outcomes. Research and theory do not give rise to a universal educational blueprint that will be a panacea for all training ills, although they may point strongly in certain directions. Two further dangers are that the 'not invented here syndrome' can be responsible for a failure to adapt and adopt successful practices, and that poor knowledge of the many complex areas of relevance (only some of which are touched on in this volume) can lead to fruitless efforts and much re-invention.

It may be that contextualized simulation can offer means of responding to such complexity, recreating the emergent properties of unique teams of people who all bring their own histories and concerns to every case. By providing a safe experimental setting where at least some variables can be managed, simulation in the future may offer insights into behaviours that cannot be observed 'in the wild'. It may also be that acculturation into the profession (on team working, living with risk, uncertainty and stress, on communication and on surgical culture) requires greater consideration within training, and can also be at least partly addressed within contextualized simulation. These are changes of emphasis that are more than minor shifts; they are about seeing the training world in a different way.

We believe that the range of contributions in this book illustrates the depth and richness of surgical education and underpins its value as an evolving field. Each of these contributions taps into its own literature, its own traditions of enquiry and its own way of framing questions. As good research should, each raises more questions than answers.

We are of course aware that we have sampled selectively from a vast field and that different choices would have led to a different emphasis and other combinations of flavours. To us, that is simply part of engaging with a field as rich, as nuanced and as protean as ours. Our selection has been moulded by our personal and academic backgrounds, our reading and our shared experience in developing Imperial's M.Ed. in Surgical Education – an example perhaps of the inescapable interweaving of the researcher and the researched.

For us, surgical education is about researching how surgeons learn. It is about gathering evidence and developing robust, defensible theories which can be challenged and refined. These are familiar goals to any academic researcher. But surgical education is also about feeding that knowledge and understanding back into the real world of surgical training and patient care; about identifying areas that can be improved; and about establishing a community of surgeon educators, from whatever background, who will jointly explore the myriad facets of this fascinating field. This point is well made by Bleakley in this volume: 'It is important that surgical education culture of the future develops an identity from within its own cultural resources'. These cultural resources must come to encompass a broader base.

So where next for surgical education? The nineteenth century pioneers of microbiology spoke of a sense of limitless horizons, of seeing a world of unexplored complexity opening before their eyes. To them, the challenge lay not in finding something to investigate but in limiting their scope and making their enquiry manageable. To us, the constantly evolving landscape of surgical education offers a similar sense of richness and potential. We hope to have conveyed some of that excitement and challenge in this book.

References

Anderson, W. D. (2011). Outside looking in: Observations on medical education since the Flexner Report. *Medical Education, 45*(1), 29–35.

Kuhn, T. (1996). *The structure of scientific revolutions*. Chicago/London: The University of Chicago Press.

Biographies of Authors

Heather Fry is Director (Education and Participation) at the Higher Education Funding Council for England (HEFCE). Prior to joining HEFCE in 2008 she worked at universities in England and overseas, including Imperial College London, and the Institute of Education and Barts and London Medical and Dental School, both at the University of London. She also worked for many years as an education faculty at the Royal College of Surgeons of England. She has taught and researched in a number of areas, including being joint founder and co-director of the UK's first Masters in Surgical Education, at Imperial, with Roger Kneebone. Her expertise is in the policy of higher and professional education and facilitating learning in these two contexts. She has published extensively across her varied areas of interest.

Roger Kneebone is Professor in Surgical Education at Imperial College London. Roger trained first as a general surgeon, then changed course to become a general practitioner and GP trainer in a large group practice near Bath. In 2003, after completing his Ph.D. in surgical education, Roger joined Imperial College London. His current research focuses on using simulation to contextualize clinical learning, and on mapping clinical environments from a pedagogical perspective. He has developed innovative approaches to learning and assessing clinical procedures (using hybrid combinations of models and simulated patients) and is currently developing lightweight, portable yet realistic surgical environments for training and assessment. Roger publishes extensively and directs Imperial's Masters in Education (M.Ed.) in Surgical Education.

Fernando Bello is a Senior Lecturer in Surgical Graphics and Computing at Imperial College London. His main research interests are in modelling and simulation, medical virtual environments and haptic interaction. His work in the area of simulation in healthcare spans technology and education, including development of patient-specific simulation and e-learning applications for a number of surgical procedures, and exploring the integration of simulation and context via Patient Focused Simulation.

H. Fry and R. Kneebone (eds.), *Surgical Education: Theorising an Emerging Domain*, Advances in Medical Education 2, DOI 10.1007/978-94-007-1682-7,

Lesley Bentley has been a lay member of the Patient Liaison Group at the Royal College of Surgeons of England since 2005, working as chair for 2 years. She has acted as patient representative on college working groups, has spoken and written about patient issues including pathways for patients with cancer, the role of the consultant in caring for patients and communication skills for doctors.

Alan Bleakley is Professor of Medical Education at Peninsula Medical School, UK, where he runs a research programme focused on surgical teamwork. He has a background in biological sciences, psychology, psychotherapy and education. Alan is widely published, including Medical Education for the Future (Springer 2011).

Harry Brenton worked in TV, film and web design before completing a Ph.D. as a research fellow at Imperial College London. He is interested in developing and evaluating technologies to help teach anatomy, physiology and surgery.

K. Anders Ericsson is a Conradi Eminent Scholar at Florida State University, USA. He studies expert performance and how expert performers attain their superior performance by acquiring complex cognitive mechanisms through extended deliberate practice. He has edited "*Cambridge Handbook of Expertise and Expert Performance*" (2006) and "*The Development of Professional Expertise*" (2009).

Ron Epstein is Professor of Family Medicine, Psychiatry and Oncology and directs the Rochester Center to Improve Communication in Health Care and the Deans Teaching Fellowship Program at the University of Rochester Medical Center, USA.

Ray Land is Professor of Higher Education and Head of Learning Enhancement at the University of Strathclyde, Glasgow, UK. His research interests include academic development, threshold concepts and troublesome knowledge, research-teaching linkages and the development of graduate attributes and theoretical aspects of digital learning. He publishes extensively.

Lorelei Lingard is a leading researcher in the study of communication and collaboration on healthcare teams. She is Professor in the Department of Medicine and Director of the Centre for Education Research & Innovation at the Schulich School of Medicine & Dentistry, University of Western Ontario, London, Ontario, Canada.

Gunther Kress is Professor of Semiotics and Education at the Institute of Education, University of London. His interests are in meaning-making and communication in contemporary environments, with an interest in developing a social semiotic theory of multimodal communication. He is the author of numerous books on semiotics and multimodality.

Jan Meyer is Professor at the University of Queensland, Australia, formerly being the Director of the Centre for Learning, Teaching, and Research in Higher Education at the University of Durham, UK. Much of his research career has been devoted to exploring mechanisms for developing metalearning capacity in students, to the modelling of individual differences in student learning and to the construction of discipline-centred models of student learning. He publishes extensively.

Carol-anne Moulton is a hepato-pancreatico-biliary surgeon at the Toronto General Hospital and an education scientist at the Wilson Centre, University of Toronto, Canada. She was awarded a Masters of Education in 2006 and a Ph.D. in 2010 for her work in surgical judgement.

Debra Nestel is Professor of Medical Education at Gippsland Medical School, Monash University, Australia. Over 25 years, she has taught clinical communication in Hong Kong, the UK, and Australia. Specific research interests include simulation-based education in healthcare and programme evaluation methodologies.

Lambert W.T. Schuwirth is a physician and Professor at The University of Adelaide, Australia, formerly being at the Department of Educational Development and Research at Maastricht University, The Netherlands. He is involved in research and development of assessment programmes, and in teaching students and faculty.

Nick Sevdalis is an experimental psychologist and Senior Lecturer in Patient Safety in the Division of Surgery and Centre for Patient Safety and Service Quality at Imperial College London. He is an expert in developing and validating tools to capture behavioural and cognitive skills in surgery and leads research methods and statistics teaching across a range of courses in his division.

Cees P.M. van der Vleuten is a psychologist and Professor and chair of the Department of Educational Development and Research at Maastricht University, Netherlands. His work is in development, organisation and research of medical education and is widely published; he is a teacher of students and faculty.

Author Index

H. Fry and R. Kneebone (eds.), *Surgical Education: Theorising an Emerging Domain*, Advances in Medical Education 2, DOI 10.1007/978-94-007-1682-7,

Subject Index

H. Fry and R. Kneebone (eds.), *Surgical Education: Theorising an Emerging Domain*, Advances in Medical Education 2, DOI 10.1007/978-94-007-1682-7,

MIX
Papier aus verantwortungsvollen Quellen
Paper from responsible sources
FSC® C105338

If you have any concerns about our products,
you can contact us on
ProductSafety@springernature.com

In case Publisher is established outside the EU,
the EU authorized representative is:
Springer Nature Customer Service Center GmbH
Europaplatz 3, 69115 Heidelberg, Germany

Printed by Libri Plureos GmbH
in Hamburg, Germany